Acute Coronary Syndromes

Acute Coronary Syndromes

EDITED BY

David de Bono
Formerly
Professor of Cardiology
Head of the Division of Cardiology
University of Leicester
Leicester
UK

Burton E. Sobel
Amidon Professor and Chair,
Department of Medicine
University of Vermont
and Physician-in-Chief,
Fletcher Allen Healthcare
Burlington
Vermont
USA

**Blackwell
Science**

© 2001
Blackwell Science Ltd
Editorial Offices:
Osney Mead, Oxford OX2 0EL
25 John Street, London WC1N 2BS
23 Ainslie Place, Edinburgh EH3 6AJ
350 Main Street, Malden
    MA 02148-5018, USA
54 University Street, Carlton
    Victoria 3053, Australia
10, rue Casimir Delavigne
    75006 Paris, France

Other Editorial Offices:
Blackwell Wissenschafts-Verlag GmbH
Kurfürstendamm 57
10707 Berlin, Germany

Blackwell Science KK
MG Kodenmacho Building
7–10 Kodenmacho Nihombashi
Chuo-ku, Tokyo 104, Japan

Iowa State University Press
A Blackwell Science Company
2121 S. State Avenue
Ames, Iowa 50014-8300, USA

First published 2001

Set by Best-set Typesetter Ltd.,
Hong Kong
Printed and bound in Great Britain by
MPG Books Ltd, Bodmin, Cornwall

The Blackwell Science logo is a
trade mark of Blackwell Science Ltd,
registered at the United Kingdom
Trade Marks Registry

DISTRIBUTORS

Marston Book Services Ltd
PO Box 269
Abingdon, Oxon OX14 4YN
(*Orders*: Tel: 01235 465500
        Fax: 01235 465555)

USA
Blackwell Science, Inc.
Commerce Place
350 Main Street
Malden, MA 02148-5018
(*Orders*: Tel: 800 759 6102
            781 388 8250
        Fax: 781 388 8255)

Canada
Login Brothers Book Company
324 Saulteaux Crescent
Winnipeg, Manitoba R3J 3T2
(*Orders*: Tel: 204 837 2987)

Australia
Blackwell Science Pty Ltd
54 University Street
Carlton, Victoria 3053
(*Orders*: Tel: 3 9347 0300
        Fax: 3 9347 5001)

A catalogue record for this title
is available from the British Library

ISBN 0-632-05579-0

Library of Congress
Cataloging-in-Publication Data

Challenges in acute coronary syndromes/edited
by David de Bono, Burton Sobel.
    p.   cm.
    Includes bibliographical references.
    ISBN 0-632-05579-0
    1. Coronary heart disease.
    I. De Bono, D. P. (David P.)   II. Sobel, Burton
E.
    RC685.C6 C445 2000
    616.1′23 — dc21   00-060891

For further information on
Blackwell Science, visit our website:
www.blackwell-science.com

Contents

List of contributors

EDITORS

David de Bono (deceased) MB Bchir, MD, FRCP, MRCP, *formerly Professor of Cardiology and Head of the Division of Cardiology, University of Leicester, Leicester LE3 9QP, UK*

Burton E. Sobel MD, FACC, FACP (Master), *Amidon Professor and Chair, Department of Medicine, University of Vermont, and Physician-in-Chief, Fletcher Allen Healthcare, 111 Colchester Avenue, Fletcher 311, Burlington, Vermont 05401, USA*

CONTRIBUTORS

Philippe L. L'Allier MD, FRCPC, *Department of Cardiology, Montreal Heart Institute, University of Montreal, 5000 Belanger Est. Montreal, PQ, Canada HIT 1C8*

Sonia S. Anand MD, MSc, *Assistant Professor of Medicine, McMaster University, 237 Barton Street East, Hamilton, Ontario, Canada L8L 2X2*

Robert M. Bell MBBS, BSc, *Clinical Research Fellow, The Hatter Institute, University College, Grafton Way, London WC1E 6DB, UK*

Steven R. Bergmann MD, PhD, *Division of Cardiology, Department of Medicine, College of Physicians and Surgeons, Columbia University, 630 West 168th Street, New York, NY 10032, USA*

Paolo G. Camici *Professor of Cardiovascular Pathophysiology, MRC Cyclotron Unit, Imperial College School of Medicine, The Hammersmith Hospital, Du Cane Road, London W12 0NN, UK*

Graham R. Cherryman FRCR, *Professor of Radiology and Head of Department, University Department of Radiology, Leicester Royal Infirmary, Leicester LE1 5WW, UK*

Paul O. Collinson FRCPath, MD, *Department of Clinical Biochemistry, 2nd Floor, Jenner Wing, St George's Hospital, Blackshaw Road, London SW17 0QT, UK*

M. J. Davies *Professor, Cardiovascular Pathology Research Group, St George's Hospital, Cranmer Terrace, Tooting, London SW17 0RE, UK*

Mikael Dellborg MD, PhD, *Department of Medicine, Sahlgrenska University Hospital/Östra, 41685, Göteborg, Sweden*

Stephen G. Ellis MD, *Department of Cardiology, Joseph J Jacobs Center for Thrombosis and Vascular Biology, The Cleveland Clinic Foundation, 9500 Euclid Avenue, Ohio 44195,USA*

Jack Hirsh MD, *Director of Hamilton Civic Hospitals Research Centre, 711 Concession Street, Hamilton, Ontario, Canada L8V 1C3*

Juan Carlos Kaski MD, DM (Hons), FRCP, FESC, FACC, *Professor of Cardiovascular Science, St George's Hospital Medical School, Cranmer Terrace, Tooting, London SW17 0RE, UK*

Mitchell W. Krucoff MD, FACC, FCCP, *Associate Professor Medicine/Cardiology, Duke University Medical Center, Director, Ischemia Monitoring Laboratory, Duke Clinical Research Institute, Director, Cardiovascular Laboratories, Durham VA Medical Center, Durham, North Carolina, NC27710, USA*

Jan Kyst Madsen MD, DrMedSc, FESC, *Head of the Cardiac Catheterisation Laboratory,The Heart Centre, Rigspitalet, Copenhagen University Hospital, Blegdamsvej 9, DK-2100, Copenhagen, Denmark*

Hans Mickley MD, DrMedSc, *Consultant Cardiologist, Department of Cardiology, Odense University Hospital, Odense, Denmark*

Petros Nihoyannopoulos MD, FACC, FESC, *Reader and Consultant Cardiologist, Cardiology Division, Imperial College School of Medicine, The Hammersmith Hospital, Du Cane Road, London, UK*

Laurence O'Toole MRCP, MD, *Specialist Registrar, Cardiology Department, The Western General Hospital, Edinburgh EH 42XU, UK*

Ravichandran Ramasamy PhD, *Division of Cardiology, Department of Medicine, College of Physicians and Surgeons, Columbia University, 630 West 168th Street, New York, NY 10032, USA*

Nilesh J. Samani MD, FRCP, *Professor of Cardiology, Division of Cardiology, University of Leicester, Clinical Sciences Wing, Glenfield Hospital, Groby Road, Leicester LE3 9QP, UK*

David J. Schneider MD, *Associate Professor of Medicine, University of Vermont, Fletcher Allen Healthcare, 111 Colchester Avenue, Fletcher 311, Burlington, Vermont 05401, USA*

Penelope R. Sensky MRCP, *Clinical Research Fellow, Division of Cardiology, Clinical Sciences Wing, Glenfield Hospital NHS Trust, Groby Road, Leicester LE3 9QP, UK*

Ravi Singh MRCP, *Clinical Research Fellow, Division of Cardiology, University of Leicester, Clinical Sciences Wing, Glenford Hospital, Groby Road, Leicester LE3 9QP, UK*

David A. Smith BM, MRCP, *Clinical Research Fellow, Coronary Artery Research Group, St George's Hospital Medical School, Cranmer Terrace, Tooting, London SW17 0RE*

Terry J. Spinks *Physicist, MRC Cyclotron Unit, Imperial College School of Medicine, The Hammersmith Hospital, Du Cane Road, London W12 0NN, UK*

Peter J. Stubbs MRCP, MD, *Consultant Cardiologist, Mayday Hospital, Croydon, Surrey, UK*

Alan J. Tiefenbrunn MD, FACC, *Associate Professor of Medicine and Radiology, Cardiovascular Division, Washington University School of Medicine, St Louis, Missouri 63110 USA*

Eric J. Topol MD, *Chairman and Professor, Department of Cardiology, Joseph J Jacobs Center for Thrombosis and Vascular Biology, The Cleveland Clinic Foundation, 9500 Euclid Avenue, Ohio 44195, USA*

Neal G. Uren MD, MRCP, FESC, FACC, *Consultant Cardiologist, Edinburgh Royal Infirmary, Lauriston Place, Edinburgh EH3 9YN, UK*

Freek W. A. Verheugt MD, *Department of Cardiology, Heart Center, University Hospital of Nijmegen, PO Box 9101, Nijmegen, The Netherlands 6500 HB*

Derek M. Yellon PhD, DSc, MRCP, FACC, FESC, *Director of Institute and Head of Centre for Cardiology, The Hatter Institute, University College, Grafton Way, London WC1E 6DB, UK*

Preface

It has been a privilege to witness two courageous men afflicted by motor neuron disease hold audiences spellbound with their intellect, insights, and computer-assisted voice synthesizers—Stephen Hawking and David de Bono. Thus, when asked to co-edit this book that David had initiated but not lived to complete, I was eager to comply. His lovely and supportive wife, Anne, indicated that my doing so was David's wish. Fulfilling it is an honour.

Professor David de Bono made prodigious contributions to cardiology, haematology, and vascular biology. Anyone who had ever heard him lecture, participated in workshops or on task forces with him, or had the benefit of one-on one exchanges could not fail to admire his brilliance, lucidity, and wisdom. He devoted his professional life to elucidating mechanisms underlying coronary heart disease and its predilection to afflict particular ethnic groups differentially and to enhancing the quality of cardiac care, most recently in Leicester and for decades throughout the United Kingdom. His influence was international and his impact profound.

David's interests were diverse. His recent manuscripts focused on electrocardiography with emphasis on abnormal repolarization as a risk factor for sudden death in type 2 diabetes, endothelial cell function and metabolism, antiplatelet drugs, rehabilitation services, thrombolysis, restenosis, and multicentre clinical trials. Accordingly, it is not surprising that he wanted this book to authoritatively address challenging work in progress that is particularly pertinent to patients with acute coronary syndromes. The expert contributors to this volume succeeded admirably.

The material is presented in three sections: (1) physiology and pathophysiology; (2) diagnostic considerations; and (3) therapeutic approaches. The contributions of plaque instability, plaque rupture, infection, abnormalities of coronary vasomotor tone, and molecular genetics to vascular biological changes underlying acute coronary syndromes are addressed in the first section. Progress in established diagnostic methods including electrocardiography and signal averaging, stress testing, and echocardiography is considered in the second section along with thoughtful discussion of macromolecular markers of myocardial and vascular wall derangements, magnetic resonance imaging, and positron emission tomography. In the third section, advances in therapeutics with emphasis on modification of coagulation and fibrinolysis and the use of stents are addressed as are novel approaches including preconditioning and myocardial metabolic protection.

It has been a pleasure to work with the contributors and to participate in the editing of their manuscripts. David would have been very proud of what they have written. It is my hope that our readers will appreciate the material and view it as a tribute to David's memory.

Burton E. Sobel, MD
August 2000

Part 1: Pathophysiology

1: Is it all plaque rupture?

M. J. Davies

Introduction

When the pathological basis of the three acute coronary syndromes (unstable angina, acute myocardial infarction and sudden ischaemic death) is considered, it is the association of thrombosis with atherosclerosis that is paramount. Plaque rupture is only one way in which thrombosis is triggered, although it is a phenomenon that has caught the imagination of clinicians, and is much in fashion.

Coronary atherosclerosis

The starting-point for any consideration of the acute coronary syndromes has to be coronary atherosclerosis. This forms the substrate on which more than 99% of patients with acute coronary syndromes (ACS) develop symptoms. The very rare exceptions are conditions such as spontaneous coronary artery dissection; coronary spasm, caused either by cocaine abuse or spontaneous coronary arteritis; coronary emboli; coronary artery bridging; and anomalous origin of a coronary artery.

Studies of atherosclerosis in large autopsy series performed in diverse geographical areas and in subjects with diverse risk factors [1–3], have established the concept of 'plaque burden'. In a given population the average number of plaques in the coronary arteries appears to determine the incidence of ischaemic heart disease. Risk factors such as smoking and hypertension, as well as hyperlipidaemia, increase the total number of plaques that are present. For an individual subject the risk of developing the symptoms of ischaemic heart disease depends also on the nature of the plaques. One major factor associated with precipitation of thrombosis on a culprit plaque is the level of inflammatory activity—plaques with a high level of this activity are regarded as vulnerable and at a high risk of changes leading to a thrombotic episode. Individuals vary widely in the proportion of their coronary plaques that exhibit high inflammatory activity at any one point in time.

Characteristics of the plaque

The archetypal fully formed mature plaque has a core of extracellular lipid, predominantly cholesterol, enclosed in a capsule of collagenous tissue [4]. The portion of the capsule separating the core from the lumen is the plaque cap (Fig. 1.1). Many plaques are situated eccentrically, that is on the arterial wall opposite the plaque there remains a segment or arc of normal arterial wall [5]. This arc of normal wall has medial muscle fully capable of contraction and relaxation that can alter the dimensions of the lumen. Thus, in marked contrast to the earlier views, atherosclerotic coronary arteries are not rigid tubes. Variations in arterial tone can alter flow even at the site of plaques.

At some stage of their evolution, plaques often exhibit an inflammatory component, consisting largely of macrophages, many containing intracellular lipid (foam cells) [6]. These cluster around a lipid core which is formed in large part by lipid released by the foam cells undergoing death by apoptosis and necrosis. The macrophages are derived from monocytes that enter the intima by migration across the endothelial surface and then become activated macrophages. These macrophages express CD40, ligation of which induces high levels of Tissue Factor [7] and the production of metalloproteinases, interleukins and Tumour Necrosis Factor α (TNFα). Large amounts of Macrophage Chemoattractant Protein (MCP-1) [8] and Macrophage Colony Stimulating Factor (MCSF) [9] are present, maintaining the recruitment of monocytes and allowing their survival in the plaque. The accumulation of these highly activated cells is triggered by the diverse stimuli, including oxidized low density lipoprotein (LDL), which constitutes a pro-inflammatory molecule [10,11]. Plaques contain considerable numbers of T lymphocytes and some basophils. The T lymphocytes can initiate an autoimmune reaction to oxidized LDL, have a cytotoxic effect mediated by perforins and granzymes and smooth muscle and initiate migration and activation of vascular cells in

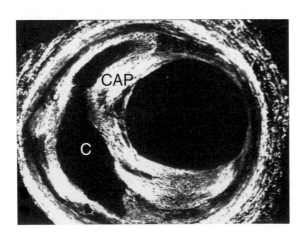

Fig.1.1 Cross-section of a human coronary artery plaque (CAP) in which only the collagen is shown by polarized light. The core (C) does not contain any collagen and if the lipid is removed becomes a space. The core is separated from the lumen by the plaque cap.

response to interferon γ [12]. Smooth-muscle cells in the plaque exhibit enhanced expression of class II MHC antigens. Thus the plaque is an inflammatory focus as active, for example, as the synovium in rheumatoid arthritis. Plaques, like rheumatoid joints, do burn out. Thus any given individual with atherosclerosis will have some lesions that, although there is a residual lipid core, have virtually no macrophages.

In the early stages of atherosclerosis before fully formed raised plaques have appeared, the intact endothelial surface prevents contact of platelets with the connective tissue matrix of the arterial wall. This is not to say that the endothelium is functionally normal. Modified LDL evokes the expression of adhesion molecules such as Vascular Cell Adhesion Molecule (VCAM) by the endothelial cell [13], a vital component influencing monocyte migration. Nitric oxide production is not normal, despite the endothelial surface being structurally intact.

Once plaque formation is established, focal areas of endothelial denudation occur [14,15]. The foci of loss of endothelial cells expose small areas of the connective tissue matrix, and some platelet adhesion occurs. This platelet deposition, although ultramicroscopic, will act to stimulate smooth muscle proliferation and therefore plaque growth. Such foci of endothelial cell loss are very common in any subject with plaques, and indicate that even in subjects with stable angina there is an element of endothelial instability. In both human and experimental-animal atheroma, endothelial loss is linked to the proximity of highly activated macrophages and is another marker of inflammation in the plaque. Results of studies with DNA synthesis markers, such as Ki67, show that endothelial replication is enhanced over plaques. Endothelial replication in normal segments is greater than that in arteries devoid of plaque.

Mechanisms of thrombosis in atherosclerosis

Studies of the pathology of atherosclerotic plaques complicated by thrombosis show that two different mechanisms exist [16]. These are endothelial erosion and plaque disruption (Fig. 1.2). Although the two processes are very different, both involve inflammatory activity [17–19].

Endothelial erosion is simply a continuation of the endothelial denudation that occurs over many plaques. The endothelial loss extends over a wider area, and the intimal surface becomes pitted with trapped activated macrophages exposed to the lumen. Red cells become trapped in the intima, and thrombus develops on the surface of the plaque. Endothelial cell loss has been associated with the induction of apoptosis related to the proximity of macrophages and with the action of proteolytic enzymes resulting in a 'cutting loose' of endothelial cells.

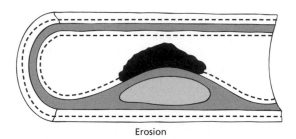

Erosion

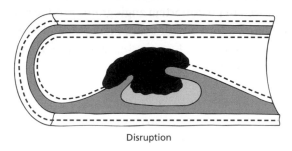

Disruption

Fig.1.2 A comparison of erosion and disruption. In erosion the thrombus is stuck on to the surface of the plaque. In disruption there is thrombus within the plaque which then protrudes into the lumen.

In contrast, plaque disruption involves the mechanical tearing of the fibrous cap of a plaque that has a lipid core [20,21]. The tear disrupts the endothelium, allowing blood to enter into the core itself where contact with Tissue Factor causes intraplaque thrombosis. The thrombus that forms distorts and expands the plaque from within, rapidly increasing the extent of stenosis. Thrombus may subsequently extend into the lumen of the artery and cause obstruction. Plaque disruption is accelerated by inflammatory activity within the plaque with weakening of the cap tissue such that it is unable to withstand the circumferential stress exerted in systole. Plaque caps are dynamic structures. The collagenous matrix, critical to mechanical strength, is constantly being replaced by smooth muscle cells [22]. Inflammatory activity can further weaken the plaque cap by causing smooth-muscle-cell apoptosis and decreasing collagen synthesis mediated by interferon γ.

Activated macrophages produce metalloproteinases (MMPS); and zymogens, inactive forms, are released into the vessel wall. These inactive zymogens can be activated by plasmin, proteinases from mast cells, or already activated MMPS. A range of metalloproteinases, including gelatinase B (MMP9), interstitial collagenase (MMP1) and stromelysin (MMP3) are produced. They can readily destroy all of the components of the connective tissue matrix of the plaque cap. Excess activity of MMPS has been demonstrated in human plaques [23].

The two mechanisms that underlie thrombosis associated with plaques have inflammation in common. They differ in that superficial endothelial erosion *per se* is not associated with thrombosis within the plaque.

The relative importance of these two mechanisms may differ between patient groups [24–26]. Plaque disruption is the dominant mechanism for thrombosis in Caucasian males with high plasma LDL and low high density lipoprotein (HDL) levels, where it is responsible for over 85% of acute coronary events. By contrast, in women and diabetic subjects, erosion may account for 50% of thrombi. The proportions in other populations are unknown.

Pathologists see the worst of everything. It has been suggested that plaque disruption is in fact rare in life. Several pieces of evidence argue against this view. Plaque disruption as visualized in post-mortem angiograms produces a highly characteristic irregular stenosis, often with overhanging or undercut edges with an intraluminal filling defect [27]. Exactly this angiographic appearance [28] is found *in vivo* in patients with unstable angina and evolving myocardial infarction, and is designated as a Type II lesion in contrast to the smooth type I lesions seen in patients with stable angina. Angioscopy demonstrates a torn plaque cap with associated thrombus *in vivo*, and intravascular ultrasound identifies ruptured plaques with intraplaque thrombus [29,30].

The pathology of specific acute coronary syndromes

Acute myocardial infarction

Typical acute myocardial infarction (Q-wave infarction) is a syndrome with consistent pathology in large areas of myocardial necrosis. An area of regional necrosis implies that flow in the artery subtending the region has been interrupted for at least several hours. The cause of myocardial infarction has, however, been argued. In the first half of this century thrombosis was considered to be the proximate cause [31], but by 1970 thrombosis was regarded in the United States as being secondary and a result of low flow secondary to stenosis and the infarction itself [32,33]. Even in retrospect it is difficult to determine what the primary precipitating cause was thought to be [34]. By 1980 thrombosis was recognized as being a causal event. This was in part because of the success of fibrinolytic agents in preventing or attenuating infarction [35].

The role of thrombosis as the cause of regional infarction was affirmed partly because it was realized that coronary thrombosis was dynamic. Results of seminal angiographic studies of DeWood [36] and Stadius [37] showed that very soon after the onset of chest pain and ECG changes indicative of infarction, the subtending artery was totally occluded. Furthermore, even without thrombolytic therapy, many arteries spontaneously reopened. The rate and number of arteries reopened could be greatly increased by the administration of thrombolytic agents, initially infused directly into the artery itself and subsequently administered intravenously.

The question of whether thrombosis was primary or secondary was answered by the work of Fulton [38,39]. He infused radiolabelled fibrinogen into subjects admitted to hospital with chest pain and evolving ECG changes indicative of infarction. Inevitably some died. In the very detailed study of the morphology of the thrombus, the element of thrombus over the plaque was found to be not radiolabelled. Thus it predated the onset of infarction. A large portion of the thrombus distal to the plaque, however, was labelled, showing that it had formed after the initial occlusion. This work showed that thrombus propagated in the artery after the onset of infarction. It countered the rather quixotic view that had been held by some in the 1970s that thrombosis was entirely a secondary phenomenon.

Despite the extensive work establishing thrombosis as a cause of infarction, this did not exclude a role for local spasm. Furthermore, it was still not clear why a thrombus should suddenly form over a plaque that had probably existed at the same site for years.

Pathology studies in which thrombus over plaque was reconstructed in its entirety led to the concept of plaque disruption and plaque erosion [40–43]. Plaque rupture, disruption, or fissuring (synonyms) exhibits a wide spectrum of severity. At one extreme it is a crack or fissure with a bilobed mass of thrombus, part in the lumen and part in the plaque, joined by thrombus in the fissure. At the other extreme the whole plaque is laid open, with exposure of the highly thrombogenic core leading to occlusion of the artery with a mass of thrombus mixed with lipid extruded from the plaque. Plaque disruption is therefore a stimulus to the development of thrombosis of variable magnitude. Patients who develop an occlusive thrombus in association with relatively minor episodes of disruption are possibly those in whom the thrombotic mechanisms are enhanced or endogenous lytic processes inefficient. Such patients are, however, readily treated with lytic drugs that often leave a relatively minor residual stenotic lesion.

In general, results of angiographic studies performed at regular intervals suggest that plaques that underlie thrombotic lesions and cause infarction are not those that have previously caused stenosis. Thrombi may occur even in an artery that appears angiographically normal. Pathology studies have suggested that about 75% of the thrombi that cause infarction are initiated by plaque disruption. Twenty-five per cent are initiated by endothelial erosion. However, these proportions reflect results in studies of populations dominated by Caucasian males. There is evidence (see above) that endothelial erosion is a more important mechanism in thrombosis in women and in diabetic subjects. When endothelial erosion gives rise to thrombi that occlude an artery, the thrombi are likely to be at points at which stenosis is already present.

Unstable angina

Unstable angina is often caused by episodes of ischaemia occurring at rest. It is a syndrome, however, with a wide spectrum of clinical features that have led to complex classification [44]. Extraneous factors such as anaemia can precipitate episodes of ischaemia in subjects with coronary stenosis. However, when such external features are excluded, unstable angina can be categorized as a form of angina in which new pain has occurred (within 48 hours of presentation) with the patient at rest. The episodes often increase in severity and frequency (crescendo angina, Braunwald type III). Alternatively, crescendo angina may follow rest pain that occurred in the more remote past, which then declines. Finally there are cases where there is marked worsening of angina in a subject who has previously had stable angina. Crescendo angina is a condition associated with considerable risk of infarction and/or sudden death. However, it may resolve itself, leaving residual stable angina or even absent angina. Crescendo type unstable angina is the form most studied by pathologists. This may have led to selection bias. Death is the worst outcome and associated with the most severe pathology. Any consideration of the autopsy pathology of unstable angina must therefore be tempered by evidence from angiography, angioscopy and atherectomy *in vivo*.

In the past, pathology studies have led to the view that unstable angina results from thrombus in a coronary artery over which antegrade flow is still occurring [21,27,45]. The underlying basis of thrombosis can be disruption or erosion. Post-mortem angiography has shown eccentric ragged stenosis to be a feature of plaque disruption; identical Type II stenoses have been found in subjects with unstable angina studied *in vivo* by angiography [46]. Progression of lesions to occlusion has been observed in those who developed infarction [28]. Post-mortem angiography can be performed with high resolution and long exposure times. It has been shown that over 75% of Type II stenoses are associated with intraluminal thrombus. With *in vivo* angiography the figure appears much lower, at around 30% [47]. Angioscopy has shown that up to 70% of the lesions responsible for unstable angina contain thrombus on a plaque [29].

However, the advent of atherectomy has led to a more complex story. A very consistent message has emerged. If the culprit lesions responsible for unstable angina are compared with lesions responsible for stable angina, with respect to tissue fragments removed, the former exhibit a far higher frequency of thrombus. However, the incidence is nowhere near 100% [48–50]. Conversely, up to a quarter of samples removed from plaques responsible for stable angina are associated with thrombotic material.

A failure to find thrombotic material in atherectomy samples from plaques thought to be responsible for unstable angina has several explanations. One is sampling error—what is taken at atherectomy is a random sample and not the whole plaque. Another consideration is the time between the procedure and the occurrence of the most recent symptoms. Plaque disruption may be followed by a healing phase in which thrombus is endogenously lysed and new smooth muscle proliferation occurs, with deposition of collagen and repair of the disrupted intima. The accelerated smooth muscle proliferation can be recognized in atherectomy samples taken from patients in whom the acute phase of unstable angina occurred some weeks earlier [50,51].

In the phase of unstable angina in which mural thrombus is present, whether related to disruption or erosion, several mechanisms can be responsible for the intermittent episodes of ischaemia. The surface of exposed thrombus is covered by a layer of activated platelets with enhanced expression of the platelet glycoprotein IIb/IIIa. Clumps of platelets are swept downstream (Fig. 1.3) as microemboli that impact on and occlude small intramyocardial arteries ranging in size from 20 to 200 μm in external diameter [45,52,53]. These microemboli are associated with microscopic foci of acute myocyte necrosis. The smaller vessels and capillaries become occluded also and are associated with foci of polymorphonuclear cell plugging. Phasic microembolization is probably a major mechanism underlying episodic pain in patients with unstable angina. Thus, elevated concentrations in urine of metabolites of thromboxane coincide with episodes of ischaemia and pain [54,55].

A second mechanism for intermittent ischaemia is arterial spasm at the site of thrombosis in an epicardial artery. Many plaques that undergo disruption are eccentric, with a normal segment of arterial wall adjacent capable of undergoing contraction. Thrombus, and in particular platelets, are powerful initiators of local arterial spasm.

A third mechanism, and one occurring largely in patients with impending infarction, is intermittent growth of the thrombus, with consequent occlusion of the artery, followed by reopening resulting from spontaneous lysis [56].

In most patients with unstable angina, intermittent ischaemic attacks either resolve or sudden death or myocardial infarction occur. For this type of patient, a culprit thrombotic lesion is present with or without associated

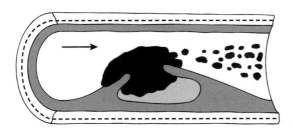

Fig.1.3 Embolization of small masses of activated platelets from the surface of thrombus projecting into the arterial lumen.

arterial spasm. More rarely, intermittent attacks of myocardial ischaemia go on for months or even years. In many such patients an ECG typical for the Prinzmetal's angina is seen and symptoms are regarded as being more related to spasm than to thrombosis. Pathology studies suggest such patients do have atherosclerosis, albeit not necessarily producing angiographically-recognized stenosis [57,58]. The sites of spasm may be very localized. They may relate to only one plaque and may persist for years. The reasons for such a localized segment being hyperactive are not clear. In one study a segment of artery was excised and confirmed to be an eccentric plaque in which microscopic foci of thrombus were present [59]. Reports of unstable angina attributable to spasm are more frequent in Japan, suggesting that ethnic features may contribute to the reactivity of the coronary arteries. Some pathology studies have linked hyperactive segments of coronary arteries to a dense periadventitial accumulation of chronic inflammatory cells [60], including basophils putatively directly influencing the periadventital nerves.

Non-Q-wave infarction

Non-Q-wave infarction is an entity that appears to lie somewhere between unstable angina and Q-wave (previously called transmural myocardial) infarction with respect to pathogenesis. In unstable angina the clinical definition excludes cases with ECG changes indicative of Q-wave infarction. Yet a considerable number of patients with this disorder do have evidence of some myocardial necrosis, as shown by elevated Troponin T levels [61–63]. These findings are in accord with the demonstration of foci of microscopic myocardial necrosis associated with platelet microemboli. Evidence for the role of platelet emboli includes the efficacy of IIb/IIIa inhibitors in preventing infarction or death in patients with unstable angina in whom Troponin T levels are initially elevated.

Non-transmural infarction is associated usually with coalescence of areas of necrosis of widely differing ages in a region of supply of an artery that has been occluded intermittently by thrombus or repeated platelet emboli. Pre-existing collateral flow to such an area is another factor that limits transmural spread of necrosis [64,65]. Nevertheless the pathogenesis of non-transmural infarction is clearly firmly rooted in thrombosis on a culprit plaque.

Sudden ischaemic death

Pathology studies of patients who die suddenly (within 6 hours of the onset of any symptoms) and in whom there is no other cause of death apart from coronary atherosclerosis causing stenosis, fall into four clear groups. There is little argument that all four groups exist, but there is considerable disagreement over their relative importance [66–68].

The groups are:

1   Arterial pathology identical to that seen with unstable angina with a non-occluding thrombus related to a plaque with disruption or erosion. Half of such cases show myocardial platelet embolization.

2   Arterial pathology identical to that seen with acute myocardial infarction with an artery occluded by thrombus due to erosion or disruption. There are no morphological changes of myocardial infarction owing to the short survival period after the onset of pain.

3   Patients with high-grade stenosis in one or more arteries due to atheroma, but no thrombus. The myocardium has old scars of prior infarction often with coexistent left ventricular hypertrophy (LVH).

4   A structurally normal myocardium without scars or hypertrophy, high-grade stenosis due to atherosclerosis, but no thrombotic lesions.

Personal experience, and that of others, indicates that groups 1 and 2 combined are responsible for over three-quarters of cases [67]. Others find these groups to be rarer. The discordance probably reflects different selection criteria [69]. Thrombotic lesions are most common in subjects with no prior history of ischaemic heart disease who have prodromal chest pain before dying suddenly. Non-thrombotic stenosis is most frequent in those who have a known history of prior heart disease and die suddenly with no prior chest pain. In sudden ischaemic death the answer to the question 'Is it all plaque rupture?' is clearly 'No', but rupture does make a major contribution.

Inflammation and coronary atherosclerosis

As previously emphasized, many atherosclerotic plaques are inflammatory lesions that are most vulnerable to an episode of erosion or disruption when high inflammatory activity coincides with a large lipid core. There has been intense interest in the levels of a wide range of inflammatory markers in the systemic circulation both in acute and chronic coronary syndromes. In both conditions the levels of markers such as C-reactive protein in blood appear to give some indication of prognosis. The similarity of the results with C-reactive protein, fibrinogen, neopterin and intercellular adhesion molecule (ICAM), to name but a minority of markers tested, are impressive and suggest that a unifying underlying phenomenon is present [70–75].

In unstable angina elevated systemic markers of inflammation could indicate that:

1   Myocardial damage has already occurred.

2   Thrombotic mechanisms and endothelial damage have been upregulated.

3   Inflammatory processes within the plaques themselves with markers have spilled into the systemic circulation.

In stable angina concentrations in blood of inflammatory markers are less high than in unstable angina, but are still indicative of risk. In the Physicians Health Study [75] although the risk of a future acute myocardial infarction differed by a factor of almost 3 between the highest and lowest quartiles of C-reactive protein and soluble ICAM, the actual concentrations in blood in individual subjects were not high and did not provide a practical prognostic marker.

A number of aspects need to be considered in this connection. One is that in the great majority of subjects with atherosclerosis there is a far greater bulk of plaques in the aorta, femoral and carotid arteries than in the coronary arteries. Exposed thrombus on aortic plaques in the abdominal aorta in subjects over 50 years of age is seen at post-mortem examination in at least 50% of individuals who have coronary disease [76]. There is a strong association between the extent of aortic atherosclerosis and coronary atherosclerosis [77]. Enhanced markers of inflammation may therefore be indicative of extensive aortic atherosclerosis and taken to be a surrogate for coronary disease. In addition there does appear to be an association between coronary thrombosis and aortic thrombosis. In one study thrombus in the aorta was far more common in subjects who died of coronary thrombosis than in those who died of non-thrombotic coronary disease. Many subjects who die with one culprit coronary plaque have others with thrombosis of lesser extent [78].

None of this precludes the concept of a vicious circle in which inflammatory mediators released by the atherosclerotic process further upregulate inflammatory activity in the plaque, thus enhancing the risk of an acute event involving erosion or disruption. Experimental evidence indicates that the injection of inflammatory agents such as endotoxin into animals with atheroma induced by high-lipid diets will elevate mRNA levels for interleukins within the plaques themselves [79]. By analogy, chronic infections such as helicobacter could upregulate inflammatory activity in human plaques and explain the link between helicobacter positive serology and risk of coronary events [80,81]. Chlamydial infection has been linked by serological studies with an increased risk of the acute coronary syndromes as well [80]. Chlamydia was found to directly colonize and live within plaques [82,83]. The mode of entry is probably via circulating monocytes that adhere to the endothelium over a plaque and are then carried in. The plaque must provide some sort of favourable milieu for the organism to replicate. Chlamydia produce heat shock protein [84] that can increase the production of TNFα and other cytokines by macrophages within the plaque and potentially increase the risk of erosion or disruption.

Conclusion

The question 'Is it all plaque rupture?' in relation to acute coronary syndromes implies that it is a sole mechanism. As far back as 1981, however, pathology studies showed it was only one of the mechanisms through which thrombosis occurred over a plaque, not the only one. Plaque disruption just happens to be fashionable today. The proximate cause of acute coronary syndromes in the great majority of cases is thrombosis. The substrate of the thrombosis is an atherosclerotic plaque. Plaques become complicated by thrombosis because of disruption or erosion. Factors that lead them to become unstable and develop disruption or erosion include inflammatory activity and the destruction of tissue. The biggest single cause of the inflammation, and indeed its initiator, is modified and oxidized low density lipoprotein derived initially from plasma lipids. However, other inflammatory agents such as Chlamydia can exacerbate the risk of plaque rupture or endothelial erosion, and thereby further increase the risk of acute coronary events.

References

1 Wissler R. An overview of the quantitative influence of several risk factors on progression of atherosclerosis in young people in the United States. *Am J Med Sci* 1995; 310: S29–S36.

2 Strong J. Atherosclerotic lesions. Natural history, risk factors and topography. *Arch Pathol Lab Med* 1992; 116: 1268–75.

3 Tracy R, Newman W, Wattigney W. Risk factors and atherosclerosis in young: autopsy findings of the Bogalusa Heart Study. *Am J Med* 1995; 310: S37–S41.

4 Stary H, Chandler A, Dinsmore R *et al*. A definition of advanced types of atherosclerotic lesions and a histological classification of atherosclerosis. A report from the Committee on Vascular Lesions of the Council on Atherosclerosis, American Heart Association. *Circulation* 1995; 92: 1355–74.

5 Saner H, Gobel F, Salomonowitz E, Erlien D, Edwards J. The disease-free wall in coronary atherosclerosis: its relation to degree of obstruction. *J Am Coll Cardiol* 1985; 6: 1096–9.

6 Ross R. Atherosclerosis —an inflammatory disease. *N Engl J Med* 1999; 340: 115–26.

7 Mach F, Schonbeck U, Bonnefoy J-Y, Pober JS, Libby P. Activation of monocyte/ macrophage functions related to acute atheroma complication by ligation of CD-40-induction of collagenase, stromelysin and tissue factor. *Circulation* 1997; 96: 396–9.

8 Nelken N, Coughlin S, Gorden D, Wilcox J. Monocyte chemoattractant protein-1 in human atheromatous plaques. *J Clin Invest* 1991; 88: 1121–7.

9 Rosenfeld M, Yla-Herttuala S, Lipton B, Ord V, Witztum J, Steinberg D. Macrophage colony-stimulation factor mRNA and protein in atherosclerotic lesions of rabbits and man. *Am J Pathol* 1992; 140: 291–300.

10 Quinn M, Parthasarathy S, Fong L, Steinberg D. Oxidatively modified low density lipoprotein: potential role in recruitment and retention of monocyte/ macrophage during atherogenesis. *Proc Natl Acad Sci USA* 1987; 84: 2995–8.

11 Yla-Herttuala S, Palinski W, Rosenfeld M *et al*. Evidence for the presence of oxidatively modified low density lipoprotein in atherosclerotic lesions of rabbit and man. *J Clin Invest* 1989; 84: 1086–95.

12 Hansson G, Jonasson L, Seifert P, Stemme S. Immune mechanisms in atherosclerosis. *Arteriosclerosis* 1989; 9: 567–78.

13 O'Brien K, Allen M, McDonald T *et al*. Vascular cell adhesion molecule-1 is expressed in human coronary atherosclerotic plaques. Implications for the

mode of progression of advanced coronary atherosclerosis. *J Clin Invest* 1993; 92: 945–51.

14 Davies M, Woolf N, Rowles P, Pepper J. Morphology of the endothelium over atherosclerotic plaques in human coronary arteries. *Br Heart J* 1988; 60: 459–64.

15 Burrig K. The endothelium of advanced atherosclerotic plaques in humans. *Arterioscl Thromb* 1991; 11: 1678–89.

16 Davies M. Stability and Instability. Two Faces of Coronary Atherosclerosis: Paul Dudley White Lecture 1995 *Circulation* 1996; 94: 2013–20.

17 Van der Wal A, Becker A, van der Loos C, Das P. Site of intimal rupture or erosion of thrombosed coronary atherosclerotic plaques is characterized by an inflammatory process irrespective of the dominant plaque morphology. *Circulation* 1994; 89: 36–44.

18 Fuster V, Lewis A. Conner Memorial Lecture: Mechanisms leading to myocardial infarction: insights from studies of vascular biology. *Circulation* 1994; 90: 2126–46.

19 Falk E. Why do plaques rupture? *Circulation* 1992; 86: 11130–42.

20 Richardson P, Davies M, Born G. Influence of plaque configuration and stress distribution on fissuring of coronary atherosclerotic plaques. *Lancet* 1989; 2: 941–4.

21 Davies M, Thomas A. Plaque fissuring— the cause of acute myocardial infarction, sudden ischaemic death and crescendo angina. *Br Heart J* 1985; 53: 363–73.

22 Libby P. Molecular basis of the acute coronary syndromes. *Circulation* 1995; 91: 2844–50.

23 Gallis Z, Sukhova G, Lark M, Libby P. Increased expression of matrix metalloproteinases and matrix degrading activity in vulnerable regions of human atherosclerotic plaques. *J Clin Invest* 1994; 94: 2493–503.

24 Burke A, Farb A, Malcom G, Liang Y-H, Smialek J, Virmani R. Coronary risk factors and plaque morphology in men with coronary disease who died suddenly. *N Engl J Med* 1997; 336: 1276–82.

25 Davies M. The composition of coronary-artery plaques. *N Engl J Med* 1997; 336: 1312–13.

26 Arbustini E, Dal Bello B, Morbini P, Burke AP, Bocciarelli M, Specchia G, Virmani R. Plaque erosion is a major substrate for coronary thrombosis in acute myocardial infarction. *Heart* 1999; 82: 269–72.

27 Levin D, Fallon J. Significance of the angiographic morphology of localized coronary stenosis: histopathologic correlations. *Circulation* 1982; 66: 316–20.

28 Ambrose J, Winters S, Arora R *et al*. Coronary angiograph morphology in acute myocardial infarction: link between the pathogenesis of unstable angina and myocardial infarction. *J Am Coll Cardiol* 1985; 6: 1233–8.

29 White C, Ramee S, Collins T *et al*. Coronary thrombi increase PTCA risk. Angioscopy as a clinical tool. *Circulation* 1996; 93: 253–8.

30 Sherman C, Litvack F, Grundfest W. Coronary angioscopy in patients with unstable pectoris. *N Engl J Med* 1986; 315: 913–19.

31 Wartman W. Occlusion of the coronary arteries by hemorrhage into their walls. *Am Heart J* 1938; 15: 459–70.

32 Roberts W. Does thrombosis play a major role in the development of symptom-producing atherosclerotic plaques? *Circulation* 1973; 48: 1161–6.

33 Roberts W. Coronary thrombosis and fatal myocardial ischaemia. *Circulation* 1974; 49: 1–3.

34 Chapman I. The cause–effect relationship between recent coronary artery occlusion and acute myocardial infarction. *Am Heart J* 1974; 87: 267–71.

35 Kim C, Braunwald E. Potential benefits of late reperfusion of infarcted myocardium. The open artery hypothesis. *Circulation* 1993; 88: 2426–36.

36 DeWood M, Spores J, Notske R *et al*. Prevalence of total coronary occlusion during the early hours of transmural myocardial infarction. *N Engl J Med* 1980; 303: 897–902.

37 Stadius M, Maynard C, Fritz J. Coronary anatomy and left ventricular function in the first 12 hours of acute myocardial infarction. *The Western Washington Randomized Intracoronary Streptokinase Trial Circulation* 1985; 72. 292–301.

38 Fulton W. Pathological concepts in acute coronary thrombosis: relevance to treatment. *Br Heart J* 1993; 70: 403–8.

39 Fulton W, Sumner D. 125 I-labelled fibrinogen, autoradiography and stereoarteriography in identification of coronary

thrombotic occlusion in fatal myocardial infarction. *Br Heart J* 1976; 38: 880.

40 Constantinides P. Plaque fissures in human coronary thrombosis. *J Atheroscl Res* 1966; 6: 1–17.

41 Falk E. Plaque rupture with severe pre-existing stenosis precipitating coronary thrombosis. Characteristics of coronary atherosclerotic plaque underlying fatal occlusive thrombi. *Br Heart J* 1983; 50: 127–31.

42 Horie T, Sekiguchi M, Hirosawa K. Coronary thrombosis in pathogenesis of acute myocardial infarction. Histopathological study of coronary arteries in 108 necropsied cases using serial section. *Br Heart J* 1978; 40: 153–61.

43 Davies M, Woolf N, Robertson W. Pathology of acute myocardial infarction with particular reference to occlusive coronary thrombi. *Br Heart J* 1976; 38: 659–64.

44 Braunwald E. Unstable angina, a classification. *Circulation* 1989; 80: 410–4.

45 Falk E. Unstable angina with fatal outcome: dynamic coronary thrombosis leading to infarction and/or sudden death. *Circulation* 1985; 71: 699–708.

46 Ambrose J, Winter S, Stern A *et al*. Angiographic morphology and the pathogenesis of unstable angina pectoris. *J Am Coll Cardiol* 1981; 5: 609–16.

47 Freeman M, Williams A, Chisholm R, Armstrong P. Intracoronary thrombus and complex morphology in unstable angina. Relation to timing of angiography and in-hospital cardiac events. *Circulation* 1989; 80: 17–23.

48 Escaned J, van Suylen R, MacLeod D *et al*. Histological characteristics of tissue excised during directional coronary atherectomy in stable and unstable angina pectoris. *Am J Cardiol* 1993; 71: 1442–7.

49 Rosenschein U, Ellis S, Haudenschild C *et al*. Comparison of histopathologic coronary lesions obtained from directional atherectomy in stable angina versus acute coronary syndromes. *Am J Cardiol* 1994; 73: 508–10.

50 Mann J, Kaski J, Pereira W, Arie S, Ramires J, Pileggi F. Histological patterns of atherosclerotic plaques in unstable angina patients vary according to clinical presentation. *Heart* 1998; 80: 19–22.

51 Flugelman M, Virmani R, Correa R *et al*. Smooth muscle cell abundance and fibroblast growth factors in coronary lesions of patients with nonfatal unstable angina: a clue to the mechanism of transformation from the stable to the unstable clinical state. *Circulation* 1993; 88: 2493–500.

52 Frink R, Ostrach L, Rooney P. Coronary thrombosis. Ulcerated atherosclerotic plaques and platelet/fibrin microemboli in patients dying with acute coronary disease. A large autopsy study. *J Inv Cardiol* 1990; 2: 199–210.

53 Davies M, Thomas A, Knapman P, Hangartner R. Intramyocardial platelet aggregation in patients with unstable angina suffering sudden ischaemic cardiac death. *Circulation* 1986; 73: 418–27.

54 Fitzgerald D, Roy L, Catella F, Fitzgerald A. Platelet activation in unstable coronary disease. *N Engl J Med* 1986; 315: 983–9.

55 Fitzgerald D, Roy L, Catella F, Fitzgerald G. Platelet activation in unstable angina. *J Am Coll Cardiol* 1987; 10: 998–1004.

56 Hackett D, Davies G, Chierchia S, Maseri A. Intermittent coronary occlusion in acute myocardial infarction. Value of combined thrombolytic and vasodilator therapy. *N Engl J Med* 1987; 317: 1055–9.

57 Braunwald E. Unstable angina. An etiologic approach to management. *Circulation* 1998; 98: 2219–22.

58 Roberts W, Curry R, Isner J. Sudden death in Prinzmetal's angina with coronary spasm documented by arteriography: analysis of three necropsy cases. *Am J Cardiol* 1982; 50: 203–10.

59 Brown B. Coronary vasospasm. Observations linking the clinical spectrum of ischaemic heart disease to the dynamic pathology of coronary atherosclerosis. *Arch Intern Med* 1981; 141: 716–22.

60 Kohchi K, Takebayashi S, Hiroki T, Nobuyoshi M. Significance of adventitial inflammation of the coronary artery in patients with unstable angina: results at autopsy. *Circulation* 1985; 71: 709–16.

61 Newby L, Christenson R, Ohman M *et al*. Value of serial troponin T measures for early and late risk stratification in patients with acute coronary syndromes. *Circulation* 1998; 98: 1853–9.

62 Antman E, Tanasikevic M, Thompson B *et al*. Cardiac-specific troponin I levels to predict the risk of mortality in patients with acute coronary syndromes. *N Engl J Med* 1996; 335: 1342–9.

63 Lindahl B, Venge P, Wallentin L. Troponin T identifies patients with unstable coro-

nary artery disease who benefit from long-term antithrombotic protection. *J Am Coll Cardiol* 1997; 29: 43–8.

64 Piek J, Becker A. Collateral blood supply to the myocardium at risk in human myocardial infarction: a quantitative post-mortem assessment. *J Am Coll Cardiol* 1988; 11: 1290–6.

65 DeWood M, Stifter W, Simpson C. Coronary arteriographic findings soon after non-Q-wave myocardial infarction. *N Engl J Med* 1986; 315: 417–23.

66 Davies M, Thomas A. Thrombosis and acute coronary artery lesions in sudden cardiac ischaemic death. *N Engl J Med* 1984; 310: 1137–40.

67 Warnes C, Roberts W. Sudden coronary death: comparison of patients with to those without coronary thrombus at necropsy. *Am J Cardiol* 1984; 54: 1206–11.

68 Davies M. Anatomic features in victims of sudden coronary death. *Circulation* 1992; 85: 119–24.

69 Davies M, Bland J, Hangartner J, Angelini A, Thomas A. Factors influencing the presence or absence of acute coronary artery thrombi in sudden ischaemic death. *Eur Heart J* 1989; 10: 203–8.

70 Koenig W, Sund M, Frohlick M *et al.* C-reactive protein, a sensitive marker of inflammation, predicts future risk of coronary heart disease in initially healthy middle-aged men Results from MONICA (Monitoring Trends Determinants Cardiovascular Disease) Augsburg Cohort Study 1984–92. *Circulation* 1999; 99: 237–42.

71 Ridker P, Buring J, Shih J, Matias M, Hennekens C. Prospective study of C-reactive protein and the risk of future cardiovascular events among apparently healthy women. *Circulation* 1998; 98: 731–3.

72 Liuzzo G, Biasucci L, Gallimore J *et al.* The prognostic value of C-reative protein and serum amyloid. A protein in severe unstable angina. *N Engl J Med* 1994; 331: 417–24.

73 Gupta S, Fredericks S, Schwartzman R, Holt D, Kaski J. Serum neopterin is elevated in acute coronary syndromes. *Lancet* 1997; 349: 1252–3.

74 Ritchie M. Nuclear-factor-kB is selectively and markedly activated in humans with unstable angina pectoris. *Circulation* 1998; 98: 1707–13.

75 Ridker P, Cushman M, Stampfer M *et al.* Inflammation aspirin and the risk of cardiovascular disease in apparently healthy men. *N Engl J Med* 1997; 336: 973–9.

76 Woolf N, Sacks M, Davies M. Aortic plaque morphology in relation to coronary artery disease. *Am J Pathol* 1969; 57: 187–97.

77 McGill H. *The Geographic Pathology of Atherosclerosis.* Baltimore: Williams & Wilkins, 1968: 193.

78 Falk F, Shah P, Fuster V. Coronary plaque disruption. *Circulation* 1995; 92: 656–71.

79 Fleet J, Clinton S, Salomon R, Loppnow H, Libby P. Atherogenic diets enhance endotoxin-stimulated interleukin-1 and tumor necrosis factor gene expression in rabbit aortae. *J Nutr* 1992; 122: 294–305.

80 Danesh J, Collins R, Peto R. Chronic infections and coronary heart disease: Is there a link? *Lancet* 1997; 350: 430–6.

81 Patel P, Mendall M, Stephens J. Association of *Helicobacter pylori* and *Chlamydia pneumoniae* infections with coronary heart disease and cardiovascular risk factors. *Br Med J* 1995; 311: 711–14.

82 Grayston J, Kuo C, Coulson A. *Chlamydia pneumoniae* (TWAR) in atherosclerosis of the carotid artery. *Circulation* 1995; 92: 3397–400.

83 Muhlestein J, Hammond E, Carlquist J *et al.* Increased incidence of chlamydia species within the coronary arteries of patients with symptomatic atherosclerotic versus other forms of cardiovascular disease. *J Am Coll Cardiol* 1996; 27: 1555–6.

84 Hol A, Sukhiva GK, Lichtman AH, Libby P. Chlamydial heat shock protein 60 localizes in human atheroma and regulates macrophage tumor necrosis factor-alpha and matrix. *Circulation* 1998; 98: 300–7.

2: Plaque vulnerability and acute coronary syndromes: what are the prophylactic and therapeutic implications?

David J. Schneider and Burton E. Sobel

Mechanisms underlying atherogenesis

A conventional overview of atherosclerosis

Atherosclerosis is typified by the progression of lesions from the earliest stage, the fatty streak, to later obstructive lesions, which are made up of diverse cells and matrix with the evolution of plaques driven by growth factors and cytokines of cells activated by stimuli such as oxidized low density lipoprotein (LDL) [1,2]. The fatty streak is found commonly in children and in most young adults by the age of 20 years. It occupies 15–25% of the intimal surface of the abdominal aorta, thoracic aorta, and right coronary artery [3]. Advanced lesions, called 'fibrous plaques', are comprised of increased neointimal vascular smooth muscle cells surrounded by a connective tissue matrix and containing variable amounts of intracellular and extracellular lipid [4].

Initiation: arterial injury

Chronic, low-level injury to the arterial endothelium initiates and potentiates atherogenesis [1,5,6]. Turbulent flow at bifurcations of vessels and tortuosities results in shear stress on vascular endothelium. Hypertension increases such stress. Other factors that may contribute to endothelial cell injury and consequent acceleration of atherogenesis include: hypercholesterolaemia, use of tobacco, advanced glycation end-products, circulating vasoactive amines, homocysteinaemia, cytokines associated with inflammation, immune complexes, and infectious agents [7].

Injury to the endothelium potentiates the accumulation of lipids and monocyte-derived macrophages in the vessel wall, and an increased permeability to diverse vasculopathic factors [8]. It induces the expression of adhesive cell-surface glycoproteins, such as intercellular adhesion molecule (ICAM-1), vascular cell adhesion molecule (VCAM-1), and E-selectin, which facilitate binding of monocytes to the luminal surface of the vessel. Oxygen-centred free radicals and activation of the renin–angiotensin system can induce expression of intercellular adhesion molecules, particularly VCAM-1 [9,10]. Local expression of monocyte chemoattractant protein-1 and colony-stimulating factor attract additional monocytes to the subendothelium, as does angiotensin-II-induced increased expression of chemoattractant protein-1 [11].

Low density lipoprotein (LDL) is the major source of cholesterol that accumulates in the vessel wall. It is initially confined to foam cells (macrophages, and to a lesser extent vascular smooth muscle cells). Oxidation of LDL appears to be critical [12]. Oxidized LDL is taken up rapidly by macrophages via scavenger receptors, is a chemoattractant for macrophages and T lymphocytes, and is cytotoxic. High density lipoprotein (HDL) limits atherogenesis by inhibiting oxidation of LDL and by reverse cholesterol transport [12,13].

Progression: smooth muscle activation and inflammatory infiltration

Injury to endothelial cells and the deposition of lipids is accompanied by the infiltration of leucocytes that cause the activation of vascular smooth muscle cells. These cells then migrate into the neointima and subsequently proliferate and stimulate production of extracellular matrix. Infiltration of macrophages, T lymphocytes, and mast cells occurs [14]. Continued recruitment of macrophages and T lymphocytes appears to be mediated by the dysfunctional, injured endothelium [15]. Neovascularization of intimal plaques may stimulate and facilitate entry of inflammatory cells [16]. The progression of atherosclerosis is associated with chronic inflammation. Plaques exhibit variable amounts of inflammatory cells. In general, these cells are seen predominantly in lipid-rich lesions in the cap and shoulder regions [17].

The proliferation and migration of vascular smooth muscle cells are seminal to the progression of atherosclerosis and the genesis of the fibrous cap. The deposition of LDL in the vessel wall is associated with the activation of vascular smooth muscle cells and their migration into the intima. Vascular smooth muscle cells are present in the intima of normal human vessels. Some of the vascular smooth muscle cells found in the neointima reflect proliferation. However, the disruption of the internal elastic lamina and depletion of the media at the base of atherosclerotic plaques facilitates the migration of vascular smooth muscle cells from the media to the neointima [18].

One of the principal mitogens implicated in the activation of vascular smooth muscle cells is platelet derived growth factor (PDGF) [1,2,4]. This agent is present in alpha granules of platelets and is produced by endothelial cells, monocytes, and vascular smooth muscle cells. Other growth factors and cytokines involved include basic and acidic fibroblast growth factor, insulin-like growth factor, epidermal growth factor, angiotensin II, endothelin,

5-hydroxytryptamine, thrombin, transforming growth factor-β, interleukin-1, and tumour necrosis factor-α [19]. These factors alone are not sufficient to induce a proliferative response in the vessel wall, because the extracellular matrix—and particularly the basement membrane—suppresses proliferation [20]. Thus, degradation of the basement membrane appears to be critical to the process, because diminished suppression results. Accordingly, activation of extracellular proteinases, including matrix metalloproteinases (MMPs) 2 and 9 as well as urokinase-type plasminogen activator, have been implicated in facilitating the proliferation of vascular smooth muscle cells, and hence the progression of atherosclerosis.

Extracellular proteinase activity is essential to the migration of vascular smooth muscle cells. Surface expression of plasminogen activators, both tissue-type and urokinase-type, enable vascular smooth muscle cells to migrate through extracellular matrix [21]. Matrix metalloproteinases appear to participate also, because their inhibitors (TIMPS, or tissue inhibitors of matrix metalloproteinases) limit migration [22]. Plasminogen activators may be central to the initiation of this process, because the product to which they give rise, plasmin, can activate precursors of MMPs, particularly MMPs 1, 3, 7, 9 and 12. Overexpression of the primary physiological inhibitor of plasminogen activators, plasminogen activator inhibitor type 1 (PAI-1), limits neointimal formation [23]. Accordingly, both plasminogen activators and MMPs appear to participate in the progression of atherosclerosis, because degradation of extracellular matrix, and particularly of the basement membrane, is pivotal in both the migration and proliferation of vascular smooth muscle cells.

The activation of vascular smooth muscle cells is accompanied by a phenotypic change from contractile to synthetic. Unlike cells with a contractile phenotype, vascular smooth muscle cells with the synthetic phenotype produce extracellular matrix [24]. Components of the matrix in atherosclerotic plaques resemble those present in normal arteries. However, there is an abundance of monomeric rather than polymerized collagen. A close relationship between extracellular matrix and vascular smooth muscle cell migration is reflected by the association of collagen synthesis with the migration of vascular smooth muscle cells [25].

Although perhaps paradoxical at first glance, the progression of atherosclerosis (both fibrosis and cellularity) is dependent on proteinase activity. Thus, the degradation of the basement membrane and proteinase activity necessary for the migration of vascular smooth muscle cells also stimulate the synthesis of new extracellular matrix. In addition, multiple growth factors stimulate the synthesis of collagen. Of these, the most potent is transforming growth factor-β.

An additional component of atheroma is calcium. Calcification appears to be particularly common in the lipid-rich core of plaques and is associated with the expression of osteopontin [26,27]. Thus, the composition of atherosclerotic plaque depends on: (1) deposition of lipid; (2) infiltration of leucocytes; (3) the proliferation and migration of vascular smooth muscle cells; (4) the accumulation of extracellular matrix; and (5) calcification.

A recent paradigm shift

The conventional view that high-grade, occlusive, stenotic coronary lesions represent the final step in a continuum that begins with fatty streaks and culminates in high-grade stenosis resulting in acute coronary syndromes has now had to be modified, since it has been found that thrombotic occlusion is commonly the result of the rupture of minimally stenotic plaques. As many as two-thirds of lesions responsible for acute coronary syndromes are minimally obstructive (less than 50% stenotic) before plaque rupture [28,29]. Disruption of 'vulnerable' plaques and subsequent thrombosis can lead to intermittent, sudden plaque growth and acute coronary syndromes [17,30]. Accordingly, the role of the specific components described above must be reassessed in this context. For example, the migration of vascular smooth muscle cells associated with the production of extracellular matrix may contribute to the growth of atherosclerotic plaques, but may be paradoxically protective by reinforcing the fibrous cap and preventing rupture [31–33].

Proteinase activity in atherogenesis appears to have diverse and, at times, opposite functions. Increased vascular smooth muscle cell proteinase activity, particularly surface expression of plasminogen activators, may contribute to the generation of stable, as opposed to vulnerable (to rupture), plaques. By contrast, decreased vascular smooth muscle cell proteinase activity may contribute to the generation of thin fibrous caps predisposing to plaque rupture. Subsequent proteinase (MMP activity) activated by and in macrophages in advanced plaques can degrade relatively acellular plaques with thin fibrous caps. The plaque rupture that ensues can initiate acute coronary syndromes.

Phenomena in subjects with type II diabetes who experience a 3- to 5-fold increased incidence of myocardial infarction indicate the consequences of these considerations. Overexpression of PAI-1 in the vessel wall appears likely to inhibit plasminogen activator activity and consequently the migration of vascular smooth muscle cells and their production of extracellular matrix [21,31–33]. The apparent result is the formation of plaques with thin fibrous caps that are particularly prone to rupture. This may account, in part, for the high incidence of acute coronary syndromes in diabetic subjects.

Proteinase activity

The role of proteinase activity in the generation of fibrous lesions and in the rupture of vulnerable plaques belies the fact that proteinase activity is neither universally protective nor universally deleterious. We believe that preservation of vascular smooth muscle cells' proteinases (plasminogen activator and plasmin mediated MMP activation) can lead to the generation of stable plaques. By contrast, excessive proteinase activity on vascular smooth muscle cells can predispose to rapid progression of stenosis — albeit in plaques that are less prone to rupture. Conversely proteinase activity, particularly MMP activity induced by macrophages, can precipitate plaque rupture, especially in a relatively smooth-muscle-poor vulnerable plaque.

The nature of atherosclerotic plaques

Atherosclerotic plaques can be categorized according to morphological characteristics, as described by the American Heart Association classification [34]. This categorization reflects the recognition that atherosclerotic occlusion of an artery is not necessarily the result of a sequential progression, but instead often entails sudden changes secondary to plaque rupture.

Lipid deposition is the dominant feature in phase 1 lesions, particularly in early lesions. Initially, lipid deposition is in macrophages and vascular smooth muscle cells, so called 'foam cells' (type I lesions). In later-stage phase 1 lesions, extracellular deposition of lipids and fibrils occurs (type II and III lesions). Traditionally, type II lesions have been termed 'fatty streaks'.

Phase 2 lesions are characterized by a high content of lipid, cells, and extracellular matrix. Plaques in this phase are not necessarily stenotic, but may be prone to rupture. Two types of lesion have been described. In the first, lipid deposition is dominant, cellularity is reduced, and lesions are characterized by a lipid core covered by a fibrous cap (type IV lesions). Type IV lesions display characteristics of vulnerable plaques. In the second type of a phase II lesion, cellular proliferation is dominant and the lesion is characterized by a confluent cellular region, fibrosis, and calcification, in association with extracellular lipid (type V lesion).

The rupture or erosion of phase 2 lesions leads to the development of a complicated plaque in which thrombosis can be either clinically silent or precipitate an acute coronary syndrome (type VI lesions). Subsequent organization of the thrombus and its incorporation into the vessel wall can lead to rapid, incremental plaque growth.

We have characterized the evolution of plaques from a related but somewhat different perspective, focusing on fibrinolytic system protein content, lipid content, and complexity [35]. We quantified PAI-1 and plasminogen activators in proteins extracted from atherosclerotic arteries. Fatty-streak lesions had a high content of PAI-1. By contrast, we have found that phase 2 lesions contain a high content of plasminogen activators. Phase 3 lesions are characterized by a high content of both PAI-1 and plasminogen activators. These observations support the notion that plasminogen activator activity is critical for the migration of vascular smooth muscle cells leading to morphology typical of phase 2 lesions.

Stable atherosclerotic plaques

The AHA classification system distinguishes two types of intermediate atherosclerotic plaques, stable and unstable. Stable atherosclerotic plaques (Fig. 2.1) are characterized by slow growth (reflecting the gradual migration and proliferation of vascular smooth muscle cells), the synthesis of extracellular matrix, and the accumulation of lipid. Ultimately, such plaques become obstructive and lead to myocardial ischaemia manifested by angina with exertion, that is, stable angina. Stable angina is generally a relatively benign process with a good prognosis as long as thrombotic complications can be prevented. However, in an individual patient the clinical syndrome (i.e. stable angina) may not accurately reflect the morphology of the underlying culprit atherosclerotic lesion [36]. Stable lesions are characterized by extensive fibrosis, calcification, and non-inflammatory cell (predominantly vascular smooth muscle cell) encapsulation of a lipid core.

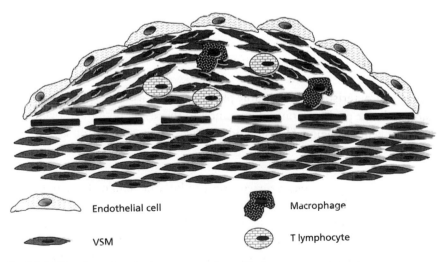

Endothelial cell   Macrophage

VSM   T lymphocyte

Fig. 2.1 Stable atherosclerotic plaques are at a low risk of rupture. Morphological characteristics include a low lipid content (< 40% of plaque volume) and an overlying cap that is rich in vascular smooth muscle (VSM) cells and supporting extracellular matrix.

Unstable atherosclerotic plaques

Features of atherosclerotic plaques (Fig. 2.2) that predispose to rupture include a necrotic lipid core occupying more than 40% of the plaque volume, a thin fibrous cap, decreased numbers of vascular smooth muscle cells, and the accumulation of macrophages at the edge or so-called shoulder of the plaque [17,30,37–49]. An atheromatous core of plaques contributes to vulnerability to rupture. The core of a vulnerable plaque is relatively devoid of supporting collagen, avascular, and hypocellular [41]. Although difficult to prove conclusively, it is likely that the predominant benefit of lipid-lowering therapy in decreasing the incidence of coronary events is mediated by a reduction in the lipid content of vulnerable plaques. Thus, minimal or no reduction in the extent of stenosis has been associated paradoxically with a marked reduction in the incidence of subsequent myocardial infarction [42]. By contrast, the high incidence of acute coronary syndromes typical of vulnerable plaques in patients with type 2 diabetes is associated with relative acellularity of plaques, an excess of lipid in lesions, and impaired vessel-wall proteolysis [31–33].

Activated vascular smooth muscle cells produce connective-tissue proteins such as collagen, elastin, and glycosaminoglycans. Thus, a reduction in the number of vascular smooth muscle cells in plaques is also associated with a reduction in the amount of connective tissue in the overlying cap. Disruption of fibrous caps frequently occurs in a shoulder region containing activated

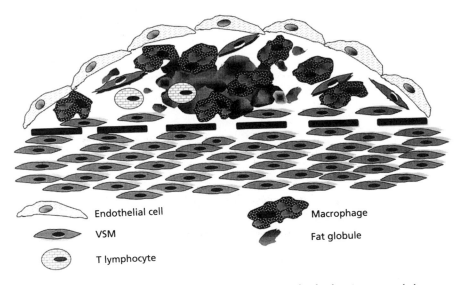

Endothelial cell   Macrophage

VSM   Fat globule

T lymphocyte

Fig. 2.2 Unstable atherosclerotic plaques are prone to rupture that leads to incremental plaque growth and acute coronary syndromes. These plaques are characterized by a necrotic lipid core that occupies greater than 40% of the plaque volume. The overlying cap has a paucity of vascular smooth muscle cells and limited supporting extracellular matrix.

macrophages [38]. The release by macrophages of proteinases, particularly MMPs such as collagenase, gelatinase, and stromelysin, trigger plaque rupture (see below).

Mechanisms underlying plaque rupture

As noted already, the rupture of atherosclerotic plaques, particularly vulnerable plaques, is a proximate cause of acute coronary syndromes. Mechanisms responsible entail those intrinsic and extrinsic to the plaque itself (Fig. 2.3). Intrinsic factors involved include compositional and structural features of the plaque. Extrinsic factors include mechanical forces.

In addition to the characteristics typical of plaques that predispose to rupture (necrotic lipid core occupying more than 40% of the plaque volume, a thin fibrous cap, decreased numbers of vascular smooth muscle cells and the accumulation of macrophages at the edge or so-called shoulder of the plaque), mechanical forces and biological features play important roles.

Mechanical forces

The pulsatile flow of blood through the arterial tree exerts stress on the arterial wall. Stress can be either perpendicular to the vessel wall or parallel. Those forces that are parallel to the endothelial surface constitute shear stress. Richardson and colleagues found that increased stress was concentrated at the edge of the fibrous cap adjacent to the normal intima, the 'shoulder region' of the plaque [43]. Similarly, Cheng and colleagues determined the magnitude of wall stress in plaques from individuals who died because of acute coronary thrombosis and compared the results with those in plaques from subjects who died from other causes. They found that mechanical stress was greater in rup-

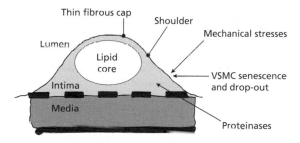

Fig. 2.3 Rupture of vulnerable plaques is precipitated by external mechanical forces and biological features of the plaque. Wall stress is concentrated on the shoulder region. Vascular smooth muscle cell senescence can lead to limited proliferation and production of extracellular matrix. Apoptosis of vascular smooth muscle cells can reduce further the cellularity overlying the lipid core. Inflammatory cell infiltration can precipitate rupture through MMP-mediated degradation of the fibrous cap.

tured plaques than in non-ruptured plaques [44]. In fact, shear stress appears to contribute directly to plaque rupture [45,46]. Accordingly, control of blood pressure is pivotal in the prevention of plaque rupture.

Despite differences observed when results from each group were compared, plaques that rupture were not found uniformly to be in areas with greatest stress. This observation underscores the role of features intrinsic to the plaque.

Increased severity of stenosis is associated with a decrease in wall stress distally [47]. Thus, wall stress is likely to play a greater role in the rupture of plaques in arteries with moderate rather than severe stenosis.

Vascular smooth muscle cells and plaque rupture

A striking morphological feature of atherosclerotic plaques that are particularly prone to rupture is a thin cap with a paucity of vascular smooth muscle cells. The activation (conversion to synthetic phenotype) of vascular smooth muscle cells renders them capable of producing extracellular matrix. Further, their migration is associated with synthesis of extracellular matrix. It can be argued that both the lack of migration of vascular smooth muscle cells into the neointima and the lack of production of extracellular matrix, particularly collagen type I and III, contribute to a predisposition to plaque rupture.

Vascular smooth muscle cell senescence and plaque rupture

Vascular smooth muscle cells that participate in the development of atherosclerotic lesions appear to be the progeny of an initially small number of cells [48,49]. The evidence supporting clonal expansion suggests that vascular smooth muscle cells that participate in the formation of atherosclerotic plaques may be transformed [50,51]. The clonal expansion of a single cell line over many years often leads to senescence [52]. Accordingly, reduced cellularity and limited fibrosis may be the result, in part, of senescence of vascular smooth muscle cells. A reduction in the reparative capacity of vascular smooth muscle cells may contribute to vulnerability of plaques. Thus, in contrast to the conventional wisdom, a mitogenic stimulus may reinvigorate the reparative function of neointimal vascular smooth muscle cells. Percutaneous angioplasty can be viewed as this type of stimulus. In fact, the iatrogenic injury induced by angioplasty is known to promote the proliferation of vascular smooth muscle cells and may stabilize a ruptured plaque. This may explain why, even though angioplasty may be followed by restenosis, the restenosis only rarely gives rise to an acute coronary syndrome. Thus, the restenotic lesion in a non-diabetic subject may be the antithesis of a vulnerable plaque [31–33]. Restenotic lesions in diabetic subjects have limited cellularity compared with those in non-diabetic subjects [53], consistent with the predominance of PAI-1 in lesions in such subjects [31–33].

Vascular smooth muscle cell apoptosis and plaque rupture

Vascular smooth muscle cells present in atherosclerotic lesions may exhibit high susceptibility to programmed cell death (apoptosis) [54–58]. Apoptosis may contribute to a reduction in the number of vascular smooth muscle cells and to the formation of a thin fibrous cap.

Growth factors, inhibitors and plaque rupture

The progression of atherosclerosis is associated with a loss of endothelial cells in the lesions [59]. This is likely to account for decreased production of endothelial-cell-derived cytokines and growth factors, particularly platelet derived growth factor (B chains). Mitogenic effects on vascular smooth muscle cells are limited by prostaglandins, nitric oxide, interferon-γ and transforming growth factor-β, all of which can be elaborated by endothelial cells. Prostaglandins increase intracellular concentrations of cAMP [60,61]. Nitric oxide increases intracellular concentrations of cGMP [61,62]. Both of these cyclic nucleotides inhibit the proliferation of vascular smooth muscle cells and vascular-smooth-muscle-cell-dependent production of extracellular matrix [61,63,64]. Interferon-γ and transforming growth factor-β inhibit the proliferation of vascular smooth muscle cells as well [65,66]. Thus, decreased production of these mediators may influence plaque morphology and stability by altering proliferation of vascular smooth muscle cells.

Inflammation and plaque rupture

The presence of leucocytes, particularly T cells and macrophages, in the shoulder regions of plaques underlying rupture has led to the hypothesis that inflammatory cells contribute to plaque rupture [67]. Lymphocytes are a primary source of the inhibitory mediators described above. Thus, their presence may promote the formation of unstable plaques by limiting the proliferation of vascular smooth muscle cells and vascular-smooth-muscle-cell-dependent production of robust fibrous caps. Low density lipoproteins (LDL), and particularly oxidized LDL, are chemoattractant factors for lymphocytes [68].

The presence of macrophages in atherosclerotic plaques, particularly in the shoulder region, has been recognized increasingly to be destabilizing [67,69]. Lipid-laden macrophages (foam cells) constitutively express MMPs [69]. Of interest, lipid-laden macrophages from cholesterol-fed rabbits spontaneously produce and release MMPs, whereas alveolar macrophages from

the same animals exhibit only limited expression of MMPs [69]. Local proteinase activity can be expected to be increased when both macrophage
content and lipid content of plaques are high [70]. Proteinase activity combined with a paucity of vascular smooth muscle cells and a thin fibrous cap are
likely to precipitate plaque rupture.

Activated mast cells have been identified at sites of plaque disruption [71].
Their numbers are low, yet they may participate in the genesis of plaque rupture by secreting tryptase and chymase. These proteinases can activate inactive zymogens of MMPs (pro-MMPs) released by macrophages and zymogens
of other proteins, including angiotensin II.

Thus, infiltration of atherosclerotic plaques with inflammatory cells can
predispose to plaque rupture. Lymphocytes limit the proliferation of vascular
smooth muscle cells and their production of extracellular matrix. Lipid-laden
macrophages release MMPs, and mast cells release proteinases that can activate MMP zymogens released by macrophages. Non-specific manifestations
of inflammation, such as the elevation of concentrations in the blood of C-
reactive protein (CRP), interleukin-6, and fibrinogen, may be a reflection of
and a contributor to inflammatory processes within the vessel wall.

Proteinase activity and plaque rupture

Proteinase activity appears to be seminal in both the formation of atherosclerotic plaques and the rupture of vulnerable atherosclerotic plaques. Vascular
smooth muscle cells synthesize and release both plasminogen activators and
MMPs. Whereas the expression of proteinases by vascular smooth muscle
cells can lead to the progression of atherosclerosis, it may also lead to the
formation of stable as opposed to vulnerable plaques. Surface expression of
plasminogen activators and consequent plasmin-mediated-MMP activity
promote the activation and migration of vascular smooth muscle cells as well
as the production of extracellular matrix. By contrast, the lack of vascular
smooth muscle cell proteinase activity appears likely to predispose to the formation of unstable plaques, with a limited number of vascular smooth muscle
cells in the cap region and a limited production of extracellular matrix, leading
to the formation of a thin cap.

The production and activation of proteinases by inflammatory cells
(macrophages and mast cells) can lead to the degradation of all the components of the fibrous cap [72]. Macrophages synthesize and release interstitial
collagenase (MMP-1), stromelysin (MMP-3), and gelatinases (MMP-2 and
MMP-9) [70,73]. The activation of MMPs appears to be a salient cause of
plaque rupture.

Metalloproteinases are secreted as proenzyme/inhibitor complexes.
They are activated in the extracellular space at neutral pH [72]. Their enzy-

matic activity is dependent on two Zn^{2+} molecules and a Ca^{2+} molecule that serves to stabilize the complex. Cleavage of the N-terminal domain results in activation. The C-terminal domain and catalytic domain participate in binding to receptors and specificity of substrate recognition. Tissue inhibitors (TIMPs) bind to catalytic sites with 1 : 1 stoichiometry. MMP activity is substrate specific, but overlap among MMPs is evident.

The activation of MMPs can occur via several mechanisms. Plasmin (generated by plasminogen activator activity on plasminogen) and tryptase and chymase (released by mast cells) can activate MMPs, as can reactive oxygen species [74]. LDL is a potent stimulus for release of MMPs. In addition, cytokines such as interferon-γ, interleukin-1, and tumour necrosis factor-α stimulate the production and release of MMPs [75]. Oxidized LDL, interferon-γ, interleukin-1, and tumour necrosis factor-α increase the expression of MMP-1 by endothelial cells, which, in turn, can activate pro-MMP-2 [76]. Thus, endothelial cells may participate in the activation of MMPs, thereby accelerating plaque rupture.

Further definition of the role of proteinase activity in both atherogenesis and the rupture of vulnerable plaques is required. Inflammatory cell expression of MMPs is highly likely to be an important mediator of plaque rupture. Atherosclerotic plaques within any given subject reflect diverse stages of evolution. Thus, it seems unlikely that the ubiquitous inhibition of MMP activity will be an effective therapy. Although MMP-induced plaque rupture may be prevented by such a strategy in some plaques, vulnerable plaques may be generated as a result in other regions.

The role of plaque rupture and thrombosis in acute coronary syndromes

Evidence for plaque rupture

The pathological role of thrombosis complicating atherosclerotic plaque rupture was first postulated by Herrick in 1912 [77], but later rejected. Thrombosis as the aetiology of acute myocardial infarction received little attention until the 1970s. Over the past 25 years, thrombosis overlying plaque rupture has been seen in autopsy studies, at angiography and surgery, and with angioscopy. Furthermore, the efficacy of coronary thrombolysis in aborting acute myocardial infarction and limiting infarct size [78,79] establishes the deleterious contribution of thrombosis to acute coronary syndromes.

In 1976, Davies and his colleagues analysed autopsy material in the hearts of 500 patients who had succumbed to myocardial infarction [80]. In 469 cases, myocardial lesions were localized in a single coronary artery. In hearts with these infarcts, an occlusive thrombus was seen in 95%.

Clinically-silent plaque rupture has been observed as well. Asymptomatic disrupted coronary plaques are seen in 9% of apparently healthy subjects and 22% of patients with diabetes or hypertension [81]. Multiple disrupted plaques are found frequently in the coronary arteries of subjects who die as a result of ischaemic heart disease [82,83].

Coronary angiography has confirmed the role of coronary thrombosis as the predominant mechanism responsible for acute myocardial infarction. When angiography is performed within 6 hours of the onset of symptoms, approximately 80% of patients exhibit the angiographic criteria of thrombus [84]. This observation has been confirmed by surgical exploration in many instances.

Coronary angioscopy demonstrates that not only acute myocardial infarction but also unstable angina is associated with intracoronary thrombi. Mizuna and colleagues found that 29 of 31 patients studied with either myocardial infarction or unstable angina had thrombus in the culprit vessel [85]. Results in recent studies have shown that thrombosis is persistent up to 1 month after an acute myocardial infarction in most patients [86]. Thus, the vast majority of subjects with acute coronary syndromes have thrombosis associated with plaque rupture. Plaque rupture can be clinically silent. Yet, sudden incremental plaque growth may result from thrombosis after plaque rupture. Accordingly the thrombotic response to plaque rupture is an important determinant not only of progression of but also of the catastrophic consequences of atherosclerosis.

Thrombosis and plaque rupture

The extent of thrombosis in response to plaque rupture depends upon factors potentiating thrombosis (prothrombotic factors), factors limiting thrombosis (antithrombotic factors), and local fibrinolytic system capacity, reflecting a balance between activity of plasminogen activators and their primary physiological inhibitor PAI-1. Plasminogen activators lead to the generation of plasmin from plasminogen. The activity of plasmin is limited by inhibitors such as α_2 antiplasmin and α_2 macroglobulin. If thrombosis is limited, localized mural thrombus may be the sole complication of rupture of a vulnerable atherosclerotic plaque and lead to clinically-silent growth of the lesion. If thrombosis is exaggerated, an occlusive thrombus can result from plaque rupture and give rise to an acute coronary syndrome.

The principal components of thrombi are fibrin and platelets. Plasma proteins and white blood cells are incorporated to a variable extent. Rupture of an atherosclerotic plaque leads to local coagulation and adhesion of platelets. Coagulation is initiated by Tissue Factor, a membrane-bound glycoprotein [86–88]. Tissue Factor binds coagulation factor VII/VIIa to form the extrinsic 'tenase' complex that activates both factors IX and X. Subsequent assembly of the 'prothrombinase' complex leads to the generation of thrombin. Thrombin in turn cleaves fibrinogen to form fibrin. The generation of thrombin is sustained and amplified greatly by its activation of factor VIII and facilitated activation of factor IX by factor Xa leading to the formation of the intrinsic 'tenase' complex.

Thrombin participates also in limiting thrombosis. Thrombin can bind to thrombomodulin on the surface of endothelial cells. This complex activates protein C (Ca) that, in combination with protein S, cleaves (inactivates) coagulation factors Va and VIIIa. Thus, thrombin formation begets thrombin, but also limits diffuse propagation of clot. The extrinsic Xase complex is inhibited by tissue factor pathway inhibitor (TFPI) present in the circulation. The relative balance of activation and inhibition determines the extent of thrombosis.

Exposure of platelets to the subendothelium after plaque rupture leads to their adherence mediated by exposure to both collagen and to von Willebrand factor [89,90]. The exposure of platelets to agonists, including collagen, von Willebrand factor, ADP (released by damaged red blood cells and activated platelets), and thrombin, leads to activation of platelets. Activation is a complex process that includes shape change (pseudopod extension that increases the surface area of the platelet), activation of the surface glycoprotein IIb-IIIa, release of products from granules (including dense and alpha granules, and lysosomes), and a change in the platelet membrane that promotes binding and assembly of coagulation factors amplifying the rate of coagulation by more than 300 000-fold. The activation of the surface glycoprotein IIb-IIIa results in a conformational change in the glycoprotein that exposes a binding site for fibrinogen on the activated conformer [91]. Each molecule of fibrinogen can bind two platelets, thereby leading to aggregation of platelets. Degranulation of dense granules leads to the release of calcium, serotonin, and nucleotides such as ADP. Degranulation of alpha granules leads to the release of proteins such as coagulation factors (platelet factor V/Va, pivotal in initial prothrombinase activity, and fibrinogen), and growth factors. After activation, the plasma membrane of platelets exposes negatively-charged phospholipids on its outer surface that markedly facilitate the assembly and subsequently the activity of the tenase and prothrombinase complexes, with consequently massive acceleration of generation of thrombin [88].

Platelets participate in thrombosis by: (1) contributing to the haemostatic plug (shape change, adherence to the vascular wall and aggregation); (2) supplying coagulation factors and calcium (release of alpha and dense granule contents); (3) providing platelet factor V/Va, and hence facilitating initial prothrombinase activity; (4) providing a surface for the assembly of coagulation factors; and (5) stimulating vasoconstriction. Increased platelet reactivity has been associated with a greater than 3-fold increase in cardiovascular mortality in apparently healthy subjects and in young survivors of myocardial infarction [92,93]. Thus, increased platelet reactivity is a risk factor for acute coronary syndromes.

Thrombosis complicated by plaque rupture can result in luminal occlusion, or, when limited, accelerated stenosis. Mechanisms by which thrombi can contribute to plaque growth include the incorporation of the organized thrombus into the vessel wall [94] and exposure of vessel-wall constituents to clot-associated mitogens and cytokines. Fibrin and fibrin-degradation products promote the migration of vascular smooth muscle cells and are chemotactic for monocytes [95]. Thrombin and growth factors released from platelet alpha granules, such as platelet-derived growth factor and transforming growth factor beta, activate vascular smooth muscle cells, potentiating their migration and proliferation [96–98]. The pivotal role of platelets has been demonstrated by a reduction in the proliferation of vascular smooth muscle cells after mechanical arterial injury in thrombocytopenic rabbits with atherosclerosis [99].

As noted already, the balance between the activity of prothrombotic and antithrombotic factors, as well as fibrinolytic system capacity, are important determinants of the thrombotic response to plaque rupture. Both local and systemic factors influence thrombosis. The morphology and composition of the plaque are powerful influences. Atheromatous plaques with substantial lipid content predispose to thrombosis more than do normal vessel walls, fatty streaks, sclerotic plaques or fibrolipid plaques [100]. The severity of injury and the extent of plaque rupture determine the extent of exposure of blood to the subendothelium and consequent thrombogenicity. Endothelial dysfunction potentiates vasoconstriction and thrombosis.

Tissue Factor antigen and activity are present in atherosclerotic plaques and are likely to contribute to thrombogenicity associated with plaque rupture [101]. Plaque morphology influences local shear stress that potentiates the activation of platelets [102,103]. Hypertension, by increasing shear stress, can potentiate activation of platelets as well. Additional systemic factors that potentiate thrombosis and its persistence include increased concentrations of fibrinogen in the blood [104,105], coagulation factor VII [105], and PAI-1 [106–108]. Increased concentrations of PAI-1 in the blood decrease endogenous fibrinolytic capacity and thereby promote accelerated thrombosis and persistence of thrombi. Increased platelet reactivity promotes thrombogenicity and is a descriptor of future cardiac events in patients with a previous myocardial infarction and in apparently healthy subjects [92,93]. Emotional stress and other conditions that increase concentrations of circulating catecholamines that potentiate platelet activation through alpha adrenergic receptors can promote thrombosis [109,110]. Thus, both local and systemic factors can potentiate thrombosis, limit fibrinolysis, and thereby predispose to exaggerated thrombosis, vessel occlusion, and the occurrence of an acute coronary syndrome.

Implications regarding therapy

In some instances, understanding of the genesis of plaque rupture has supported the implementation of treatments that have already been previously empirically shown to prevent acute coronary syndromes. In others, advances in mechanistic understanding have suggested novel treatment options that are currently being tested in clinical trials. An improved definition of the mechanisms responsible for plaque rupture and for acute thrombosis should facilitate the development of effective treatment strategies aimed at preventing plaque rupture and thereby decreasing the incidence of acute coronary syndromes. Examples include the following.

Lipids

A reduction in the concentration of cholesterol, and particularly LDL cholesterol, markedly reduces the incidence of cardiac events in subjects with or without previous myocardial infarction [111,112]. The reduction is consistent with the role of cholesterol in the genesis of vulnerable plaques and their rupture. When the cholesterol content exceeds 40% of plaque composition, the plaque is more vulnerable to rupture. Furthermore, LDL cholesterol is chemotactant for inflammatory cells and a stimulant to the release of MMPs. Thus, an increased deposition of LDL cholesterol in the vessel wall can promote rupture, by destabilizing the plaque and degrading the fibrous cap as a result of increased activity of MMPs. This view is consistent with the paradoxical lack of 'regression' of coronary artery stenoses seen by angiography in trials of lipid-lowering therapy in the face of a decreased incidence of events. Thus, despite a marked reduction in the incidence of myocardial infarction, there appears to be limited reduction in the extent of stenosis [113]. The predominant benefit of cholesterol-lowering in this setting appears to be stabilization of atherosclerotic plaques.

High density lipoprotein (HDL) is responsible for 'reverse' transport of cholesterol, that is from the periphery to the liver. Optimal treatment for plaque stabilization should decrease LDL cholesterol and increase HDL cholesterol. Unfortunately, limited options are available for increasing HDL cholesterol. Nevertheless, the potential value of even modest increases in HDL cholesterol is suggested by a recently reported study from the Veterans Affairs High-Density Lipoprotein Cholesterol Intervention Trial Study Group [114]. The importance of modest changes in HDL cholesterol supports the use of niacin- and fibric-acid derivatives to increase HDL cholesterol.

The content of triglycerides *per se* in atherosclerotic plaques has not been associated with vulnerability of the lesions. Nevertheless, increased concentrations of triglycerides in the blood, particularly in combination with hypercholesterolaemia, have been associated with an increase in cardiac events [115]. Potential mechanisms responsible include the inverse relationship between hypertriglyceridaemia and low concentrations in blood of HDL cholesterol (attributable to activity of the cholesterol ester exchange protein and lipoprotein lipase activity on hyperlipidated HDL) and the effects of triglycerides on expression of PAI-1. Thus, the effect of hypertriglyceridaemia *per se* cannot be differentiated easily from the effects of HDL cholesterol and PAI-1.

Triglycerides, and their constituent free fatty acids, can directly augment expression of PAI-1 [116–118]. Overexpression of PAI-1 may potentiate the formation of unstable atherosclerotic plaques and exuberant thrombosis in response to plaque rupture. Thus, the reduction in event rates in patients treated with fibric-acid derivatives [114,119] may be secondary to both the increase in HDL cholesterol and the reduction in expression of PAI-1. Gemfibrozil *in vitro* inhibits the expression of PAI-1 [120]. Accordingly, the use of fibric-acid derivatives in patients with hypertriglyceridaemia may promote the stabilization of vulnerable plaques.

Hypertension and wall stress

Hypertension is a well established risk factor for ischaemic heart disease. Its treatment decreases the incidence of subsequent cardiac events [121]. One mechanism responsible may be a decrease in the rupture of vulnerable plaques as a result of a decrease in wall stress.

Treatment with beta adrenergic blocking agents decreases the incidence of subsequent cardiac events in patients with previous myocardial infarction [122]. Beta adrenergic blocking agents decrease blood pressure. In addition, they decrease wall stress by decreasing the rate of rise of pulse pressure (dp/dt). Subjects who have experienced a myocardial infarction are likely to harbour other vulnerable plaques. Thus, beneficial effects derived from treatment with beta-blocking agents may be secondary, in part, to the decreased blood-vessel-wall stress associated with their use.

Oxygen-centred free radicals

Oxidation and oxygen-centred free radicals appear to contribute to plaque rupture. Oxidized LDL is taken up by the scavenger receptor that is refractory to down-regulation, despite extensive exposure to its ligands. Thus, oxidized LDL leads to continued uptake of LDL, cell death, and ultimately to the accumulation of an extracellular pool of lipids. Reactive oxygen species potentiate the release of MMPs as well as their activation. Accordingly, oxidative stress is likely to predispose to the generation of vulnerable plaques and to plaque rupture. Clinical trials with antioxidants such as vitamins C and E have yielded mixed results [123]. Nevertheless, antioxidant therapy (particularly vitamin E) may benefit subjects who are at high risk for the generation and rupture of unstable plaques.

Inflammation

The presence of macrophages, T lymphocytes and mast cells destabilizes atherosclerotic plaques. MMPs released by macrophages appear to precipitate plaque rupture. Thus, inhibition of inflammation should decrease the incidence of atherosclerotic plaque rupture. Although MMPs appear to mediate plaque rupture, it seems unlikely that ubiquitous inhibition of MMP activity is an appropriate therapeutic target, because MMP activity can contribute to the evolution of stable as opposed to unstable plaques by promoting vascular smooth muscle cell migration. Because plaque evolution is likely to be at diverse stages in a given individual at any time, the ubiquitous inhibition of MMP activity could promote the formation of unstable plaques even while decreasing the likelihood of rupture of others. One could envisage that the beneficial effects may be offset by the generation of other unstable plaques that are prone to rupture in response to stimuli such as mechanical stress.

A reduction in the infiltration of inflammatory cells is an attractive target for the suppression of proteinase activity within already vulnerable plaques. Trials designed to suppress inflammatory and immune mediated responses are being undertaken.

Systemic infections with agents such as *Chlamydia pneumoniae*, *Helicobacter pylori*, and cytomegalovirus have been associated with atherosclerotic disease [124–127]. Yet infection has not been linked conclusively to the progression of atherosclerosis. Nevertheless, it may contribute to plaque rupture augmented by inflammatory cell infiltration. Trials designed to test the potential role of macrolide antibiotics in preventing acute myocardial infarction are ongoing.

Platelet reactivity

Increased platelet reactivity is associated with an increased incidence of cardiovascular mortality in apparently healthy individuals and in survivors of myocardial infarction. Treatment with aspirin decreases the incidence of myocardial infarction in diverse subjects [128]. The mechanisms by which aspirin prevents myocardial infarction are not yet completely understood. Aspirin acetylates cyclooxygenase I, and thereby prevents the formation of thromboxane A_2, a platelet-agonist released when platelets are activated [129]. Thus, aspirin limits the recruitment of additional activated platelets. When one considers the potency and abundance of other platelet agonists such as thrombin, the effects of aspirin on platelet function appear modest. This observation leads to two speculations. First, aspirin may confer beneficial effects by mechanisms other than by affecting platelets (such as anti-inflammatory effects). Second, the combination of aspirin and other more powerful inhibitors of platelet function may be indicated in subjects with highly reactive platelets.

Through acetylation of proteins, aspirin is known to inhibit the production of prostaglandins. Prostaglandins can theoretically promote the genesis of unstable plaques by limiting the proliferation of vascular smooth muscle cells and the production of extracellular matrix. Accordingly, the aspirin-mediated inhibition of synthesis of prostaglandins may promote the formation of stable rather than unstable plaques. This may account, in part, for the beneficial effects of aspirin in preventing myocardial infarction in patients who present with unstable angina and in those in secondary prevention trials.

Potent antiplatelet therapy with GP IIb/IIIa inhibitors and ADP receptor antagonists in combination with aspirin may be particularly useful in the treatment of patients with increased platelet reactivity. Implementation of therapy for these subjects is limited by the lack of availability of accurate bedside assays of platelet function and the variability of the response of platelets to given concentrations of antagonists under different circumstances [130,131]. The value of long-term treatment with a combination of antiplatelet agents is currently being tested (e.g. in an ongoing study of clopidogrel plus aspirin).

Cytokines and growth factors, and the renin–angiotensin system

Multiple growth factors and cytokines can contribute to the genesis of unstable plaques. Because cytokines and growth factors have ubiquitous effects, it is unlikely that altering the expression of these factors will be safe unless therapy can be targeted to atherosclerotic lesions. The use of angiotensin-converting enzyme inhibitors reduces the incidence of myocardial infarction [132]. This effect may be secondary to the inhibition of direct effects of angiotensin II on the endothelium and vascular wall. In addition, beneficial effects may be mediated through the inhibition of stimulatory effects of angiotensin IV, a breakdown product of angiotensin II, on expression of PAI-1 [133].

Diabetes

Type 2 diabetes confers a 3- to 5-fold increase in the risk of myocardial infarction [134]. The increase is independent of frequent coexistent risk factors such as hypertension and hyperlipidaemia. The mechanisms responsible are undoubtedly multifactorial. Deranged metabolism of glucose and lipids contribute. Hyperglycaemia leads to glycosylation of proteins that can potentiate endothelial damage [135,136]. The atherogenic effects of the advanced glycosylation end-products (AGE) that accumulate in vascular tissue include chemotaxis for monocytes; increased production of growth factors and cytokines such as platelet-derived growth factor, tumour necrosis factor α, and interleukin-1; and the stimulation of vascular smooth cell proliferation. The presence of AGE in the arterial wall increases the binding and deposition of LDL [136].

Derangements in lipid metabolism lead to the production of VLDL remnants implicated in the development of atherosclerosis in subjects with type II diabetes [137]. Increased VLDL potentiates the production of LDL and small, dense LDL through its intermediary metabolite, IDL [138]. In addition, diabetes has been associated with an increase in the oxidation of LDL known to promote atherogenesis [139].

Type 2 diabetes is a disease of insulin resistance. This, in turn, leads to hyperinsulinaemia, particularly during early phases and for as long as one to two decades before the diagnosis of frank diabetes can be established [140]. Increased concentrations of insulin, and precursors such as proinsulin and split proinsulin, may accelerate atherosclerosis directly. This possibility is consistent with the observed high incidence of atherosclerosis in subjects manifesting insulin-resistant states other than type 2 diabetes, including those with obesity and subsets of patients with hypertension [141–143]. A positive correlation has been observed between concentrations of immunoreactive insulin in the blood and the development of complications of atherosclerosis [142,143].

Increased expression of PAI-1 may predispose to the development of vulnerable plaques. Patients with type 2 diabetes have a 4-fold increase in the concentration of PAI-1 in blood that is paralleled by increased PAI-1 in atheroma from the vessel wall [31]. The combination of hyperinsulinaemia, hyperglycaemia, and hyperlipaemia (particularly VLDL and free fatty acids) increases expression of PAI-1 [144]. Thus, the combined metabolic and hormonal abnormalities typical of diabetes appear to accelerate atherosclerosis and contribute to the generation of vulnerable plaques.

Treatment of type 2 diabetes must focus on control of metabolic abnormalities without exacerbating hormonal abnormalities. Thus, insulin-sensitizing agents, such as the glitazones that control metabolic abnormalities without promoting hyperinsulinaemia, are likely to be advantageous for the treatment of patients with type 2 diabetes [79,145]. Agents such as metformin (a biguanide) diminish hyperinsulinaemia by decreasing hepatic gluconeogenesis and can be insulin-sparing as well. The potential value of insulin-sparing therapy is anticipated to be tested in the BARI II trial.

Conclusions and some counter-intuitive implications

The identification of the mechanisms responsible for the vulnerability of atherosclerotic plaques to rupture is critical for defining therapies that can prevent myocardial infarction and death. Features responsible for rupture of atherosclerotic plaques include morphology, biochemical composition, and the mechanical forces exerted. Reductions of the lipid content of plaques and the mechanical stress to which they are exposed have already been proved to be beneficial. The promotion of vascular smooth muscle cell migration into the neointima and associated elaboration of matrix protein (such as the reduction of elevated vessel wall PAI-1), measures that are paradoxical at first glance, may facilitate the stabilization of plaques. If they can be applied without accelerating stenosis, they may well prove to be beneficial as well.

References

1 Ross R, Glomset JA. The pathogenesis of atherosclerosis. *N Engl J Med* 1976; 295: 369–77, 420–5.

2 Ross R. The pathogenesis of atherosclerosis—an update. *N Engl J Med* 1986; 314: 488–500.

3 Pathobiological determinants of atherosclerosis in youth (PDAY) research group. Natural history of aortic and coronary atherosclerotic lesions in youth: Findings from the PDAY study. *Arterioscler Thromb* 1993; 13: 1291–8.

4 Ross R, Wight TN, Strandnes E, Thiele B. Human atherosclerosis. I. Cell constitution and characteristics of advanced lesions of the superficial femoral artery. *Am J Pathol* 1984; 78: 175–90.

5 Ross R. The pathogenesis of atherosclerosis: a perspective for the 1990s. *Nature* 1993; 362: 801–9.

6 Fuster V, Badimon L, Badimon JJ, Cheseboro JH. The pathogenesis of coronary artery disease and the acute coronary syndrome. *N Engl J Med* 1992; 326: 310–18.

7 Strong JP, for the Pathobiological Determinants of Atherosclerosis in Youth (PDAY) Research Group. Natural history and risk factors for early human atherogenesis. *Clin Chem* 1995; 41: 134–8.

8 Hansson GK, Bonjers G, Bylock A, Hjalmarsson L. Ultrastructural studies on the localization of IgG in the aortic endothelium and subendothelial intima of atherosclerotic and non-atherosclerotic rabbits. *Exp Mol Pathol* 1980; 33: 302–15.

9 Tummala PE, Chen XL, Sundell CL, Laursen JB, Hammes CP, Alexander RW, Harrison DG, Medford RM. Angiotensin II induces vascular cell adhesion molecule-1 expression in rat vasculature: a potential link between the renin–angiotensin system and atherosclerosis. *Circulation* 1999; 100: 1223–9.

10 Khan BV, Harrison DG, Olbrych MT, Alexander RW, Medford RM. Nitric oxide regulates vascular cell adhesion molecule 1 gene expression and redox-sensitive transcriptional events in human vascular endothelial cells. *Proc Natl Acad Sci USA* 1996; 93: 9114–19.

11 Chen XL, Tummala PE, Olbrych MT, Alexander RW, Medford RM. Angiotensin II induces monocyte chemoattractant protein-1 gene expression in rat vascular smooth muscle cells. *Circ Res*, 1998; 83: 952–9.

12 Steinberg D, Witztum JL. Lipoproteins and atherogenesis. Current concepts. *J Am Med Assoc* 1990; 264: 3047–56.

13 Badimon L, Badimon JJ, Fuster V. Regression of atherosclerotic lesions by high density lipoprotein plasma fractions in the cholesterol-fed rabbit. *J Clin Invest* 1990; 85: 1234–41.

14 Gown AM, Tsukada T, Ross R. Human atherosclerosis. II. Immunocytochemical analysis of the cellular composition of human atherosclerotic lesions. *Am J Pathol* 1986; 125: 191–207.

15 Munro JM, Cotra RS. The pathogenesis of atherosclerosis. Atherogenesis and inflammation. *Lab Invest* 1988; 58: 249–61.

16 O'Brien KD, McDonals TO, Chait A, Allen M, Alpers CE. Neovascular expression of E-selectin, intercellular adhesions molecule-1 and vascular adhesion molcule-1 in human atherosclerosis and their relation to intimal leukocyte content. *Circulation* 1996; 93: 672–82.

17 Davies MJ, Richardson PD, Woolf N, Kratz DR, Mann J. Risk of thrombosis in human atherosclerotic plaques: role of extracellular lipid, macrophage, and smooth muscle content. *Br Heart J* 1993; 69: 377–81.

18 Davies MJ, Woolf N. *Atherosclerosis in Ischaemic Heart Disease. The Mechanisms* London: Science Press, 1990.

19 Newby AC, George SJ. Proposed role for growth factors in mediating smooth muscle proliferation in vascular pathologies. *Cardiovasc Res* 1993; 27: 1173–83.

20 Southgate KM, Davie M, Booth RFG, Newby AC. Involvement of extracellular matrix degrading proteinases in rabbit aortic smooth muscle cell proliferation. *Biochem J* 1992; 288: 93–9.

21 Reidy M, Irvin C, Lindner V. Migration of arterial wall cells. Expression of plasminogen activators inhibitors in injured rat arteries. *Circ Res* 1996; 78: 405–14.

22 Kempo N, Koyama N, Kenagy R, Lea H, Clowes A. Regulation of vascular smooth muscle cell migration and proliferation *in vitro* and injured rat arteries by a synthetic matrix metalloproteinase inhibitor. *Arterioscler Thromb Vasc Biol* 1996; 16: 28–33.

23 Carmeliet P, Moons L, Lijnen R *et al.* Inhibitory role of plasminogen activator inhibitor-1 in arterial wound healing and neointimal formation. A gene targeting and gene transfer study in mice. *Circulation* 1997; 96: 3180–91.

24 Ang AH, Tachas G, Campbell JH, Bateman JF, Campbell GR. Collagen synthesis by cultured rabbit aortic smooth muscle cells. *Biochem J* 1990; 265: 461–9.

25 Rocnik EF, Chan BM, Pickering JG. Evidence for a role of collagen synthesis in arterial smooth muscle cell migration. *J Clin Invest* 1998; 101: 1889–98.

26 Shanahan CM, Cary NR, Metcalfe JC, Weissberg PL. High expression of genes for calcification-regulating proteins in human atherosclerotic plaques. *J Clin Invest* 1994; 93: 2393–402.

27 Fitzpatrick LA, Severson A, Edwards WD, Ingram RT. Diffuse calcification in human coronary arteries. Association of osteopontin with atherosclerosis. *J Clin Invest* 1994; 94: 1597–604.

28 Ambrose JA, Tannenbaum AM, Alexpoulos D, Hjemdahl-Monsen CE, Leavy J, Weiss M, Borrico S, Gorling R, Fuster V. Angiographic progression of coronary artery disease and the development of myocardial infarction. *J Am Coll Cardiol* 1988; 12: 56–62.

29 Little WC, Constantinescu M, Applegate RJ, Kutcher MA, Burrows MT, Kahl FR, Santamore WP. Can coronary angiography predict the site of a subsequent myocardial infarction in patients with mild-to-moderate coronary artery disease? *Circulation* 1988; 78: 1157–66.

30 Falk E, Shah PK, Fuster V. Coronary plaque disruption. *Circulation* 1995; 92: 657–71.

31 Sobel BE, Woodcock-Mitchell J, Schneider DJ, Holt RE, Marutsuka K, Gold H. Increased plasminogen activator inhibitor type-1 in coronary artery atherectomy specimens from type 2 diabetic compared with nondiabetic patients: a potential factor predisposing to thrombosis and its persistence. *Circulation* 1998; 97: 2213–21.

32 Sobel BE. Increased plasminogen activator inhibitor type 1 and vasculopathy. A reconcilable paradox. *Circulation* 1999; 99: 2496–8.

33 Sobel BE. The potential influence of insulin and plasminogen activator inhibitor type 1 on the formation of vulnerable atherosclerotic laques associ-

ated with type 2 diabetes. *Proc Assoc Am Physicians* 1999; 111: 313–18.

34 Stary HC, Chandler AB, Dinsmore RE, Fuster V, Glagov S, Insull W, Rosenfeld ME, Schwartz CJ, Wagner WD, Wissler RW. A definition of advanced types of atherosclerotic lesions and a histological classification of atherosclerosis: a report from the Committee on Vascular Lesions of the Council on Arteriosclerosis, American Heart Association. *Circulation* 1995; 92: 1355–74.

35 Schneider DJ, Ricci MA, Taatjes DJ, Baumann PQ, Reese JC, Leavitt BJ, Absher M, Sobel BE. Changes in arterial expression of fibrinolytic system proteins in atherogenesis. *Arterioscler Thromb Vasc Biol* 1997; 17: 3294–301.

36 van der Wal AC, Becker AE, Koch KY, Piek JJ, Teeling P, van der Loos CM, David GK. Clinically stable angina is not necessarily associated with histologically stable atherosclerotic plaques. *Heart* 1996; 76: 112–17.

37 Davies MJ, Woolf N, Rowles P, Richardson PD. Lipid and cellular constituents of unstable human aortic plaques. *Basic Res Cardiol* 1994; 89: 33–9.

38 Lendon CL, Davies MJ, Born GVR, Richardson PD. Atherosclerotic plaque caps are locally weakened when macrophage density is increased. *Atherosclerosis* 1991; 87: 87–90.

39 Davies MJ, Woolf N, Katz DR. The role of endothelial denudation injury, plaque fissuring and thrombosis in the progression of human atherosclerosis. *Atheroscler Rev* 1991; 23: 105–13.

40 Libby P. Molecular basis of the acute coronary syndromes. *Circulation* 1995; 91: 2844–50.

41 Davies MJ. A macro and micro view of coronary vascular insult in ischemic heart disease. *Circulation* 1990; 80 (Suppl. II): 38–46.

42 Levine GN, Kearney JF, Vita JA. Cholesterol reduction in cardiovascular disease. *N Engl J Med* 1995; 332: 1354–63.

43 Richardson PD, Davies MJ, Born GVR. Influence of plaque configuration and stress distribution on fissuring of the coronary atherosclerotic plaques. *Lancet* 1989; 2: 941–4.

44 Cheng GC, Loree HM, Kamm RD, Fishbein MC, Lee RT. Distribution of circumferential mechanical stress in rup-

tured and stable atherosclerotic lesions. a structural analysis with histopathological correlation. *Circulation* 1993; 87: 1179–87

45 Gertz SD, Roberts WC. Hemodynamic shear force in rupture of coronary arterial atherosclerotic plaques. *Am J Cardiol* 1990; 66: 168–72.

46 Vito RP, Whang MC, Giddens DP, Zarins CK, Glagov S. Stress analysis of the diseased arterial cross-section. *ASME Adv Bioeng Proc* 1990; 19: 273–8.

47 Loree HM, Kamm RD, Stringfellow RG, Lee RT. Effects of fibrous cap thickness on peak circumferential stress in model atherosclerotic vessels. *Circ Res* 1992; 71: 850–8.

48 Benditt EP, Benditt JM. Evidence for a monoclonal origin of human atherosclerotic plaques. *Proc Natl Acad Sci USA* 1973; 70: 1753–6.

49 Murry C, Gipaya C, Bartosek T, Benditt E, Schwartz S. Monoclonality of smooth muscle cells in human atherosclerosis. *Am J Pathol* 1997; 151: 697–705.

50 Penn A, Garte SJ, Warren L, Nesta D, Mindich B. Transforming gene in human atherosclerotic plaque DNA. *Proc Natl Acad Sci USA* 1986; 83: 7951–5.

51 Parks JL, Cardell RR, Hubbard FC *et al.* Cultured human atherosclerotic plaque smooth muscle cells retain transforming potential and display enhanced expression of the myc protooncogene. *Am J Pathol* 1991; 138: 765–75.

52 Moss N, Benditt E. Human atherosclerotic plaque cells and leiomyoma cells. *Am J Pathol* 1975; 78: 175–90.

53 Moreno PR, Fallon JT, Murcia AM, Leon MN, Simosa H, Fuster V. Tissue characteristics of restenosis after percutaneous transluminal coronary angioplasty in diabetic patients. *J Am Coll Cardiol* 1999; 34: 1045–9.

54 Bennett MR, Evan GI, Schwartz SM. Apoptosis of human vascular smooth muscle cells derived from normal vessels and coronary atherosclerotic plaques. *J Clin Invest* 1995; 95: 2266–74.

55 Isner JM, Kearney M, Bortman S, Passeri J. Apoptosis in human atherosclerosis and restenosis. *Circulation* 1995; 91: 2703–11.

56 Geng YJ, Libby P. Evidence for apoptosis in advanced human atheroma — colocalization with interleukin-1-beta-

converting enzyme. *Am J Pathol* 1995;
147: 251–66.

57 Kockx MM, Muhring J, Bortier H,
Demeyer GRY, Jacob W. Biotin-conjugat-
ed or digoxigen-conjugated nucleotides
bind to matrix vesicles in atherosclerotic
plaques. *Am J Pathol* 1996; 148: 1771–7.

58 Kockx MM, Muhring J, Bortier H,
Demeyer GRY. RNA synthesis and splic-
ing interferes with DNA in situ end label-
ing techniques used to detect apoptosis.
Am J Pathol 1998; 152: 885–8.

59 Masuda J, Ross R. Atherogenesis during
low level hypercholesterolemia in the
nonhuman primate. 2. Fatty streak conversion to fibrous plaque. *Arterioscler*
1990; 10: 178–87.

60 Kerr L, Olashaw N, Matrisian L. Transforming growth factor β1 and cAMP inhibit transcription of epidermal growth
factor- and oncogene-induced transin
RNA. *J Biol Chem* 1988; 26:
16999–7005.

61 Assender JWA, Southgate KM, Hallett
MB, Newby AC. Inhibition of proliferative but not Ca^{2+} mobilization by cAMP
and cGMP in rabbit aortic smooth muscle cells. *Biochem J* 1992; 288: 527–32.

62 Garg UC, Hassid A. Nitric oxide-
generating vasodilators inhibit mitogene-
sis and proliferation of BALB/C 3T3
fibroblasts by a cyclic GMP-dependent
mechanism. *Biochem Biophys Res
Commun* 1990; 171: 474–9.

63 Yu H, Gallagher AM, Garfin PM, Printz
MP. Prostacyclin release by rat cardiac
fibroblasts—Inhibition of collagen expression. *Hypertension* 1997; 30:
1047–53.

64 Kolpakov V, Gordon D, Kulik T. Nitric
oxide-generating compounds inhibit
total protein and collagen-synthesis in
cultured vascular smooth muscle cells.
Circ Res 1995; 76: 305–9.

65 Polyak K. Negative regulation of cell
growth by TGFβ. *Biochim Biophys Acta*
1996; 1242: 185–99.

66 Hansson GK, Hellstrand M, Rymo L,
Rubia L, Gabbiani G. Interferon-gamma
inhibits both proliferation and expression of differentiation specific alpha-
smooth muscle actin in arterial smooth
muscle cells. *J Exp Med* 1989; 170.
1595–608

67 van der Wal AC, Becker AE, van der Loos
CM, Das PK. Site of intimal rupture or
erosion of thrombosed coronary atherosclerotic plaques is characterized by an
inflammatory process irrespective of the
dominant plaque morphology. *Circulation* 1994; 89: 36–44.

68 Palinski W, Miller E, Witztum J. Immu-
nization of low-density-lipoprotein
(LDL) receptor deficient rabbits with
homologous malondialdehyde-
modified LDL reduces atherogenesis.
Proc Natl Acad Sci USA 1995; 92:
821–5.

69 Galis ZS, Sukhova GK, Kranzhofer R,
Clark S, Libby P. Macrophage foam cells
from experimental atheroma constitutively produce matrix degrading proteinases. *Proc Natl Acad Sci USA* 1995;
92: 402–6.

70 Galis ZS, Sukhova GK, Lark MW, Libby
P. Increased expression of matrix metalloproteinases and matrix degrading
activities in vulnerable regions of human
atherosclerotic plaques. *J Clin Invest*
1994; 94: 2493–503.

71 Kovanen PT, Kaartinen M, Paavonen T.
Infiltrates of activated mast cells at the
site of coronary atheromatous erosion or
rupture in myocardial infarction. *Circulation* 1995; 92: 1084–8.

72 Dollery CM, McEwan JR, Henney AM.
Matrix metalloproteinases and cardiovascular disease. *Circ Res* 1995; 77:
863–8.

73 Henney A, Wakely P, Davies MJ *et al.*
Localization of stromelysin gene expres
sion in atherosclerotic plaques by *in situ*
hybridization. *Proc Natl Acad Sci USA*
1991; 88: 8154–8.

74 Rajagopalan S, Meng XP, Ramasamy S,
Harrison DG, Galis ZS. Reactive oxygen
species produced by macrophage-derived
foam cells regulate the activity of vascular matrix metalloproteinases *in vitro*.
J Clin Invest 1996; 98: 2572–9.

75 Rajagopalan S, Meng XP, Ramasamy S,
Harrison DG, Galis ZS. Reactive oxygen
species produced by macrophage-derived
foam cells regulate the activity of vascular matrix metalloproteinases *in vitro*.
Implications for atherosclerotic plaque
stability. *J Clin Invest* 1996; 98: 2572–9.

76 Rajavashisth TB, Liao JK, Galis ZS,
Tripathi S, Laufs U, Tripathi J, Chai NN,
Xu XP, Jovinge S, Shah PK, Libby P. Inflammatory cytokines and oxidized low
density lipoproteins increase endothelial

cell expression of membrane type 1-matrix metalloproteinase. *J Biol Chem* 1999; 274: 11924–9.

77 Herrick JB. Clinical features of sudden obstruction of the coronary arteries. *J Am Med Assoc* 1912; 59: 2015–20.

78 Tiefenbrunn AJ, Sobel BE. The impact of coronary thrombolysis on myocardial infarction. *Fibrinolysis* 1989; 3: 1–15.

79 Sobel BE. Coronary artery disease and fibrinolysis: From the blood to the vessel wall. *Thromb Haemost* 1999; 82: 8–13.

80 Davies MJ, Woolf N, Robertson WB. Pathology of acute myocardial infarction with particular reference to occlusive coronary thrombi. *Br Heart J* 1976; 38: 659–64.

81 Davies MJ, Bland JM, Hangartner JRW, Angelini A, Thomas AC. Factors influencing the presence of absence of acute coronary artery thrombi in sudden ischemic death. *Eur Heart J* 1989; 10: 203–8.

82 Falk E. Plaque rupture with severe preexisting stenosis precipitating coronary thrombosis. Characteristics of coronary atherosclerotic plaques underlying fatal occlusive thrombi. *Br Heart J* 1983; 50: 127–34.

83 Davies MJ, Thomas A. Thrombosis and acute coronary-artery lesions in sudden cardiac ischemic death. *N Engl J Med* 1984; 310: 1137–40.

84 DeWood MA, Spores J, Hensley GR, Simpson CS, Eugster GS, Sutherland KI, Grunwald RP, Shields JP. Coronary arteriographic findings in acute transmural myocardial infarction. *Circulation* 1983; 68: 39–49.

85 Mizuna K, Satomura K, Miyamoto A, Arakawa K, Shibuya T, Arai T, Kurita A, Nakamura H, Ambrose JA. Angioscopic evaluation of coronary-artery thrombi in acute coronary syndromes. *N Engl J Med* 1992; 326: 287–91.

86 Nemerson Y. Tissue factor and hemostasis. *Blood* 1988; 71: 1–8.

87 Rand MD, Lock JB, Veer CV, Gaffney DP, Mann KG. Blood clotting in minimally altered whole blood. *Blood* 1996; 88: 3432–45.

88 Monroe DM, Roberts HR, Hoffman M. Platelet procoagulant complex assembly in a tissue factor-initiated system. *Br J Haemotol* 1994; 88: 364–71.

89 Staatz WD, Rajpara SM, Wayner EA, Carter WG, Santoro SA. The membrane glycoprotein Ia-IIa (VLA-2) complex mediates the Mg^{+2}-dependent adhesion of platelets to collagen. *J Cell Biol* 1989; 108: 1917–21.

90 Kroll MH, Harris TS, Moake JL, Handin RI, Schafer AI, Von Willebrand Factor binding to platelet GP, Ib initiates signals for platelet activation. *J Clin Invest* 1991; 88: 1568–73.

91 Sims PJ, Ginsberg MH, Plow EF, Shattil SJ. Effect of platelet activation on the conformation of the plasma membrane glycoprotein IIb-IIIa complex. *J Biol Chem* 1991; 266: 7345–52.

92 Trip MD, Cats VM, van Capelle FJL, Vreeken J. Platelet hyperreactivity and prognosis in survivors of myocardial infarction. *N Engl J Med* 1990; 322: 1549–54.

93 Thaulow E, Erikssen J, Sandvik L, Stormorken H, Cohn PF. Blood platelet count and function are related to total and cardiovascular death in apparently healthy men. *Circulation* 1991; 84: 613–17.

94 Schwartz CJ, Valente AJ, Kelley JL, Sprague EA, Edwards EH. Thrombosis and the development of atherosclerosis: Roditansky revisited. *Semin Thromb Hemost* 1988; 14: 189–95.

95 Stirk CM, Kochhar A, Smith EB, Thompson WD. Presence of growth-stimulating fibrin-degradation products containing fragment E in human atherosclerotic plaques. *Atherosclerosis* 1993; 103: 159–69.

96 Scharf RE, Harker LA. Thrombosis and atherosclerosis: Regulatory role of interactions among blood components and endothelium. *Blut* 1987; 55: 131–44.

97 Bar-Shavit R, Hruska KA, Kahn AJ, Wilner GD. Hormone-like activity of human thrombin. *Ann NY Acad Sci* 1986; 485: 335–48.

98 Jawien A, Bowen-Pope DF, Lindner V, Schwartz SM, Clowes AW. Platelet-derived growth factor promotes smooth muscle migration and intimal thickening in a rat model of balloon angioplasty. *J Clin Invest* 1992; 89: 507–11.

99 Friedman RJ, Stemerman MB, Wenz B, Moore S, Gauldie J, Gent M, Tiell ML, Spaet TH. The effect of thrombocytopenia on experimental arteriosclerotic lesion formation in rabbits. Smooth muscle

proliferation and re-endothelialization. *J Clin Invest* 1977; 60: 1191–1201.

100 Fernandez-Ortiz AJ, Badimon JJ, Falk E, Fuster V, Meyer B, Mailhac A, Weng D, Shah PK, Badimon LL. Characterization of relative thrombogenicity of atherosclerotic plaque components: Implications for consequences of plaque rupture. *J Am Coll Cardiol* 1994; 23: 1562–9.

101 Wilcox JN, Smith KM, Schwartz SM, Gordon D. Localization of tissue factor in normal vessel wall and atherosclerotic plaque. *Proc Natl Acad Sci USA* 1989; 86: 2839–43.

102 Dalal JJ, Griffiths BE, Lewis MJ, Sheridan DJ, Henderson AH. Effect of coronary artery disease and myocardial ishaemia on transmyocardial platelet aggregability. *Eur Heart J* 1982; 3: 463–8.

103 Moake JL, Turner NA, Stathopoulos NA, Nolasco LH, Hellums JD. Involvement of large plasma von Willebrand factor multimers and unusually large vWF forms derived from endothelial cells in shear stress-induced platelet aggregation. *J Clin Invest* 1986; 78: 1456–61.

104 Ernst E. Plasma fibrinogen—independent cardiovascular risk factor. *J Int Med* 1990; 277: 365–72.

105 Meade TW, Mellows S, Brozovic M, Miller GJ, Chakrabarti RR, North WR, Stirling Y, Thompson SG. Hemostatic function and ischaemic heart disease: Principal results of the Northwick Park Heart Study. *Lancet* 1986; ii: 533–7.

106 Cortellaro M, Cofrancesco E, Boschetti C, Mussoni L, Donati MB, Cardillo M, Catalano M, Gabrielli L, Lombardi B, Specchia G. Increased fibrin turnover and high PAI-1 activity as predictors of ischemic events in atherosclerotic patients. A case-control study. The PLAT Group. *Arterioscl Thromb* 1993; 13: 1412–17.

107 Malmberg K, Bavenholm P, Hamsten A. Clinical and biochemical factors associated with prognosis after myocardial infarction at a young age. *J Am Coll Cardiol* 1994; 24: 592–9.

108 Wieczorek I, Ludlam CA, Fox KAA. Tissue-type plasminogen activator and plasminogen activator inhibitor activities as predictors of adverse events in unstable angina. *Am J Cardiol* 1994; 74: 424–9.

109 Haft JI, Kranz PD, Albert FJ, Fani K. Intravascular platelet aggregation in the heart induced by norepinephrine: Microscopic studies. *Circulation* 1972; 46: 698–708.

110 Levine SP, Towell BL, Suarez AM, Knieriem LK, Harris MM, George JN. Platelet activation and secretion associated with emotional stress. *Circulation* 1985; 71: 1129–34.

111 Scandinavian Simvistatin Survival Study Group. Randomised trial of cholesterol lowering 4444 patients with coronary heart disease: the Scandinavian Simvistatin Survival Study (4S). *Lancet* 1994; 344: 1383–9.

112 Shepherd J, Cobbe SM, Ford I, Isles CG, Lorimer AR, MacFarlane PW, McKillop JH, Packard CJ. Prevention of coronary heart disease with pravastatin in men with hypercholesterolemia: West of Scotland Coronary Prevention Study Group. *N Engl J Med* 1995; 333: 1301–7.

113 Waters D. Review of cholesterol-lowering therapy: coronary angiographic and event trials. *Am J Med* 1996; 101 (Suppl. 4A): 34S–9S.

114 Rubins HB, Robins SJ, Collins D, Fye CL, Anderson JW, Elam MB, Faas FH, Linares E, Schaefer FJ, Schectman G, Wilt TJ, Wittes J. Gemfibrozil for the secondary prevention of coronary heart disease in men with low levels of high-density lipoprotein cholesterol. Veterans Affairs High-Density Lipoprotein Cholesterol Intervention Trial Study Group. *N Engl J Med* 1999; 341: 410–18.

115 Assmann G, Schulte H, von Eckardstein A. Hypertriglyceridemia and elevated lipoprotein (a) are risk factors for major coronary events in middle-aged men. *Am J Cardiol* 1996; 77: 1179–84.

116 Mussoni L, Mannucci L, Sirtori M, Camera M, Maderna P, Sironi L, Tremoli E. Hypertriglyceridemia and regulation of fibrinolytic activity. *Arterioscl Thromb* 1992; 12: 19–27.

117 Sironi L, Mussoni L, Prati L, Baldassarre D, Camera M, Banfi C, Tremoli E. Plasminogen activator inhibitor type-1 synthesis and mRNA expression in HepG2 cells are regulated by VLDL. *Arterioscler Thromb Vasc Biol* 1996; 16: 89–96.

118 Schneider DJ, Sobel BE. Synergistic augmentation of expression of PAI-1 induced by insulin, VLDL, and fatty acids. *Coron Artery Dis* 1996; 7: 813–17.

119 Manninen V, Elo MO, Frick MH, Haapa K, Heinonen OP, Heinsalmi P, Huttunen JK, Kaitaniemi P, Koskinen P *et al.* Lipid alterations and decline in the incidence of coronary heart disease in the Helsinki Heart Study. *JAMA* 1988; 260: 641–51.

120 Fujii S, Sobel BE. Direct effects of gemfibrozil on the fibrinolytic system. Diminution of synthesis of plasminogen activator inhibitor type 1. *Circulation* 1992; 85: 1888–93.

121 O'Donnell CJ, Kanel WB. Cardiovascular risks of hypertension: lessons from observational studies. *J Hypertens* 1998; 16 (Suppl.): S3–7.

122 Roberts R, Rogers WJ, Mueller HS, Lambrew CT, Diver DJ, Smith HC, Willerson JT, Knatterud GL, Forman S, Passamani E *et al.* Immediate versus deferred beta-blockade following thrombolytic therapy in patients with acute myocardial infarction. Results of the Thrombolysis in Myocardial Infarction (TIMI) II-B study. *Circulation* 1991; 83: 422–37.

123 Rimm EB, Stampfer MJ. The role of antioxidants in preventive cardiology. *Curr Opin Cardiol* 1997; 12: 188–94.

124 Saikku P, Leinonen M, Mattila KJ, Ekman MR, Nieminen MS, Makela PH, Huttunen JK, Valtonen V. Serological evidence of an association of novel *Chlamydia*, TWAR, with chronic coronary heart disease and acute myocardial infarction. *Lancet* 1988; 2: 983–6.

125 Gupta S, Leatham EW, Carrington D, Mendall MA, Kaski JC, Camm AJ. Elevated *Chlamydia pneumoniae* antibodies, cardiovascular events, and azithromycin in male survivors of myocardial infarction. *Circulation* 1997; 96: 404–7.

126 Melnick JL, Adam E, Debakey ME. Possible role of cytomegalovirus in atherogenesis. *JAMA* 1990; 263: 2204–7.

127 Mendall MA, Goggin PM, Molineaux N *et al.* Relation of *Helicobacter pylori* infection and coronary heart disease. *Br Heart J* 1994; 71: 437–9.

128 Roth GJ, Calverley DC. Aspirin, platelets, and thrombosis: theory and practice. *Blood* 1994; 83: 885–98.

129 Roth GJ, Majerus PW. The mechanism of the effect of aspirin on human platelets: I. acetylation of a particulate fraction protein. *J Clin Invest* 1975; 56: 624–9.

130 Holmes MB, Sobel BE, Schneider DJ. Variable responses to inhibition of fibrinogen binding induced by tirofiban and eptifibatide in healthy subjects. *Am J Cardiol* 1999; 84: 203–7.

131 Holmes MB, Sobel BE, Cannon CP, Schneider DJ. Increased platelet reactivity in patients given orbofiban after an acute coronary syndrome. An OPUS-TIMI 16 substudy. *Am J Cardiol* (In press).

132 Ferrari R. Effect of ACE inhibition on myocardial ischaemia. *Eur Heart J* 1998; 19 (Suppl. J): J30–5.

133 Brown NJ, Agirbasli MA, Williams GH, Litchfield WR, Vaughan DE. Effects of activation and inhibition of the renin-angiotensin system on plasma PAI-1. *Hypertension* 1998; 32: 65–71.

134 Uusitupa MI, Niskanen LK, Siitonen O, Voutilainen E, Pyorala K. 5-Year incidence of atherosclerotic vascular disease in relation to general risk factors, insulin level, and abnormalities in lipoprotein composition in non-insulin-dependent diabetic and nondiabetic subjects. *Circulation* 1990; 82: 27–36.

135 Brownlee M. Glycation and diabetic complications. *Diabetes* 1994; 43: 836–41.

136 Vlassara H. Recent progress on the biologic and clinical significance of advanced glycosylation end products. *J Lab Clin Med* 1994; 124: 19–30.

137 Manninen V, Tenkanen L, Koskinen P, Huttunen JK, Manttari M, Heinonen OP, Frick MH. Joint effects of serum triglyceride and LDL cholesterol and HDL cholesterol on coronary heart disease risk in the Helsinki Heart Study. Implications for treatment. *Circulation* 1992; 85: 37–45.

138 Dejager S, Bruckert E, Chapman MJ. Dense low density lipoprotein subspecies with diminished oxidative resistance predominate in combine hyperlipidemia. *J Lipid Res* 1993; 34: 295–308.

139 Bucala R, Makita Z, Zoschinsky T, Cerami A, Vlassara H. Lipid advanced glycosylation: pathway for lipid oxidation *in vivo. Proc Natl Acad Sci USA* 1993; 90: 6434–8.

140 Warram JH, Martin BC, Krolewski AS, Soeldner JS, Kahn CR. Slow glucose removal rate and hyperinsulinemia precede the development of type II diabetes in the

offspring of diabetic parents. *Ann Int Med* 1990; 113: 909–15.

141 Fontbonne A, Tchobroutsky G, Eschwege E, Richard JL, Claude JR, Rosselin GE. Coronary heart disease mortality risk: Plasma insulin level is a more sensitive marker than hypertension or abnormal glucose tolerance in overweight males. The Paris prospective study. *Int J Obes* 1988; 12: 557–65.

142 Pyorala K, Savolainen E, Kaukola S, Haapakoski J. Plasma insulin as coronary heart disease risk factor: Relationship to other risk factors and predictive value during $9\frac{1}{2}$-year follow-up of the Helsinki Policemen Study Population. *Acta Med Scand* 1985; 701 (Suppl.): 38–52.

143 Cullen K, Stenhouse NS, Wearne KL, Welborn TA. Multiple regression analysis of risk factors for cardiovascular disease and cancer mortality in Busselton, Western Australia—13-year study. *J Chronic Dis* 1983; 36: 371–7.

144 Calles-Escandon J, Mirza S, Sobel BE, Schneider DJ. Induction of hyperinsulinemia combined with hyperglycemia and hypertriglyceridemia increases plasminogen activator inhibitor type-1 (PAI-1) in blood in normal human subjects. *Diabetes* 1998; 47: 290–3.

145 Ginsberg H, Plutzky J, Sobel BE. A review of metabolic and cardiovascular effects of oral antidiabetic agents: Beyond glucose-level lowering. *J Cardiovasc Risk* 1999; 6: 337–46.

3: What is the role of infection in the pathogenesis of acute coronary syndromes?

David A. Smith and Juan Carlos Kaski

Results of epidemiological studies of biochemical and molecular markers (sero-epidemiological studies) and the publication of two small antibiotic secondary prevention trials [1,2] have fuelled interest in the hypothesis that chronic infections play a causal role in atherogenesis, and that antibiotic treatment may have beneficial effects on its progression and outcome. In particular, *Chlamydia pneumoniae, Helicobacter pylori*, cytomegalovirus and pathogens associated with chronic dental sepsis have been associated with atherosclerotic disease. Among these pathogens, *C. pneumoniae* appears to be the most plausible candidate for playing a causative role in atherogenesis [3]. *Chlamydia pneumoniae* is a recently recognized and characterized pathogen, and is distinct from other chlamydial species [4–6]. Since 1988, when Saikku reported an association between acute *C. pneumoniae* infection and myocardial infarction [7], numerous studies have found an association between *C. pneumoniae* infection and atherosclerosis.

Evidence for the link comes from several types of research—sero-epidemiological studies, pathological studies, animal experiments and antibiotic trials. More than 20 sero-epidemiological studies have reported a positive association between *C. pneumoniae* and atherosclerosis [8]. Most, however, have been cross-sectional or case-control studies, rather than the cohort or prospective studies that are the preferred approach for examining association. A meta-analysis of 18 published epidemiological studies [9], involving over 2700 patients, indicated that a raised anti-*C. pneumoniae* antibody titre is associated with a 2- to 4-fold increased prevalence of coronary heart disease. However, as stated by the authors, it must be taken into account that most of these studies were based on small sample sizes, and made differing degrees of adjustment for potential confounders, and were therefore prone to different biases. In addition, whilst all studies have assayed IgG antibody titres (considered to represent a marker of prior infection with *C. pneumoniae*), only five prospective studies and fifteen cross-sectional studies have assayed IgA antibody titres (a marker of on-going acute or chronic infection).

To date, nine prospective serological studies have been published [10–18]. They have been inconclusive. Four studies reported no association [10–13]. The other five reported a positive association between *C. pneumoniae* seropositivity and subsequent cardiovascular disease [14–18], although conclusions in two depended on subset analysis [14,15]. Furthermore, the positive studies reported conflicting associations with respect to specific classes of antibody (Table 3.1). Three studies [14,17,18] showed a positive association with IgA antibodies, whereas two [10,15] showed a positive association only with IgG antibodies. In the recent Caerphilly prospective heart disease study [17], which followed up 1773 middle-aged men over 13 years, IgG antibody titres against *C. pneumoniae* were not related to the prevalence of ischaemic heart disease (IHD), incident IHD, or fatal IHD. By contrast, there was a

Table 3.1 Prospective serological studies investigating the association between *C. pneumoniae* and atherosclerosis.

Study	No. of cases	Sex*	Association with IgG†	Association with IgA†	Diagnostic antibody titre
Saikku 1992 [14]	103	Males only	2.2 (1.1–4 5)	2.6 (1.2–5.2)	IgG ≥ 128 IgA > 64
Miettinen 1996 [15]	162 NIDDM 40 No DM		2.44 (0.98–6.08)	No	IgG ≥ 128 IgA ≥ 40
Ossewarde 1998 [16]	54		2.8 (1.3–5.8)	No	ELISA
Nieto 1997 [10]	256		No		IgG ≥ 64
Siscovick 1998 [11]	100		No		Not stated (abstract)
Ridker 1999 [12]	343	Males only	No	No	IgG ≥ 16
Caerphilly 1999 [17]	278	Males only	No	1.83 (1.17–2.85)‡ 1.07 (0.75–1.53)**	IgG ≥ 16 IgA ≥ 16
Fagerberg 1999 [18]	84	Males only	2.69 (1.04–6.97)††	2.69 (1.04–6.97)††	IgG ≥ 512 IgA IgA ≥ 64
Danesh 1999 [13]	288		No		IgG in top third of control distribution

* Mixed sex unless stated.
† Odds ratio and 95% confidence interval.
‡For fatal ischaemic heart disease.
** For all incident ischaemic heart disease.
†† Relative risk and 95% confidence interval for any cardiovascular event.
NIDDM, non-insulin-dependent diabetes mellitus; DM, diabetes mellitus.

highly significant association between IgA antibody titres and prevalent IHD, fatal IHD, and risk of mortality.

Unfortunately, short of atherectomy, there is as yet no direct means of detecting *C. pneumoniae* infection of vascular tissue. Serology is a poorly standardized marker of systemic infection, that fails to discriminate between subjects with and without intra-arterial *C. pneumoniae* infection [19,20]. Naidu *et al.* [21] reported that *C. pneumoniae* can be detected by polymerase chain reaction (PCR) in serum samples of patients with coronary artery disease (CAD) [22]. However, *C. pneumoniae* DNA detection by PCR in circulating white cells is a particularly promising technique. In a geographical area with high seroprevalence of *C. pneumoniae* antibody, Boman *et al.* [23] found a high prevalence of *C. pneumoniae* DNA in patients with CAD and in blood donors. Recently, Wong *et al.* [24] have reported an association of CAD with circulating *C. pneumoniae* DNA in men but not in women.

The association between *C. pneumoniae* and atherosclerosis has been shown definitively in studies worldwide that have demonstrated the presence of *C. pneumoniae* organisms in atherosclerotic tissue. Shor *et al.* were the first to identify chlamydia-like structures in the walls of coronary arteries at necroscopy, with the use of electron microscopy [3]. At least 23 other publications have confirmed the presence of *C. pneumoniae* organisms in the walls of atherosclerotic coronary and major peripheral arteries [8]. The techniques used to detect *C. pneumoniae* include polymerase chain reaction (PCR), electron microscopy, immunocytochemistry, immunofluorescence, culture, enzyme immunoassay, and *in situ* hybridization. Evidence of *C. pneumoniae* has been found in 15–100% of cases [8], with only three published studies having failed to detect *C. pneumoniae* in atheromatous tissue [25–27]. In contrast, *C. pneumoniae* appears to be uncommon in non-atheromatous control vessels with only two studies reporting a similar prevalence of *C. pneumoniae* in control and diseased vessels [28,29].

Although the studies cited have proved beyond doubt that an association exists between *C. pneumoniae* and atherosclerosis, they do not tell us whether or not *C. pneumoniae* has a role in the aetiology of atherosclerosis. To establish a causative relationship between an infectious agent and a disease process, all of three conditions, known as Koch's postulates [30], must be met. First, the infectious agent must be found to be present in the majority, or all, of the patients in which the disease is manifested. Second, the infectious agent must be introduced into another subject, which then results in the new development of the proposed disease process. Third, the new subject manifesting the disease must be able to have the infectious agent recovered again. In a process as chronic and potentially deadly as atherosclerosis, it is not possible to test Koch's postulates directly on humans. Therefore animal models have been used to explore aetiological links.

Animals with *C. pneumoniae*-induced atherosclerosis

Mouse and rabbit preparations permit the study of atherosclerosis. Moazed *et al.* [31] examined the relation of infection with *C. pneumoniae* in two different types of mice. Apolipoprotein (apo) E-deficient transgenic mice which spontaneously develop atherosclerosis in a time- and age-dependent manner, and C57BL/6 J mice, which develop atherosclerosis only when on an atherogenic diet, were evaluated. After intranasal inoculation in these animals, *C. pneumoniae* was demonstrated persistently within aortic atherosclerotic lesions in the apoE-deficient mice by ICC (Immunocytochemistry) and PCR techniques, but only transiently in the C57BL/6 J mice. Further work by Moazed *et al.* [32] with apo-E-deficient mice showed that *C. pneumoniae* can accelerate atherosclerosis. Apo-E mice fed a normal chow diet and given three inoculations of *C. pneumoniae* had significantly larger lesions compared with those in uninfected mice.

Two types of rabbit are available for study of atherosclerosis. The New Zealand White (NZW) rabbit develops atherosclerosis if fed a cholesterol-rich diet, whereas the Watanabe heritable hyperlipidaemic (WHHL) rabbit develops spontaneous atherosclerosis. The WHHL rabbit is less susceptible to *C. pneumoniae* infection than is the NZW rabbit [33]. Thus NZW rabbits on normal or high-cholesterol diets have been studied. Fong *et al.* [34] reported results from a small study of NZW rabbits infected nasally with *C. pneumoniae*. Two of eleven animals exhibited early and intermediate histological lesions of atherosclerosis, results corroborated by Laitinen *et al.* [35] who induced inflammatory changes in the aortas of six out of nine NZW rabbits infected nasally with *C. pneumoniae*. Only one study has failed to induce inflammatory lesions in the aortas of NZW rabbits [33], despite the presence of inflammatory changes in the lungs and spleens that were seen in these animals.

Animal preparations have also been used to study the effects of antimicrobial intervention on the progression of atherosclerosis. Muhlestein *et al.* [36] nasally innoculated 30 NZW rabbits and fed them a modestly cholesterol-enhanced diet. The animals were then randomized to a 7-week course of azithromycin or no treatment. Intranasal *C. pneumoniae* infection accelerated intimal thickening compared with that seen in the uninfected animals, but treatment with azithromycin prevented accelerated intimal thickening, strengthening the aetiological link between *C. pneumoniae* and atherosclerosis. Interestingly, however, the *C. pneumoniae* vascular antigen was detected by immunofluorescence in the aortas of treated rabbits as frequently as in those from untreated animals.

Studies *in vitro*

Recent studies have helped to elucidate how *C. pneumoniae* may interact with the known risk factors of atherosclerosis at the cellular level to cause or accelerate the progression of atheroma. *Chlamydia pneumoniae* can infect most of the types of cells involved in atherosclerosis, including smooth muscle cells, endothelial cells, and macrophages [37–39]. Airenne *et al.* [40] have shown that *C. pneumoniae* remains metabolically active in human monocytes for as long as 7 days, as evidenced by chlamydial mRNA synthesis detected by RT-PCR. Molestina *et al.* [41] demonstrated that *C. pneumoniae* promotes the transendothelial migration of neutrophils and monocytes via upregulation of monocyte chemotactic protein-1 (MCP-1) and interleukin-8. Intriguingly, Kalayoglu *et al.* [42] found that human macrophages infected with *C. pneumoniae* and incubated with low density lipoprotein were transformed into foam cells (cells characteristic of early atheroma) within 22 h.

Mechanisms of vascular disease seen with *C. pneumoniae* infection: cell-mediated bacteraemia and macrophage activation

How *C. pneumoniae* enters atheromatous plaques, and whether it has a direct causal role in the pathogenesis of atherosclerosis, remains speculative. Mice have been used for investigating the mechanism of dissemination of the organism from the primary site of infection in the lungs to the atheromatous plaque. *Chlamydia pneumoniae* was found in blood monocytes but not in plasma, demonstrating that cell-associated bacteraemia occurred during acute infection [43]. The passive transfer of infected macrophages from mice inoculated intranasally or intraperitoneally with *C. pneumoniae,* to naïve mice by intraperitoneal inoculation, resulted in the dissemination of infection to the lung, thymus, spleen, and/or abdominal lymph nodes. Thus macrophages may mediate dissemination from the lung to other sites by either haematogenous or lymphatic routes. The macrophages adhere to sites of endothelial damage and can then contribute, via various mechanisms, to further damage. Alternatively, the organism may simply reside in the macrophage without causing any harmful effects, and any association between *C. pneumoniae* residing in coronary tissue and consequent damage may be purely coincidental [44].

Chronic infection of macrophages and their activation may contribute to local inflammation and the development of atheromatous plaques, as suggested by results in animals with infection-induced atherosclerosis described above [31,32,34–36]. *Chlamydia pneumoniae* infection can induce a chronic immune activation (mediated by cytokines such as IL-6, and TNF alpha [39]) that contributes to direct chronic endothelial cell damage. It can stimulate the synthesis of acute-phase proteins such as fibrinogen [45] and C-reactive protein (CRP) [46]. However, two recent prospective sero-epidemiological trials have not shown these phenomena. Ridker *et al.* [12] did not find a relationship between IgG anti-*C. pneumoniae* antibody titres and CRP, and the Caerphilly study group [17] found no relationship between either IgG or IgA antibody titres and fibrinogen levels.

Atherogenic lipid profile

Chlamydia pneumoniae infection may directly affect cholesterol metabolism and lipid oxidation, resulting in the creation of an atherogenic lipid profile. Several studies have shown an association between *C. pneumoniae* infection and lipid levels [17–49], although early studies largely ignored the potential influence of confounding factors, such as smoking, body mass index, and socioeconomic status [47,48]. Murray *et al.* [49] recently demonstrated a robust association between IgG anti-*C. pneumoniae* antibodies and an atherogenic lipid profile. In both males and females total cholesterol was increased. Infected men had lower HDL cholesterol concentrations compared with uninfected men. Differences in women did not reach statistical significance, but both total and HDL cholesterol were higher in sero-positive than in sero-negative individuals. As the authors stated, more work is required to determine whether the atherogenic profile is sustained or recurs with repeated infection sufficiently often to alter long-term cardiovascular risk.

Hypercoagulable state

Infection may lead to a local or a generalized hypercoagulable state, or both, by increasing tissue factor expression, following activation and recruitment of monocytes [50]. Cardiovascular risk factors (blood levels of fibrinogen, factor VIIa, leucocytes and C-reactive protein) are associated with elevated anti-*C. pneumoniae* antibody titres [51,52]. Infection of endothelial cells by *C. pneumoniae* can alter thrombin generation on the cell surface, increase platelet accumulation, induce leucocyte adhesion molecule expression, and reduce prostacyclin secretion [53].

Antigenic mimicry

An auto-immune hypothesis has recently been suggested, evolving from evidence that the immune response is involved in the pathogenesis of atherosclerosis. During chronic, persistent infection, *Chlamydia pneumoniae* expresses a heat shock protein (HSP 60) that shows close homology with human and mycobacterial heat shock proteins (mHSP) [54,55]. Birnie *et al.* [56] found that antibodies to HSP 65 correlated with the severity and extent of coronary artery disease, even after control for confounding factors. They also showed a significant reduction in HSP 65 titres after the successful eradication of *Helicobacter pylori*. Recently, Kol *et al.* [57] showed that chlamydial HSP 60 co-localizes with human HSP 60 within plaque macrophages, and that HSP 60 from both species can induce the production of tumour necrosis factor-α (TNF-α) and collagen-matrix-degrading metalloproteinases when incubated with mouse macrophages. With the use of Western blot analyses and competitive enzyme-linked immunosorbent assays (ELISAs), Mayr *et al.* [58] showed that serum antibodies against HSP 65/60 cross-react with human HSP 60, chlamydial HSP 60 and *Escherichia coli* HSP. The antibodies against HSP 60/65 correlated with the presence of anti-*C. pneumoniae* IgG antibodies, and also markedly enhanced complement-mediated endothelial cytotoxicity on stressed human umbilical vein endothelial cells. These findings have confirmed and expanded the results from earlier work that suggested a role for HSP 60/65 in atherogenesis [59]. These results thus support the hypothesis that *C. pneumoniae* and other microorganisms induce an immune response to bacterial HSP 60/62/65, and that the antibodies produced cross-react with the human HSP 60 [60], thereby initiating or contributing to a local inflammatory and auto-immune process.

Reactive oxygen species

The superoxide radical has been implicated in mediating vascular damage and plaque disruption. The direct and indirect attack of reactive oxygen species on polyunsaturated fatty acids (essential constituents of biological membranes) result in the formation of lipid breakdown products (lipid peroxidation), that can induce permanent cell damage [61]. All three major cell types in arterial lesions—endothelial cells, smooth muscle cells and macrophages—are capable of elaborating reactive oxygen species [62,63]. Intriguingly, *Chlamydia pneumoniae* has been shown to replicate *in vitro* in these cell types [37–39] and may increase lipid peroxidation, although this potential mechanism remains speculative.

Studies with antibiotics

Following the demonstration of the association between *C. pneumoniae* and atherosclerosis, secondary prevention studies in humans evaluating the effect of treatment with antibiotics on cardiovascular events have begun to capture the interest of investigators around the world. The results from pilot studies that have been performed (Table 3.2) and of several large-scale prospective intervention studies that are currently in progress are of interest.

Table 3.2 Secondary prevention antibiotic trials of C. *pneumoniae* and atherosclerosis.

Study	Patient group	Antibiotic regimen	Clinical endpoints	Inflammatory markers	Cp antibody titres
Gupta 1997 [1]	Post-MI males	Azithromycin 500 mg for 3 days	4-fold decrease in cardiovascular events	Fall in fibrinogen, WCC, monocyte activation ($P < 0.05$)	Fall in IgG titre ($P = 0.02$)
ROXIS 1997 [2]	Non-Q-wave acute coronary syndromes	Roxithromycin 150 mg bd for 30 days	2% antibiotic group (9% placebo group)*	Non-significant fall in CRP	No change in titres
Sinisalo 1998 [67]	Males with previous CABG	Doxycycline 100 mg od for 4 months	Not studied	No change in, fibrinogen, NO production and thrombin fragments†	No change in titres
ACADEMIC 1999 [66]	Chronic IHD	Azithromycin 500 mg for 3 days then 500 mg per week for 3 months	No difference between antibiotic and placebo groups at 6 months‡	Fall in CRP, IL-1, IL-6 and TNF-α at 6 months ($P = 0.011$)	No change in titre
Torgano 1999 [68]	Chronic IHD	Clarithromycin 500 mg bd for 14 days	Not studied	Fall in fibrinogen in antibiotic group ($P < 0.01$)	Fall in IgG titre ($P < 0.001$)

* Incidence of triple endpoint (death, acute myocardial infarction and recurrent ischaemia) at 30 days.
† Nitric oxide production assessed by forearm blood flow responses.
‡ Clinical endpoint evaluation awaited at 2-year follow-up.
CABG, coronary artery bypass graft; Cp, *Chlamydia pneumoniae*; NO, nitric oxide; WCC, white cell count.

The first reported antibiotic prevention study was by Gupta *et al.* [1] in our institution, who conducted a randomized, placebo-controlled trial of azithromycin in a series of male survivors of myocardial infarction with stable elevated anti-C. *pneumoniae* antibody titres. The primary aim of the study was to determine whether changes in serum and monocyte markers of inflammation were paralleled by hypercoagulation [64]. An assessment was also made of whether an elevated anti-C. *pneumoniae* antibody titre predicted future cardiovascular events in 213 consecutive post-myocardial infarct (MI) males, stratified according to antibody titres, at a mean 18 months of follow-up. The incidence of future cardiovascular events in those patients with elevated titres (IgG $\geq$ 1:64) randomized to azithromycin (single course of 500 mg/day for 3 days, $n = 28$; or a double course, $n = 12$) or placebo ($n = 20$) was also assessed. A 4-fold increase in risk of experiencing adverse cardiovascular events was seen in the group with elevated C. *pneumoniae* titres compared with that in the group with negative serology. For the high-titre group treated with antibiotics, the adjusted odds ratio was the same as that in the seronegative group. Subjects given azithromycin had a significant fall in levels of serum and monocyte activation markers (monocyte integrins CD11b/CD11c, fibrinogen and leucocyte count). In addition, patients receiving azithromycin were more likely to have decreased anti-C. *pneumoniae* antibody titres after 6 months compared with titres in the placebo group.

In the Roxithromycin in Ischaemic Syndromes study (ROXIS) [2] the aim was to determine whether the macrolide antibiotic, roxithromycin (150 mg twice a day, for 30 days), could decrease the incidence of recurrent ischaemic events in 205 patients presenting with acute coronary syndromes, irrespective of C. *pneumoniae* antibody status. There was a significant reduction in combined ischaemic events (recurrent ischaemia, plus MI, plus ischaemic death) at day 31 in the patients randomized to roxithromycin, compared with the incidence in the placebo group. Unlike the Gupta trial, in which persistent beneficial effects were shown in the antibiotic treatment group, the beneficial effects of roxithromycin on combined ischaemic events were not statistically significant at 3 or 6 months [65]. Furthermore, no reduction in antibody titres was seen in the roxithromycin-treated group.

More recently, results from the ACADEMIC study [66] (Azithromycin in Coronary Artery Disease: Elimination of Myocardial Infection with Chlamydia) involving 302 IHD patients sero-positive for C. *pneumoniae* (IgG > 1 : 16), who were randomized to a 3-month course (500 mg/day for 3 days followed by 500 mg/week for 3 months) of azithromycin or placebo, were reported. Overall, 89% of the patients were male, with 60% having suffered a previous MI. The study was designed to evaluate both laboratory and clinical endpoints over a 2-year period. No differences in clinical events or anti-C. *pneumoniae* antibody titres were reported at 6 months, although concentrations of circulating markers of inflammation (C-reactive protein (CRP), interleukin-1 (IL-1), IL-6 and TNF-α) were reduced significantly in the antibiotic-treatment group. The clinical endpoint evaluation is not yet available. However, as noted by the authors, the study is powered for laboratory endpoints. Thus a much larger study would be needed to detect a clinical 'protective effect' of azithromycin.

Two small, laboratory, endpoint, antibiotic-treatment studies have been reported. Sinisalo *et al.* [67] treated 34 non-smoking males with previous coronary artery bypass surgery (CABG) with 4 months of doxycycline (100 mg/day) or placebo. No significant differences in anti-C. *pneumoniae* antibody titres, lipids, fibrinogen or nitric oxide production (as evidenced by forearm blood flow responses) were noted. Torgano *et al.* [68] performed a single, blind randomized prospective trial to investigate the effect of a 2-week course of antibiotics (clarithromycin 500 mg twice/day) on fibrinogen levels in 84 IHD patients seropositive for *H. pylori* and/or *C. pneumoniae*. They demonstrated a significant reduction in fibrinogen levels 6 months after treatment with clarithromycin, with the greatest reductions seen in those seropositive for both *H. pylori* and *C. pneumoniae*. A significant reduction in IgG anti-*C. pneumoniae* antibody titres was also seen in the treated group, in keeping with the results in the Gupta study.

Further evidence, albeit indirect, for a beneficial effect of antibiotics in patients with IHD has come recently from a case-control study by Meier *et al.* [69] They used a computerized general practice database to define the history of antibiotic usage in the 3 years before a first MI in 3315 patients. For each case, four controls were matched for age, sex, general practice attended, and calendar date. The main finding was that patients who had sustained MI, compared with controls, were less likely to have been taking tetracycline or quinolone antibiotics in the past. No such association was found for macrolide antibiotics — although the main macrolide in use was erythromycin, which is not very effective against *C. pneumoniae*. Although the results of this study support the hypothesis that certain antibiotics may prevent a first MI, they are also paradoxically consistent with MI cases having had fewer infections requiring antibiotics than controls. Jackson *et al.* [70] have reported a similar study design looking at the use of antibiotics over a 5-year period before a first MI. In contrast to Meier *et al.* [69] they found no association between the use of erythromycin, tetracycline, or doxycycline and the risk for first MI, although the cumulative duration of antibiotics in this study was short, with only 9% of subjects treated for more than 28 days of antibiotics over the 5-year period.

It is possible that the beneficial clinical effects seen in some of the above studies are independent of an antimicrobial effect, and instead attributable to the anti-inflammatory effects of macrolide antibiotics. This view is supported by results from the ROXIS study [2], in which short-term benefit (up to 30 days) of roxithromycin was demonstrated in patients, irrespective of their *C. pneumoniae* antibody titre levels. Macrolide antibiotics may: (1) suppress macrophage activity by blockade of the large conductance potassium channel, which appears to be involved in cytokine-mediated and adherence-mediated macrophage activation [71]; (2) suppress active oxygen generation and chemotaxis of neutrophils [72]; (3) suppress the response of phagocytic cells to bacterial pathogens after a therapeutic dose [73]; and (4) down-modulate antigen presentation [74].

After the publication of results from the early antibiotic trials, larger secondary prevention trials were initiated. Undoubtedly others are being designed. The WIZARD study (Weekly Intervention with Zithromax Against Atherosclerotic-Related Disorders) is a double-blind, placebo-controlled trial in post-MI patients with positive anti-*C. pneumoniae* serology (IgG ≥ 1 : 16). More than 3300 patients have been recruited for randomization to treatment with either a 3-day course of azithromycin (600 mg/day) followed by a 3-month treatment with the antibiotic (600 mg/week) or placebo. The primary aim is to determine whether azithromycin reduces total cardiovascular events over a 2.5-year follow-up period. However, the study may not be able to differentiate between any non-antimicrobial action of the antibiotic and antibacterial effects, because only seropositive patients are involved.

The duration of antibiotic treatment is presently arbitrary, albeit based on a logical rationale. An acute course of azithromycin may treat any possible acute inflammatory process caused by active *C. pneumoniae* infection. There are, however, two additional scenarios that may require antibacterial intervention. If *C. pneumoniae* is able to 'infect' an already established atherosclerotic plaque, it may trigger a burst in inflammation that ultimately leads to plaque rupture. Alternatively, the immune response to a remote infection may cause a burst of cytokine-mediated inflammation that could trigger instability in the plaque. In either case, a continuous course of antibiotics may prevent this deleterious process from leading to coronary events.

In the second scenario, the chlamydial pathogen may lie dormant within the arterial lesion as a 'persistent body'. It is possible that an antibiotic that works by inhibiting protein synthesis will not be able to exert its effect on a stage of the lifecycle of Chlamydia that is metabolically quiescent. As a consequence, it may be necessary to keep a level of drug available that will kill the organism—if and when it becomes active. This approach conforms to that of the antituberculous model, in which antibiotic is provided for a prolonged period of time in order to catch the bacillus when its synthetic pathways are most vulnerable.

The MARBLE study (Might Azithromycin Reduce Bypass List Events) is a UK-based prospective, placebo-controlled trial of azithromycin in patients awaiting CABG surgery. Patients will be randomized to 3 months of treatment (as in the WIZARD study design), irrespective of *C. pneumoniae* serology. The aim is to determine whether total cardiovascular events will be reduced in this high-risk group, by administration of azithromycin during the period of waiting for the operation. Coronary atheroma samples will be obtained from some patients who undergo coronary endarterectomy, and examined for the presence of *C. pneumoniae*. The MARBLE study may therefore provide important data on the relationship between *C. pneumoniae* infection and the effects of antibiotic treatment on organisms and phenomena within coronary arteries. This study, if positive, could have major ramifications regarding the political and medical issues pertinent to CABG waiting lists in the United Kingdom and elsewhere.

For the ACES trial (Azithromycin Coronary Events Study) 4000 patients with evidence of CAD will be treated, irrespective of antibody status. The treatment period will be 1 year, with a planned 4-year observation period. In the STAMINA study (South Thames Antibiotics in Myocardial Infarction and Angina) 600 patients with acute coronary syndromes will be randomized to an azithromycin-based regimen, an amoxycillin-based regimen, or placebo. The aim is to treat both *H. pylori* and *C. pneumoniae* and assess effects on serological markers of infection, markers of inflammation (fibrinogen, CRP and IL-6) and cardiovascular events.

Summary and conclusion

Although it is an intriguing and exciting hypothesis, there is as yet no conclusive evidence that *C. pneumoniae* causes atherosclerosis or precipitates acute coronary syndromes. However, evidence from pathological studies, animal models and antibiotic secondary prevention trials suggests that *C. pneumoniae* infection may exacerbate atherosclerosis. The mechanisms responsible remain speculative. *Chlamydia pneumoniae* is often found in atheromatous blood-vessels throughout the body, but not in normal vessels. Whether these findings reflect a causal association with atherosclerosis is unknown. *Chlamydia pneumoniae* could play a role in the initiation of atherosclerosis, in the progression of the disease, or in precipitating complicating events [75]. The results of eradication studies are eagerly awaited, as they may help to elucidate the role of *C. pneumoniae* in atherogenesis. The issues of optimal antibiotic therapy, duration of therapy, patient selection, re-infection rates and effects of other infections require further clarification. In conjunction with the prospect of prolonged courses of broad-spectrum antibiotics, the spectre of community antibiotic resistance merits careful risk–benefit analysis [76].

Atherosclerosis is a multifactorial disease. We believe that it is unrealistic to expect that chronic bacterial infection can explain all incident cases of IHD. It is unlikely that antibiotics will have a beneficial effect in all patients with the disease, although some may benefit. Who will benefit most, if any, will be established only with further study.

Antibiotics may reduce the incidence of cardiovascular events in patients with atherosclerotic disease. If so, it is possible that the cause will be anti-inflammatory action rather than antibacterial action [2]. Alternatively, the drugs may act against a pathogen other than *C. pneumoniae*. On the other hand, if antibiotics fail to reduce events, the possibility that *C. pneumoniae* plays a role in the initiation and progression of atherosclerosis will not have been excluded. Nevertheless, if antibiotics are shown to significantly reduce the incidence of events in CAD patients, the finding may constitute an important advance in the fight against the Western world's biggest killer.

References

1 Gupta S, Leatham EW, Carrington D *et al.* Elevated *Chlamydia pneumoniae* antibodies, cardiovascular events and azithromycin in male survivors of myocardial infarction. *Circulation* 1997; 96: 404–7.

2 Gurfinkel E, Bozovich G, Darococa A *et al.* Randomised trial of roxithromycin in non-Q wave coronary syndromes: ROXIS pilot study. *Lancet* 1997; 350: 404–7.

3 Shor A, Kuo CC, Patten DL *et al.* Detection of *Chlamydia pneumoniae* in coronary arterial fatty streaks and atheromatous plaques. *S Afr Med J* 1992; 82: 158–61.

4 Grayston JT, Kuo CC, Wang SP *et al.* A new *Chlamydia pssitaci* strain TWAR, isolated in acute respiratory tract infections. *N Eng J Med* 1986; 315: 161–8.

5 Grayston JT. Infections caused by *Chlamydia pneumoniae* strain TWAR. *Clin Infect Dis* 1992; 165: 757–61.

6 Aldous MB, Grayston JT, Wang SP *et al.* Sero-epidemiology of *Chlamydia pneumoniae* TWAR infection in Seattle families. 1966–79. *J Infect Dis* 1992; 166: 646–9.

7 Saikku P, Leinonen M, Mattila K *et al.* Serologic evidence of an association of a novel *Chlamydia*, TWAR, with chronic coronary heart disease and acute myocardial infarction. *Lancet* 1988; 2: 983–6.

8 Wong Y-K, Gallagher PJ, Ward ME. *Chlamydia pneumoniae* and atherosclerosis. *Heart* 1999; 81: 232–8.

9 Danesh J, Collins R, Peto R. Chronic infections and coronary heart disease: is there a link? *Lancet* 1997; 350: 430–6.

10 Nieto FJ, Folsom A, Sorlie P *et al. Chlamydia pneumoniae* infection and incident coronary heart disease: the atherosclerosis in communities (ARIC) study (Abstract). *Am J Epidemiol* 1997; 145: 331.

11 Siscovick DS, Schwartz SM, Corey L *et al.* Antibody to *Chlamydia pneumoniae*, Herpes simplex virus type I, cytomegalovirus and incident myocardial infarction and coronary heart disease death: the cardiovascular health study (Abstract). *Circulation* 1998; 97: 2.

12 Ridker PM, Kundsin RB, Stampfer PJ *et al.* Prospective study of *Chlamydia pneumoniae* IgG seropositivity and risks of future myocardial infarction. *Circulation* 1999; 99: 1161–4.

13 Danesh J, Wong Y, Ward M *et al.* Chronic infection with *Helicobacter pylori*, *Chlamydia pneumoniae*, or Cytomegalovirus: population based study of coronary heart disease. *Heart* 1999; 81: 245–7.

14 Saikku P, Leinonen M, Tenkanen L *et al.* Chronic *Chlamydia pneumoniae* infection as a risk factor for coronary heart disease in the Helsinki heart study. *Ann Intern Med* 1992; 116: 273–8.

15 Miettinen H, Lehto S, Saikku P *et al.* Association of *Chlamydia pneumoniae* and acute coronary heart disease events in non-insulin dependent diabetic and non-diabetic subjects in Finland. *Eur Heart J* 1996; 17: 682–8.

16 Ossewarde JM, Feskens EM, deVries A *et al. Chlamydia pneumoniae* is a risk factor for coronary heart disease in symptom free elderly men, but *Helicobacter pylori* and cytomegalovirus are not. *Epidemiol Infect* 1998; 120: 93–9.

17 Strachan DP, Carrington D, Mendall MA *et al.* Relation of *Chlamydia pneumoniae* serology to mortality and incidence of ischaemic heart disease over 13 years in the Caerphilly prospective heart disease study. *Br Med J* 1999; 318: 1035–40.

18 Fagerberg B, Gnarpe J, Gnarpe H *et al. Chlamydia pneumoniae* but not cytomegalovirus antibodies are associated with future risk of stroke and cardiovascular disease: a prospective study in middle-aged to elderly men with treated hypertension. *Stroke* 1999; 30: 299–305.

19 Maass M, Krause E, Engel PM *et al.* Endovascular presence of *Chlamydia pneumoniae* in patients with haemodynamically effective carotid artery stenosis 1997; 48: 699–706.

20 Chiu B, Viira E, Tucker W *et al. Chlamydia pneumoniae*, cytomegalovirus, and herpes simplex virus in atherosclerosis of the carotid artery. *Circulation* 1997; 96: 2144–8.

21 Naidu BR, Ngeow YF, Kannan P *et al.* Evidence of *Chlamydia pneumoniae* infection obtained by the polymerase chain reaction (PCR) in patients with acute myocardial infarction and coronary heart disease (Letter). *J Infect* 1997; 35: 199–200.

22 Boman J, Petersen E, Persson K *et al.* Failure to detect *Chlamydia pneumoniae* DNA by nested PCR in serum samples of patients with infra-renal abdominal aortic aneurysms. In: Stephens RS, Byrne GI, Christiansen G, Clark I, Grayston JT, Hatch T, Ridgeway G, Saikku P, Schachter J, Stamm WE. eds. *Chlamydial Infections. Proceedings of the Ninth International*

Symposium on Human Chlamydial Infection International Chlamydia Symposium, San Francisco 1998: 211–14.

23 Boman J, Soderberg S, Forsberg J *et al.* High prevalence of *Chlamydia pneumoniae* DNA in peripheral blood mononuclear cells in patients with cardiovascular disease and in middle-aged blood donors. *J Infect Dis* 1998; 178: 274–7.

24 Wong YK, Dawkins K, Ward ME. Detection of *C. pneumoniae* DNA circulating in the blood of patients attending for cardiac angiography: preliminary clinical and serological correlates. In: Stephens RS, Byrne GI, Christiansen G, Clark I, Grayston JT, Hatch T, Ridgeway G, Saikku P, Schachter J, Stamm WE. eds. *Chlamydial Infections. Proceedings of the Ninth International Symposium on Human Chlamydial Infection International Chlamydia Symposium, San Francisco,* 1998: 227–30.

25 Weiss SM, Roblin P, Gaydos CA *et al.* Failure to detect *Chlamydia pneumoniae* in coronary atheromas of patients undergoing atherectomy. *J Inf Dis* 1996; 173: 957–62.

26 Lindholt JS, Ostergard L, Henneberg EW *et al.* Failure to demonstrate *Chlamydia pneumoniae* in symptomatic abdominal aortic aneurysms by a nested polymerase chain reaction (PCR). *Eur J Vasc Endovasc Surg* 1998; 15: 161–4.

27 Paterson DL, Hall J, Rasmussen SJ *et al.* Failure to detect *Chlamydia pneumoniae* in atherosclerotic plaques of Australian patients. *Pathology* 1998; 30: 169–72.

28 Wong Y, Thomas M, Gallagher PJ *et al.* The prevalence of *Chlamydia pneumoniae* in atherosclerotic and normal blood vessels of patients undergoing redo and first time coronary artery bypass surgery. *J Am Coll Cardiol* 1999; 33: 152–6.

29 Ong G, Thomas BJ, Mansfield AO *et al.* Detection and widespread distribution of *Chlamydia pneumoniae* in the vascular system and its possible implications. *J Clin Path* 1996; 49: 102–6.

30 Koch R. Uber bakteriologische studien. In: Schwelbe J, Gaffky GP, Fuhl E eds. *Gesammelte Werke Von Robert Koch*, Vol 1 Leipzig: George Thieme, 1912: 650.

31 Moazed TC, Kuo CC, Grayston JT *et al.* Murine models of *Chlamydia pneumoniae* infection and atherosclerosis. *J Infect Dis* 1997; 175: 883–90.

32 Moazed TC, Campbell LA, Rosenfeld ME *et al. Chlamydia pneumoniae* infection accelerates the progression of atherosclerosis in apoE-deficient mice. In: Stephens RS, Byrne GI, Christiansen G, Clark I, Grayston JT, Hatch T, Ridgeway G, Saikku P, Schachter J, Stamm WE. eds. *Chlamydial Infections*. Berkeley: University of California Printing Services, 1998: 426–9.

33 Moazed TC, Kuo C-C, Grayston JT *et al.* An experimental rabbit model of *Chlamydia pneumoniae* infection. *Am J Path* 1996; 148: 667–76.

34 Fong IW, Chiu B, Viira E *et al.* Rabbit model for *Chlamydia pneumoniae* infection. *J Clin Microbiol* 1997; 35: 48–52.

35 Laitinen K, Laurila A, Pyhala L *et al. Chlamydia pneumoniae* infection induces inflammatory changes in the aortas of rabbits. *Infection Immunity* 1997; 65: 4832–25.

36 Muhlestein JB, Anderson JL, Hammond EH *et al.* Infection with *Chlamydia pneumoniae* accelerates the development of atherosclerosis and treatment with azithromycin prevents it in a rabbit model. *Circulation* 1998; 97: 633–6.

37 Gaydos CA, Summersgill JT, Sahney NN *et al.* Replication of *Chlamydia pneumoniae in vitro* in human macrophages, endothelial cells and aortic artery smooth muscle cells. *Infection Immunol* 1996; 64: 1614–20.

38 Godzik KL, O'Brien ER, Wang SK *et al.* In vitro susceptibility of human vascular wall cells to infection with *Chlamydia pneumoniae*. *J Clin Microbiol* 1995; 33: 2411–14.

39 Kaukoranta-Tolvanen SS, Teppo AM, Laitinen K *et al.* Growth of *Chlamydia pneumoniae* in cultured human blood mononuclear cells and induction of a cytokine response. *Microbiol Pathog* 1996; 21: 215–21.

40 Airenne S, Surcel H-M, Alakarpa H *et al. Chlamydia pneumoniae* infection in human monocytes. *Infection Immunity* 1999; 67: 1445–9.

41 Molestina RE, Miller RD, Ramirez JA *et al.* Infection of human endothelial cells with *Chlamydia pneumoniae* stimulates trans endothelial migration of neutrophils and monocytes. *Infection Immunity* 1999; 76: 1323–30.

42 Kalayoglu MV, Byrne GI. Induction of macrophage foam cell formation by

Chlamydia pneumoniae. J Infect Dis 1998; 177: 725–9.

43 Moazed TC, Kuo CC, Grayston JT *et al.* Systemic dissemination of *Chlamydia pneumoniae* infection via macrophages. *J Infect Dis* 1998; 177: 1322–5.

44 Gupta S, Camm AJ. *Chlamydia pneumoniae* and coronary heart disease: Coincidence, association, or causation? *Br Med J* 1997; 314: 1778–9.

45 Patel P, Carrington D, Strachan DP *et al.* Fibrinogen: a link between chronic infection and coronary heart disease. *Lancet* 1994; 343: 1634–5.

46 Mendall MA, Patel P, Ballam L *et al.* C-reactive protein and its relation to cardiovascular risk factors: a population based cross sectional study. *Br Med J* 1996; 312: 1061–5.

47 Laurila A, Bloigu A, Nayha A *et al.* *Chlamydia pneumoniae* antibodies and serum lipids in Finnish men: cross sectional study. *Br Med J* 1997; 314: 14546–7.

48 Laurila A, Bloigu A, Nayha S *et al.* Chronic *Chlamydia pneumoniae* infection is associated with a serum lipid profile known to be a risk factor for atherosclerosis. *Arterioscler Thromb Vasc Biol* 1997; 17: 2810–13.

49 Murray LJ, O'Reilly DPJ, Ong GML *et al.* *Chlamydia pneumoniae* antibodies are associated with an atherogenic lipid profile. *Heart* 1999; 81: 239–44.

50 Leatham EW, Bath PM, Tooze JA *et al.* Increased monocyte tissue factor expression in coronary disease. *Br Heart J* 1995; 73: 10–13.

51 Patel P, Mendall MA, Carrington D *et al.* Association of *Helicobacter pylori* and *Chlamydia pneumoniae* infections with coronary heart disease and cardiovascular risk factors. *Br Med J* 1995; 311: 711–14.

52 Toss H, Gnarpe J, Siegbahn A *et al.* Increased fibrinogen levels are associated with persistent *Chlamydia pneumoniae* infection in unstable coronary artery disease. *Eur Heart J* 1998; 19: 570–7.

53 Visser MR, Tracey PB, Vercellotti GM *et al.* Enhancing thrombin generation and platelet binding on herpes simplex virus-infected endothelium. *Proc Natl Acad Sci USA* 1988; 85: 8227–30.

54 Morrison RP, Belland RJ, Lyng K, Caldwell HD. Chlamydial disease pathogenesis. The 57-kD *Chlamydial*

hypersensitivity antigen is a stress response protein. *J Exp Med* 1989; 170: 1271–83.

55 Beatty WL, Byrne GI, Morrison RP. Morphologic and antigenic characterization of interferon gamma-mediated persistent *Chlamydia trachomatis* infection *in vitro*. *Proc Natl Acad Sci USA* 1993; 90: 3998–4002.

56 Birnie DH, Holme ER, McKay IC *et al.* Association between antibodies to heat shock protein 65 and coronary atherosclerosis. *Eur Heart J* 1998; 19: 387–94.

57 Kol A, Sukhova GK, Lichtman AH, Libby P. Chlamydial heat shock protein 60 localises in human atheroma and regulates macrophage tumour necrosis factor-α and matrix metalloproteinase expression. *Circulation* 1998; 98: 300–7.

58 Mayr M, Metzler B, Kiechl S *et al.* Endothelial cytotoxicity mediated by serum antibodies to heat shock proteins of *Escherichia coli* and chlamydia pneumoniae: immune reactions to heat shock proteins as a possible link between infection and atherosclerosis. *Circulation* 1999; 99: 1560–6.

59 Wick G, Kleindienst R, Schett G *et al.* Role of heat shock protein 65/60 in the pathogenesis of atherosclerosis. *Int Arch Allergy Immunol* 1995; 107: 130–1.

60 Kaski JC, Cox I. Chronic infection and atherogenesis. *Eur Heart J* 1998; 19: 366–7.

61 Fujita T, Fujimoto Y. Formation and removal of active oxygen species and lipid peroxides in biological systems. *Nippon Yakurigaku Zasshi* 1992; 99 (6): 381–9.

62 Steinbrecher UP, Parathasarathy S, Leake DS *et al.* Modification of low density lipoprotein by endothelial cells involves lipid peroxidation and degradation of low density lipoprotein phospholipids. *Proc Natl Acad Sci USA* 1984; 81: 3883–7.

63 Morel DW, DiCorleto PE, Chisholm GM. Endothelial and smooth muscle cells alter low density lipoprotein in vitro by free radical oxidation. *Arteriosclerosis* 1984; 4: 357–64.

64 Gupta S, Leatham EW, Carrington D *et al.* The effect of azithromycin in post myocardial infarction patients with elevated *Chlamydia pneumoniae* antibody titres (Abstract). *J Am Coll Cardiol* 1997; 755: 209.

65 Gurfinkel E, Bozovich G, Beck E *et al*. Treatment with the antibiotic roxithromycin in patients with acute non-Q-wave coronary syndromes. The final report of the ROXIS study. *Eur Heart J* 1999; 20: 121–7.

66 Anderson JL, Muhlestein JB, Carlquist J *et al*. Randomised secondary prevention trial of azithromycin in patients with coronary artery disease and serological evidence for *Chlamydia pneumoniae* infection: the Azithromycin in Coronary Artery Disease: Elimination of Myocardial Infection with *Chlamydia* (ACADEMIC) study. *Circulation* 1999; 99: 1540–7.

67 Sinsalo J, Mattila K, Nieminen MS *et al*. The effect of prolonged doxycycline therapy on *Chlamydia pneumoniae* serological markers, coronary heart disease risk factors and forearm basal nitric oxide production. *J Antimicrob Cheother* 1998; 41: 85–92.

68 Torgano G, Cosentini R, Mandelli C *et al*. Treatment of *Helicobacter pylori* and *Chlamydia pneumoniae* infections decreases fibrinogen plasma levels in patients with ischaemic heart disease. *Circulation* 1999; 99: 1555–9.

69 Meier CR, Derby LE, Jick SS *et al*. Antibiotics and risk of subsequent first-time acute myocardial infarction. *JAMA* 1999; 281: 427–31.

70 Jackson LA, Smith NL, Heckbert SR *et al*. Lack of association between first myocardial infarction and past use of cry thromycin, tetracycline, or doxycycline. *Emerg Infect Dis* 1999; 5: 281–4.

71 Martin D, Bursill J, Qui MR, Breit S, Campbell T. Alternative hypothesis for efficacy of macrolides in acute coronary syndromes (letter). *Lancet* 1998; 351: 1858–9.

72 Sugiura Y, Ohashi Y, Nakai Y. Roxithromycin stimulates the mucociliary activity of the Eustachian tube and modulates neutrophil activity in the healthy guinea pig. *Acta Otolaryngol Suppl* 1997; 531: 34–8.

73 Wenisch C, Parschalk B, Zedtwitz-Liebenstein K, Weihs A, el Menyawi I, Graninger W. Effect of single oral dose of azithromycin, clarithromycin, and roxithromycin on polymorphonuclear leucocyte function assessed *ex vivo* by flow cytometry. *Antimicrob Agents Chemother* 1996; 40: 2039–42.

74 Ohshima A, Tokura Y, Wakita H, Furukawa F, Takigawa M. Roxithromycin down modulates antigen-presenting and interleukin-1-beta-producing abilities of murine Langerhans cells. *J Dermatol Sci* 1988; 17: 214–22.

75 Grayston JT. Antibiotic treatment trials for secondary prevention of coronary artery disease events. *Circulation* 1999; 99: 1538–9.

76 Gupta S, Kaski JC, Camm AJ. Antibiotic therapy in coronary heart disease: hype versus hope. *Br J Cardiol* 1998; 5: 65–6.

4: What is the role of coronary tone in acute coronary syndromes?

Laurence O'Toole and Neal G. Uren

Introduction

The manifestations of ischaemic heart disease are based on the development and progression of atherosclerotic coronary disease — a condition characterized by intimal thickening and lipid-rich deposits in the epicardial coronary artery, which encroach on the coronary lumen, once adaptive remodelling is exhausted [1]. Increasing atherosclerotic plaque load leads to progressive flow limitation, and, as the limit of adaptive vasodilatation of the coronary resistive vessels is reached, transient episodes of myocardial ischaemia occur at times of increased myocardial oxygen demand. This produces the symptoms of classical stable angina pectoris. However, in the acute coronary syndromes the two main clinical entities of coronary blood flow limitation and plaque instability overlap. Plaque instability with acute plaque rupture can lead to acute thrombotic coronary occlusion and the clinical event of myocardial infarction. When there is plaque erosion, or less extensive dissection, with non-occlusive thrombosis and inadequate collateralization from other epicardial vessels, the acute coronary syndromes of unstable angina and non-Q-wave myocardial infarction may occur, with a combination of recurrent coronary flow limitation and dynamic thrombosis at the site of plaque erosion. The development of an eroded fibrous cap, intraplaque haemorrhage or mural thrombus at the site of a fibrous plaque is a highly unpredictable event. Therefore, the progression of atherosclerosis is not linear; rather there is a dominant role of very localized alterations in coronary architecture. For instance, over 70% of coronary segments responsible for acute myocardial infarction (MI) are less than 50% stenosed beforehand [2]. Thus, although the symptoms of ischaemic heart disease are more likely to be manifest in those with more extensive atherosclerosis, a poor correlation exists between the extent of obstructive atherosclerosis and acute ischaemic manifestations. This suggests a major role of transient stimuli, such as the response to local inflammation, platelet aggregability, thrombin generation and, possibly, coronary vasoconstriction in the genesis of the acute ischaemic syndromes.

Dynamic coronary tone as a clinical entity

In 1910, Osler [3] proposed spasm of the coronary artery to explain the occurrence of spontaneous episodes of angina, but in later times it was thought, on the basis of post-mortem observations, that the coronary arteries of patients with angina were so fibrotic and calcified that vasoconstriction was not possible [4–6], and the concept of coronary artery spasm went out of fashion. Thereafter, until the mid 1970s, the diagnosis of coronary artery spasm as a mechanism for variable onset angina was often felt to be a last resort of the 'diagnostically destitute'. In 1959, Prinzmetal and colleagues challenged the traditional view, proposing that increased tone at the site of a coronary plaque was the probable cause of a 'variant' form of angina [7]. Gensini and colleagues [8] reported episodes of coronary artery spasm witnessed during angiography. In 1972 Oliva *et al.* [9] produced the first clear angiographic evidence of recurrent occlusive coronary arterial spasm in an otherwise angiographically normal right coronary artery. The spasm was associated with severe chest pain and ST segment elevation on the ECG, and was relieved by sublingual nitrate. The next year MacAlpine *et al.* [10] proposed transient spastic occlusion of the coronary artery as the mechanism of variant angina in a series of 20 patients with focal atherosclerotic stenoses and preserved exercise capacity. In 1976, Maseri *et al.* [11] widened the concept and argued that many non-variant cases of angina at rest were caused by a transient reduction in coronary blood flow, and not just increased myocardial oxygen demand. In the mid-1980s, the concept of an episodic increase in vasomotor tone as the cause of not only variant angina, but also as a significant pathogenic factor in other more common angina syndromes, began to gain wider acceptance [12–14]. It is now widely accepted that there is an important role for increased coronary artery tone in clinical manifestations of the acute coronary syndromes.

The generation and control of coronary tone

The epicardial coronary arteries are large elastic distensible vessels with a contractile media containing vascular smooth muscle cells between the intima and fibrous adventitia. The calibre of the epicardial coronary arteries is controlled by the dynamic-flow-mediated release of nitric oxide through shear stress and pressure-mediated changes in myogenic tone. These intrinsic mechanisms are modulated by neurohumoral controls. This autoregulatory process allows wall shear stress and lumen diameter to be kept within narrow limits as flow and pressure vary. Epicardial vessels act as conduits with capacitance function and under normal conditions have negligible pressure drop along their length down to a diameter of 500 μm. The pattern of branching and tapering minimizes blood kinetic energy losses.

During systole, epicardial coronary arteries increase their blood volume by as much as 25%, due to anterograde flow from the aorta and retrograde flow from intramyocardial vessels. This elastic energy is turned into kinetic energy in early diastole and increases diastolic coronary flow. With an increase in myocardial demand, coronary-flow-mediated vasodilatation increases the coronary capacitance and reduces shear stress, accommodating a larger volume of blood during systole. Myogenic regulation of coronary tone occurs in response to changes in aortic perfusion pressure, acting to maintain a constant coronary blood flow [15]. The endothelial lining of these arteries constantly acts as a sensori-effector mechanism that responds to increased shear stress by increasing the release of nitric oxide, bradykinin and other factors, resulting in vasodilatation. Thus, epicardial vessels intrinsically regulate coronary tone by the release of locally produced autocoids with paracrine and autocrine function.

The resistive vessels match myocardial blood flow to variable myocardial energy requirements, and to myocardial demand when the coronary perfusion pressure varies, such that myocardial oxygen extraction is virtually constant over a wide range of cardiac work and perfusion pressures. Coronary resistance is influenced both by extrinsic factors such as myocardial compression (intramyocardial wall tension) and by intrinsic factors such as tissue metabolism and neural and humoral influences. The former influence means that coronary blood flow ceases when the perfusion pressure is low but still substantially above coronary venous pressure [15]. Although it was first considered that most resistance to coronary flow resided in arterioles < 100 μm, much resistance is present in larger arterioles/small arteries up to 300 μm in diameter (90% in vessels < 300 μm) [16]. In the cat, 50% of coronary resistance is in vessels > 100 μm (25% in vessels > 170 μm) under basal conditions [17]. As 10% of resistance is in the venous compartment, this leaves about 40% of resistance in the vessels < 100 μm. Thus, coronary resistance coexists in different arteriolar compartments, and this changes depending on the perfusion pressure and local metabolic environment.

The resistive vessels comprise two general groups [18,19]. The arteriolar vessels (< 100 μm) respond to local tissue metabolism and maintain the extracellular environment within optimal biochemical limits for myocardial contractile function, modulated primarily by tissue oxygen tension. Flow is dependent on inherent arteriolar tone and the perfusion pressure at their origin. The latter is determined by the prearteriolar vessels (100–350 μm), which are influenced by coronary perfusion pressure and flow, by myogenic tone and by neurogenic influences [18]. With an increase in myocardial oxygen demand and arteriolar vasodilatation, a pressure drop occurs across the prearteriolar vessels with subsequent flow-mediated vasodilatation, thus coordinating the vascular response to physiological stress to meet tissue needs. Washout of metabolites leads to a relative vasoconstriction of arterioles, increasing the pressure head in the prearterioles, which, through a greater myogenic responsiveness counteracting even-flow-mediated vasodilatation, would limit this increase [19]. With increasing aortic pressure, arteriolar pressure may be maintained by pre-arteriolar constriction through increased myogenic tone. A marked decrease in aortic pressure leads to dilatation of all resistive vessels [20]. Vasoconstriction, or a failure of pre-arteriolar vessels to dilate, would lead to a reduction in flow in the arteriolar bed, despite maximal dilatation in response to tissue metabolism. There is considerable evidence to suggest that coronary resistive vessel dysfunction is highly prevalent in patients with coronary artery disease [21]. However, in the acute coronary syndromes, it seems most likely that it is an abnormal coronary vasomotor tone in an epicardial vessel adjacent to an eroded plaque that contributes principally to the clinical syndrome of myocardial ischaemia at rest, as a result of a primary reduction in myocardial oxygen supply.

Evaluation of changes in the coronary vasomotor tone is to some extent complicated by the distribution of resistance and capacitance among the different segments of the same epicardial artery, by variations in intramyocardial pressure in the different myocardial layers and by the effect of heart rate. In the coronary circulation, the arterioles, prearterioles and large arteries are modulated principally by oxygen consumption, flow and pressure, respectively. The effects of constrictor and dilator stimuli on epicardial tone are influenced by segmental basal tone and local mechanisms of control of tone, by α- and β-adrenoreceptor density and their distribution, both on the endothelium and on smooth muscle, and by the reactivity of the vessels to constrictor stimuli. In epicardial conductive arteries, basal tone is set at an intermediate level, as on average these vessels exhibit similar percentage dilatation and constriction to a variety of dilator and constrictor stimuli, and those that dilate more readily, appear to constrict less readily and vice versa [22]. Both dilator and constrictor responses are also greater in distal (< 1.5 mm) vessels than in proximal arteries. Considerable variability exists in the vasomotor response to vasoactive stimuli, depending on the segment of coronary artery exposed and the strength of the stimulus. Furthermore, secondary changes in vascular tone may occur downstream. For example, low doses of nitrate cause maximal dilatation of epicardial coronary arteries, with minimal increases in coronary flow. Acetylcholine and serotonin may dilate conduit arteries at low doses and constrict at higher doses. Similarly, differences occur in vasoactive response to a variety of differing agents depending on microvessel size [23] and position [24].

Possible roles of coronary tone in the acute coronary syndromes

Fixed stenosis

Fixed epicardial coronary stenoses begin to have significant effects on hyper-aemic coronary blood flow when the stenosis exceeds 40% [25]. Resistance to flow, measured as the drop in pressure across a lesion, is determined primarily by the minimal lumen diameter and also by the length of the lesion. Flow may also be influenced by the presence of other stenoses in series, and by energy loss due to turbulence caused by luminal irregularities (friction loss). Pulsatile flow and a post-stenotic increase in capacitance (expansion loss) further compli-cate calculation of the effects of a stenosis on myocardial blood flow, as does the variable degree of collateral supply. The rise in resistance to flow is highly non-linear, for example, tripling as the diameter stenosis increases from 80% to 90% [26]. Experimental studies in anaesthetized dogs indicate that a 90% reduction in diameter (99% reduction in vessel area) is required to reduce coronary flow at rest [27], although collateral supply can maintain normal basal myocardial blood flow in the presence of a 100% stenosis (occlusion) in man [25]. The fall in coronary perfusion can initially be compensated for by progressive dilatation of resistive vessels (metabolic autoregulation) up to a diameter stenosis of 90%. However, this vasodilatory compensation requires the use of an increasing fraction of the coronary flow reserve. Thus, as resistive vessels dilate to maintain resting flow, the available coronary flow reserve is re-duced in proportion to the fall in post-stenotic pressure.

Occlusive coronary artery spasm

Normal coronary arteries respond to a variety of differing constrictor stimuli with a modest (10–20%) reduction in diameter. No constrictor stimulus has yet been identified that can cause segmental occlusive spasm in normal epicar-dial coronary arteries [28]. As demonstrated in aortic strips from cholesterol-fed rabbits, hypersensitivity to constrictor stimuli such as serotonin and ergonovine (of up to 3 orders of magnitude) will occur in atherosclerotic ves-sels, but without much hyperreactivity (~30% increase in maximal response) [29]. Thus, the abnormal response to vasoconstrictor stimuli will not in itself cause occlusive spasm. However, in patients with variant angina, severe local coronary hyperreactivity (~80% reduction in coronary diameter) occurs both spontaneously, and with provocation at doses of agonists similar to those which cause mild vasoconstriction (~15% reduction in coronary diameter) in other coronary segments from the same patients, or in patients without vasospastic angina [30]. Thus, hyperreactivity but not hypersensitivity occurs in these coronary arteries. The cause of this phenomenon is unknown. The miniature swine model of coronary artery spasm partially mimics this effect with coronary occlusion in response to serotonin and histamine, but not ergonovine in atherosclerotic arterial segments that have undergone endothelial denudation 3 months previously [31]. The features of the arterial repair process that renders the coronary segment hyperreactive in this model are unknown.

The physiological constrictor response to intracoronary ergonovine is a luminal reduction of less than 30%. Rarely, severe segmental, or even (in less than 2% of cases) diffuse, spasm to ergonovine is observed [32]. This may be seen in patients with no clinical or ECG evidence of variant angina. Between the extremes of the mild physiological response and severe spasm of variant angina, dynamic coronary vasoconstriction may occur in patients with chronic stable and unstable angina. Its significance depends on the underlying extent of stenosis and persisting vasomotor potential of the coronary segment. It will be most significant in a severe lesion in which changes in coronary diameter are most difficult to measure angiographically with any accuracy. Occlusive epicardial spasm, as observed in the syndrome of variant (Prinzmetal) angina, is usually localized and readily separated from lesser degrees of coronary vasoconstriction. The syndrome is rare, with an incidence of perhaps 1% of subjects referred for coronary angiography [33]. Local coronary hyperreactivity to a variety of normal constrictor stimuli has been shown to be the mechanism, but the exact cause remains unclear [34]. Features of variant angina include the fact that spasm can be induced by a wide variety of drugs in the same patient: spasm can be induced by raising the arterial pH (hyperventilation), by handgrip, and by the cold pressor test in some patients, but it also occurs in transplanted hearts excluding a purely neurogenic mechanism. These features suggest a postreceptor signalling alteration as the primary mechanism, presumably in the presence of local endothelial dysfunction. The exaggerated local response can persist unchanged for years, or wax and wane over a few weeks. Segmental coronary constriction in patients with variant angina may result in total occlusion and dysrhythmia, myocardial infarction and sudden death [35,36].

Severe spasm to intracoronary ergonovine may occur in other coronary syndromes. Bertrand et al. [37] performed an ergometrine provocation test in 1089 patients undergoing coronary angiography. Occlusive spasm was induced in 1% of patients with atypical chest pain, 4% of those with chronic stable angina and 6% of those with old MI, but in 38% of patients with unstable angina and 20% of those with recent MI. Thus, local coronary hyperreactivity occurs more frequently in subjects with an acute plaque rupture. This is consistent with the presence of contraction bands at the plaque site at post-mortem examination of patients with unstable angina [38], and with reports of spasm persisting *post mortem* [39,40]. Occlusive artery spasm has been reported following coronary artery bypass surgery and in aorto-coronary bypass grafts [41]. Occlusive spasm has been shown also in subjects with sudden cardiac death or fatal myocardial infarction [42,43]. These data suggest a significant role of coronary tone in at least a proportion of patients with an acute coronary syndrome.

Dynamic modulation of a plaque stenosis

Occlusive coronary spasm is probably a rare phenomenon compared with dynamic coronary vasoconstriction, which may contribute to the majority of acute coronary syndromes, as well as to variable-workload stable angina; and these two phenomena should be considered separate entities [44]. As discussed above, an acute reduction of epicardial coronary diameter of the order of 90% is required to cause subendocardial ischaemia and ST-segment depression at rest [15], although the presence of anaemia, hypoxia or myocardial hypertrophy will result in ischaemia at lesser degrees of lumen reduction. The 'ischaemic potential' of a coronary plaque is dependent not only on its ability to create a fixed impediment to flow but also its thrombotic and vasomotor potential. This is compensated in part by the extent of collateral coronary circulation distal to the stenosis. The degree of vasoconstriction required to induce ischaemia at a 70% diameter stenosis will, of course, be much less than that at the site of a 50% stenosis. The morphology and composition of a plaque provides an indication of its vasomotor potential [45]. Concentric stenoses are generally fibrotic, and, when severe, are often associated with considerable smooth muscle atrophy in the medial layer. In contrast, eccentric stenoses with smooth borders often have a disease-free arc of wall with preserved smooth muscle. Thus, the residual lumen area may be modified by vasomotor stimuli more readily. Eccentric lesions with irregular borders at angiography usually correspond to complex lesions with recent plaque fissuring or mural thrombus. Irregular stenoses, recently formed from the organization of mural thrombus, are likely to retain an arc of preserved media and significant vasomotor potential, whereas multichannelled recanalized thrombi are unlikely to have any vasomotor potential due to their dense fibrous nature. The relationship between disease-free arc and severity of stenosis is very variable, however. Frequently more than 30% of the free wall is preserved in lesions causing between 70% and 80% area stenosis [46]. Thus, when the plaque occupies a large percentage of the vessel wall, when the constrictor stimuli are strong (e.g. in the presence of activated platelets) and where the coronary segment remains compliant, alterations in coronary tone can induce rest pain. After thrombolytic therapy, many recently recanalized infarct-related stenoses show a marked potential to dilate following the administration of intracoronary nitrate, confirming significant dynamic modulation of the unstable plaque stenosis and a role of coronary tone in the pathogenesis of myocardial infarction [47].

The influence of atheromatous endothelial dysfunction on the role of coronary tone in acute coronary syndromes is not clear. Intra-coronary acetylcholine dilates normal, epicardial, human coronary arteries, but causes no response, or even constriction, in an atherosclerotic section of a coronary artery, as a result of an unopposed muscarinic effect on vascular smooth muscle [48]. Similarly, the dilatory effect of bradykinin is blunted in atherosclerotic segments of coronary arteries [49]. In acute coronary syndromes, a defective vasodilator response will potentiate ischaemia and enhance a local thrombotic tendency [50]. The response of the human coronary artery tends toward vasoconstriction with increasing age (increasing risk-factor status) and with atherosclerosis. The significance of this is uncertain, as the maximal extent of inducible constriction in most human coronary arteries is modest. Also, the frequent presence of asymptomatic coronary atherosclerosis in the general population suggests that coronary endothelial dysfunction is not necessarily associated with clinical manifestations of ischaemic heart disease [29].

Resistive vessel function

The tone of the smaller coronary arteries and larger coronary resistive vessels (pre-arterioles) is under considerable neural influence; under some circumstances neural mediation of coronary tone can result in myocardial ischaemia. Vascoconstrictor centres in the hypothalamus activate the sympathetic nervous system and can induce coronary constriction and reduce coronary blood flow. Coronary blood flow varies 2-fold during sleep [51]. In animal studies, coronary vasoconstriction has been induced in response to anger caused by watching other dogs eat their food [52]. Studies in experimental animals indicate that constriction of coronary resistive vessels can impair flow in the absence of coronary stenosis. This is inferred by the presence of ischaemia occurring during infusion of pharmacological agents, in the absence of visible angiographic coronary artery spasm, for example the infusion of endothelin into the left anterior descending coronary artery of dogs [53], or the tripeptide N-formyl-L-leucyl-L-phenylamine into rabbit coronary arteries [54]. These ischaemic effects occur evenly across the myocardial wall, contrasting with the predominantly subendocardial effect of epicardial coronary stenoses.

The influence of distal coronary artery tone on the genesis of myocardial ischaemia received little attention until relatively recently [55]. Few data are available regarding its influence in the acute coronary syndromes [56]. Infusion of neuropeptide Y, which acts on vessels of less than 500 µm diameter, or of high doses of acetylcholine, into the coronary arteries of angiographically normal humans, causes ischaemia with extremely slow visible dye flow, but without epicardial artery constriction [57]. In patients with coronary stenosis, intracoronary infusion of serotonin (5-HT) causes ischaemia, with only small changes in the calibre of stenotic segments, but with diffuse spasm of secondary and tertiary coronary branches [58]. The dose of serotonin that induces ischaemia is within the range found in coronary arteries during intracoronary platelet activation [59].

Further evidence of the effects of distal coronary tone is the occurrence of persisting inducible ischaemia after successful coronary angioplasty. This has been demonstrated by persisting defects of thallium uptake during stress myocardial scintigraphy [60,61] as well as by the demonstration of persisting ST-segment changes during exercise testing [62]. The mechanism is thought to be the reduced dilator response of coronary resistive vessels, subtended by the previously stenosed artery, presumably because of vascular adaptation to decreased post-stenotic pressure [63]. Reduced coronary flow response to intracoronary papaverine or systemic dipyridamole has been shown by Doppler flow-wire measurements and positron emission tomography (PET) perfusion studies, in which, in the majority of patients, coronary flow reserve gradually returned to normal over the first 3 months following angioplasty [64,65]. The reduced response could not be improved by intracoronary nitroprusside, indicating that the mechanism is not simply impaired endothelial nitric oxide production in resistive vessels. This response is not seen in all patients following angioplasty; it may persist or regress, and it may be present in areas of myocardium supplied by a non-stenosed artery [66], indicating that it may represent a more general dysfunction of resistive vessel function exacerbated by the presence of stenosis. Thus, alterations in distal coronary artery tone may be an explanation for the variable relationship between the severity of coronary stenosis, the impairment of coronary flow reserve and anginal symptoms. The site of distal coronary constriction remains unclear, but could be at the small artery or pre-arteriolar levels, and could be attributable to inadequate flow-mediated dilatation, abnormal neurogenic vasoconstriction or even organic alterations, such as medial hypertrophy or perivascular fibrosis.

Collateral support and coronary tone

In experimental animal studies, collaterals develop within hours of the development of coronary stenosis by the dilatation of preformed anastamotic connections and the formation of new connections under the stimulus of myocardial ischaemia. Full collateral development takes a few months, and varies greatly between different individuals. The extent of myocardial infarction or severity of ischaemia in unstable angina is critically dependent on the extent of distal collateral circulation. Factors determining the development of collateral circulation are poorly understood, but there is evidence that collateral support may be subject to dynamic changes in vasomotor tone, and such changes could be very important in determining outcome in acute coronary syndromes. Studies in patients with single-vessel occlusion, but no evidence of myocardial infarction, have been performed to evaluate collateral circulatory support. In such subjects, changes in coronary flow reserve can be modulated only by constriction of vessels supplying or receiving collateral flow [67]. Pupita *et al.* found a marked difference in ischaemic threshold on exercise treadmill testing in such patients when testing was repeated in association with the administration of constrictor (ergonovine) or dilator (nitroglycerin) drugs [68]. Ambulatory monitoring suggested that most episodes of ischaemia occurred at much lower heart rates than occurred at the onset of ischaemia during treadmill testing, and administration of ergonovine during coronary arteriography caused a marked reduction in collateral filling with no evidence of epicardial artery spasm [68]. Thus, these data suggest that dynamic changes in vasomotor tone influence the development of ischaemia in chronic stable angina. How this effect relates to the unstable coronary syndromes has been little studied, but, presumably, reductions in collateral support during acute ischaemia will magnify the effects of a reduction in coronary artery flow and affect outcome.

Clinical evidence for increased coronary tone in the acute coronary syndromes

Many investigators now feel that episodic increases in coronary tone are a significant factor in the pathogenesis of acute coronary syndromes as well as in variant angina [12–14,29]. As discussed above, the degree of epicardial constriction varies greatly from mild physiological constriction observed in animal studies to the segmental occlusion observed in variant angina. The effects are proportional to the intensity of the stimulus and the reactivity of the smooth muscle, as well as the anatomic features of the stenosis and basal tone. Changes in vascular tone in the distal coronary circulation and in collateral vessels could also critically affect the response to coronary thrombosis.

It is well established that, in patients with rest angina, spontaneous episodes of acute ischaemia usually occur with no major change in heart rate or blood pressure, and that these episodes certainly occur at levels of both that are much less than the rates yielding a rate-pressure product sufficient to induce ischaemia during stress-testing [69]. Regional defects in thallium-201 uptake during ischaemia at rest in myocardial perfusion studies indicate the dominant role of a transient reduction in regional myocardial blood flow [70]. Thus, the severity of ischaemia is a product of the extent of the underlying coronary artery stenoses and the thrombotic and vasoconstrictor potential of the unstable lesion. The role of vasoconstriction is much more difficult to detect than the role of thrombosis in patients with unstable angina. Thrombi are readily visible at angiography, angioscopy and at post-mortem studies, whereas increased vasomotor tone is much less so and is best demonstrated by intravascular ultrasound.

Drug therapy in unstable angina

Nitrates, calcium-channel blockers and potassium-channel activators all reduce coronary tone by a direct action on smooth muscle and are used in unstable angina. Nitrates undoubtedly have benefit in relieving angina in unstable patients, and there is a clear dose–response effect [71]. Abrupt withdrawal of intravenous nitrate therapy in patients with unstable angina may cause rebound myocardial ischaemia [72], presumably because of an increase in epicardial coronary tone at the lesion site. However, there are no placebo-controlled studies that provide data regarding the effect of nitrate therapy on outcomes in patients with unstable angina. Nonetheless, the success of these agents in relieving ischaemic pain is clear evidence of a vasoconstrictive component in the pathogenesis of unstable angina. Whether their vasorelaxant action translates into improved survival is not clear.

After the recognition of the importance of calcium transport in the plasmalemma in the control of smooth muscle tone in coronary and systemic vessels in the late 1970s, calcium-channel blockers were developed as agents for the management of angina pectoris and hypertension [73]. The main mechanism of action is blockage of the L-type-voltage-dependent channels. Calcium-channel blockers are undoubtedly beneficial in reducing both symptomatic and silent ischaemia in patients with stable and unstable angina pectoris [74–76]. Intravenous diltiazem has been shown to be superior to intravenous nitrates in preventing ischaemia in unstable angina [77], presumably through a more effective direct vasodilating effect. However, a pooled analysis of results from trials comparing the use of calcium-channel blockers with placebo in patients with unstable angina did not show a reduction in the progression to myocardial infarction or death [78]. The total number of patients in this analysis was small (~1000 patients). Thus, a biological effect may have been missed.

Potassium channel activators, such as nicorandil, are a heterogeneous class of compounds that cause hyperpolarization of smooth muscle cells, decreased calcium permeation and inhibition of intracellular storage and release of calcium, resulting in a fall in vascular tone [79]. Nicorandil has recently been shown to be effective in reducing ischaemia in unstable angina; however, as with nitrates and calcium channel blockers, data regarding its efficacy in preventing progression to MI or death are lacking [80].

Myocardial infarction

The identification and quantification of the role of coronary tone in the pathogenesis of acute MI is difficult. Myocardial infarction is often the first manifestation of disease in apparently healthy subjects. There are multiple pathogenic mechanisms that can underlie the development of myocardial infarction following acute plaque rupture, including thrombus, spasm, embolus and distal vessel constriction; and the contribution of each will vary from patient to patient. Furthermore, there are multiple mechanisms for the production of each of these factors. Thrombotic occlusion of a major epicardial coronary artery is found in 90% of subjects presenting within the first two hours of MI, with subtotal occlusion in the remaining 10%. The coronary obstruction is frequently a dynamic process, with transient occlusion and reocclusion occurring during acute presentation [48,81]. The dominant pathogenic role of thrombus is proven by the efficacy of thrombolytic agents in promoting recanalization of the infarct-related artery. However, the residual stenosis at the time of completion of successful intracoronary thrombolysis can often be reduced by intracoronary nitrate [48], indicating that significant coronary spasm is present also. The magnitude of vasoconstriction exhibited will in part be determined by the dynamic potential of the underlying plaque. However, most myocardial infarction occurs at sites subtended by lesions of less than 50% diameter stenosis, which usually have an arc of preserved medial smooth muscle that can produce vasoconstriction. In the very early phase of infarction, balloon dilatation of the artery may not be associated with the restoration of normal flow. This may be due to diffuse distal intravascular thrombus, but distal coronary vasoconstriction may also play a role.

Variant angina

In patients with variant angina, occlusive spasm relatively rarely results in infarction. Thus, an unusually prolonged stimulus must be required in the presence of prothrombotic cofactors. Nonetheless, long-term follow up of patients with variant angina does not indicate a consistently benign course. Maseri *et al.* [82] followed 187 patients with variant angina for 5 years. Twenty patients died, most within the first year. Cipriano *et al.* [83] followed 25 patients with variant angina for over 2 years. Eleven suffered a major cardiac event. In both studies the extent of the underlying atherosclerosis strongly predicted outcome. Variant angina is a rare phenomenon. Thus, the relevance of these findings to the larger population of patients presenting with infarction is unknown. However, as Bertrand and colleagues [38] have shown, increased coronary reactivity to ergonovine is much more frequent in patients presenting with an acute coronary syndrome. The significance of this vascular hyperreactivity in acute coronary syndromes is unknown. It is possible that heightened coronary vasoreactivity is an important pathogenic factor in the progression from white platelet thrombus to occlusive red thrombus in the early stages of infarction [45].

Infarction with normal coronary arteries

Infarction distal to angiographically normal coronary arteries is well described [84,85]. This may be initiated by an intense local thrombogenic stimulus, a background prothrombotic state, local occlusive arterial spasm or severe distal vasoconstriction. Blood flow could be interrupted by the presence of intense distal vasoconstriction, possibly due to small vessel hyperreactivity to serotonin, thromboxane A_2 and other factors derived from activated platelets at the site of mural thrombus. Some munitions workers, following withdrawal of exposure to nitroglycerine, have developed infarction caused by prolonged coronary artery spasm [86]. Cocaine abuse is well recognized as a cause of acute infarction. It presumably acts through intense stimulation of coronary vasoconstriction [87]. Similarly, reports of myocardial infarction in association with betel-nut abuse [88], during dreams [89], following exposure to extremes of temperature [90] and after ergonovine administration all implicate epicardial coronary vasospasm in the pathogenesis. Thus, the contribution of coronary tone to the pathogenesis of infarction appears to vary greatly, depending on the clinical situation. It is often difficult to assess the contribution in a given instance. The relative lack of efficacy of vasodilator agents during acute infarction [78] may reflect the fact that intense spasm could initiate a cascade of events, e.g. plaque rupture, that relief of the coronary spasm alone will not alleviate.

Therapeutic trials

The success of specific therapies gives some indication of the relative importance of differing pathogenic mechanisms in acute coronary syndromes. Aspirin and heparin improve both short- and long-term prognosis in unstable angina [91–94], confirming the predominant role of platelet-derived white thrombus in pathogenesis. Similarly, fibrinolytic agents are highly effective in the early phase of acute myocardial infarction [95], but are of no benefit in unstable angina [96]. Early coronary revascularization improves outcome in higher risk subjects with unstable angina [97,98] and myocardial infarction [99,100], confirming the influence of persisting ischaemia on outcomes. Agents that act primarily by reducing coronary artery tone reduce symptoms in unstable angina, but have no clear prognostic benefit [78,101]. Overall, there is evidence of the effects of active coronary artery vasoconstriction at several sites during the acute phase of myocardial infarction. However, trials of vasodilators in acute infarction have produced disappointing results. Meta-analysis of 19 trials (~17000 patients) of the use of calcium-channel blockers in acute MI reveals no evidence of improved outcome (odds ratio vs. placebo 1.06) [78]. Similarly, the ISIS-4 trial, comparing the use of a long-acting oral nitrate preparation and placebo in patients presenting with acute MI, found no benefit from the oral nitrate drug [102]. Of note, however, is the fact that nearly 50% of patients in the placebo group received intravenous nitrate during the early phase of their infarction. This may have confounded results.

Conclusions

There is clear evidence of the effect of changes in coronary tone in epicardial coronary arteries, in resistance arteries and in the collateral circulation during the development of experimentally induced and clinically encountered myocardial ischaemia. Drugs that reduce coronary tone reduce both symptomatic and silent ischaemia in the acute phase of unstable coronary syndromes. However, this benefit has not been translated into an improved outcome. This suggests that, in most situations, coronary tone has a modest modulating influence on the clinical progression of coronary syndromes. However, a significant role for coronary tone is not excluded in certain clinical situations or in predisposed individuals. With improved understanding of the causes of increased coronary tone, and with better ways of assessing increased dynamic tone, specific treatment strategies may emerge that can modulate tone and impact favourably on clinical outcomes in patients with acute coronary syndromes.

References

1 Glagov S, Weisenberg E, Karins CK, Stankunavicius R, Kolettis GJ. Compensatory enlargement of human atherosclerotic coronary arteries. N Engl J Med 1987; 316: 1371–5.

2 Giroud D, Li JM, Urban P, Meier B, Rutihauser W. Relation of the site of acute myocardial infarction to the most severe coronary arterial stenosis at prior angiography. Am J Cardiol 1992; 69: 729.

3 Osler W. The Lumlean lecture on angina pectoris II. Lancet 1910; 1: 839–44.

4 Keefer CS, Resnik WH. Angina pectoris: a syndrome caused by anoxemia of the

myocardium. *Arch Intern Med* 1928; 41: 769–807.

5 Blumgart HL. The question of spasm of the coronary arteries. *Am J Med* 1947; 2: 129–30.

6 Pickering GW. Vascular spasm. *Lancet* 1951; 2: 845–50.

7 Prinzmetal M, Kennamer Rmerliss R, Wade T, Bor N. Angina pectoris: I. A variant form of angina pectoris: preliminary report. *Am J Med* 1959; 27: 375–88.

8 Gensini GG, DiGiorgi S, Murad-Netto S, Black A. Arteriographic demonstration of coronary artery spasm and its release after the use of a vasodilator in a case of angina pectoris and in the experimental animal. *Angiology* 1962; 13: 550–3.

9 Oliva PB, Potts DE, Pluss RG. Coronary arterial spasm in Prinzmetal angina. Documentation by coronary angiography. *N Engl J Med* 1973; 288: 745–51.

10 MacAlpine RN, Kattus AA, Alvaro AB. Angina pectoris at rest with preservation of exercise capacity: Prinzmetal's variant angina. *Circulation* 1973; 47: 946–57.

11 Maseri A, Preface. In: Maseri A, Klassen GA, Lesch M, eds. *Primary and Secondary Angina Pectoris*. New York: Grune and Stratton, 1978: xiii.

12 Epstein SE, Talbot TL. Dynamic coronary tone in preciptation, exacerbation and relief of angina pectoris. *Am J Cardiol* 1981; 48: 797–803.

13 Brown BG. Coronary vasospasm: observations linking the clinical spectrum of ischaemic heart disease to the dynamic pathology of coronary atherosclerosis. *Arch Intern Med* 1981; 141: 716–22.

14 Willerson JT, Hillis LD, Winniford M, Buja M. Speculation regarding mechanisms responsible for acute ischaemic heart disease syndromes. *J Am Coll Cardiol* 1986; 8: 245–50.

15 Klocke FJ, Mates RE, Canty JM, Ellis AK. Coronary pressure–flow relationships. Controversial issues and probable implications. *Circ Res* 1985; 56: 311–18.

16 Chilian WM, Eastham CL, Marcus ML. Microvascular distribution of coronary vascular resistance in beating left ventricle. *Am J Physiol* 1986; 251: H779– 88.

17 Chilian WM, Layne SM, Eastham CL, Marcus ML. Heterogeneous microvascular coronary alpha-adrenergic vaso-

constriction. *Circ Res* 1989; 64: 376–88.

18 Maseri A, Crea F, Kaski JC, Crake T. Mechanisms of angina pectoris in syndrome X. *J Am Coll Cardiol* 1991; 17: 499–506.

19 Kuo L, Chilian WM, Davis MJ. Interaction of pressure- and flow-induced responses in porcine coronary resistance vessels. *Am J Physiol* 1991; 261: H1706–15.

20 Kanatsuka H, Lamping KG, Eastham CL, Dellsperger KC, Marcus ML. Comparison of the effects of increased myocardial oxygen consumption and adenosine on the coronary microvascular resistance. *Circ Res* 1989; 65: 1296–1305.

21 Uren NG, Crake T. Resistive vessel function in coronary artery disease. *Heart* 1996; 76: 299–304.

22 Maseri A. The multiple ischaemic stimuli. In: Maseri A, ed. *Ischaemic Heart Disease; A Rational Basis for Clinical Practice and Research*. New York: Churchill Livingstone, 1995: 237–301.

23 Marcus ML, Chilian WM, Kanatsuka H, Dellsperger KC, Eastham CL, Lamping KG. Understanding the coronary circulation through studies at the microvascular level. *Circulation* 1990; 82: 1–7.

24 Domenech RJ, MacLellon PR. Transmural ventricular distribution of coronary blood flow during coronary beta-2 adrenergic activation in dogs. *Circ Res* 1980; 46: 29–36.

25 Uren NG, Melin JA, De Bruyne B, Wijns W, Baudhuin T, Camici PG. Relation between myocardial blood flow and severity of coronary-artery stenosis. *N Engl J Med* 1994; 330: 1782–7.

26 Klocke FJ. Measurements of coronary blood flow and degree of stenosis: Current clinical implications and continuing uncertainties. *J Am Coll Cardiol* 1983; 1: 31–4.

27 Gould KL. Pressure–flow characteristics of coronary stenoses in un-sedated dogs at rest and during coronary vasodilation. *Circ Res* 1978; 43: 242–53.

28 Maseri A. Regulation of coronary vasomotor tone. In: Maseri A, ed. *Ischaemic Heart Disease; A Rational Basis for Clinical Practice and Research*. New York, Churchill Livingstone, 1995: 105–135.

29 Henry PD, Yokoyama M. Supersensitivity of atherosclerotic rabbit aorta to ergonovine: mediated by an adrenergic mechanism. *J Clin Invest* 1980; 66: 306–13.

30 Hackett D, Larkin S, Chieria S, Davies G, Kaski JC, Maseri A. Induction of coronary artery spasm by a direct local action of ergonovine. *Circulation* 1987; 75: 577–82.

31 Shimokawa H, Tomoike H, Nabeyama S, Yamamoto H, Araki H, Nakamura M. Coronary artery spasm induced in atherosclerotic miniature swine. *Science* 1983; 221: 560–62.

32 Maseri A. Role of coronary artery spasm in symptomatic and silent myocardial ischaemia. *J Am Coll Cardiol* 1987; 9: 249–62.

33 Maseri A. Variant angina. In: *Ischaemic Heart Disease; A Rational Basis for Clinical Practice and Research*. New York: Churchill Livingstone, 1995; 559–88.

34 Freedman B, Richmond DR, Kelly DT. Pathophysiology of coronary artery spasm. *Circulation* 1982; 66: 705.

35 Maseri A, Severi S, Marzullo P. Role of coronary arterial spasm in sudden coronary ischaemic death. *Ann NY Acad Sci* 1982; 382: 204–17.

36 Nakamura M, Takeshita A, Nose Y. Clinical characteristics associated with myocardial infarction, arrhythmias and sudden death in patients with vasospastic angina. *Circulation* 1987; 75: 1110–16.

37 Bertrand ME, LaBlanche JM, Tilmant PY *et al*. Frequency of provoked coronary arterial spasm in 1089 consecutive patients undergoing coronary arteriography. *Circulation* 1982; 65: 1299–1306.

38 Factor SM, Cho S. Smooth muscle contraction bands in the media of coronary arteries: a post-mortem marker of antemortem coronary spasm? *J Am Coll Cardiol* 1985; 6: 1329–37.

39 El-Maraghi NRH, Sealey BJ. Recurrent myocardial infarction in a young man due to coronary arterial spasm demonstrated at autopsy. *Circulation* 1980; 61: 199–207.

40 Roberts WC, Curry RC, Isner JM *et al*. Sudden death in Printzmetals angina with coronary spasm documented by angiography. *Am J Cardiol* 1982; 50: 203–10.

41 Kafka H, FitzGibbon GM, Leach AJ. Aortocoronary vein graft spasm during angiography. *Can J Cardiol* 1995; 11: 211–16.

42 Dalen JE, Ockene IS, Alpert JS. Coronary artery spasm, coronary thrombosis, and myocardial infarction: a hypothesis concerning the pathophysiology of acute myocardial infarction. *Am Heart J* 1982; 104: 1119–24.

43 Myerburg RJ, Kessler K, Mallon SM *et al*. Life-threatening ventricular arrhythmia in patients with silent myocardial ischaemia due to coronary artery spasm. *N Engl J Med* 1992; 326: 1451–5.

44 Maseri A, Davies G, Hackett D, Kaski JG. Coronary artery spasm and vasoconstriction. The case for a distinction. *Circulation* 1990; 81: 1983–91.

45 Ambrose J, Winters S, Arora R. Angiographic evolution of coronary artery morphology in unstable angina. *J Am Coll Cardiol* 1986; 7: 472–8.

46 Saner HE, Gobel FL, Salomonowitz E, Erlien DA, Edwards JE. The disease-free wall in coronary atherosclerosis: its relation to degree of obstruction. *J Am Coll Cardiol* 1985; 6: 1096–9.

47 Hackett D, Davies G, Chierchia S, Maseri A. Intermittent coronary occlusion in acute myocardial infarction: value of combined thrombolytic and vasodilator therapy. *N Engl J Med* 1987; 317: 1055–9.

48 Ludmer PL, Selwyn AP, Shook TL *et al*. Paradoxical vasoconstriction induced by acetylcholine in atherosclerotic coronary arteries. *N Engl J Med* 1986; 315: 1046–51.

49 Groves PH, Kurz S, Just H, Drexler H. Role of endogenous bradykinin in human coronary vasomotor control. *Circulation* 1995; 92: 3424–30.

50 Biegelsen ES, Loscalzo J. Endothelial function and atherosclerosis. *Coron Artery Dis* 1999; 10: 241–56.

51 Vatner SF, Franklin D, Higgins CB, Patrick T, White S, Van Citters RL. Coronary haemodynamics in unrestrained conscious baboons. *Am J Physiol* 1971; 221: 1396–1401.

52 Verrier RL, Hagestad EL, Lown B. Delayed myocardial ischaemia induced by anger. *Circulation* 1987; 75: 249–54.

53 Larkin SW, Clarke JG, Keogh BE *et al*. Intracoronary endothelin induces myocardial ischaemia by small vessel con-

striction in the dog. *Am J Cardiol* 1989;
64: 956–8.

54 Gillespie MN, Booth DC, Friedman BJ,
Cunningham MR, Jay M, DeMaria A.
fMLP provokes coronary vasoconstriction and myocardial ischaemia in rabbits.
Am J Physiol 1988; 254: H481–6.

55 Epstein SE, Cannon RO III. Site of increased resistance to coronary flow in patients with angina pectoris and normal
epicardial coronary arteries. *J Am Coll
Cardiol* 1986; 8: 459–61.

56 Maseri A. Coronary vasoconstriction:
visible and invisible. *N Engl J Med* 1991;
325: 1579–80.

57 Clarke JG, Davies GJ, Kerwin R *et al.*
Coronary infusion of neuropeptide Y in
patients with angina pectoris. *Lancet*
1987; 1: 1057–9.

58 McFadden EP, Clarke JG, Davies GJ,
Haider AW, Kaski JC, Maseri A. Effect of
intracoronary serotonin on coronary vessels in patients with stable and variant
angina. *N Engl J Med* 1991; 324:
648–54.

59 McFadden EP, Bauters C, LaBlanche JM
et al. Effect of ketaserin on proximal and
distal coronary constrictor responses to
intracoronary infusion of serotonin in
patients with stable angina, patients with
variant angina and control patients.
Circulation 1992; 86: 187–95.

60 Powelson SW, De Puey EG, Roubin GS,
Berger HJ, King SB. Discordance of coronary angiography and 201-thallium
tomography early after transluminal
coronary angioplasty. *J Nucl Med* 1986;
27: 900.

61 Manyari DE, Knudtson M, Kloiber R,
Roth D. Sequential thallium-201 myocardial perfusion studies after succesful
coronary angioplasty: delayed resolution
of exercise-induced scintigraphic abnormalities. *Circulation* 1988; 77: 86–95.

62 El-Tamimi H, Davies GJ, Crea F, Sritara
P, Hackett D, Maseri A. Inappropriate
constriction of small coronary vessels as
a possible cause of a positive exercise test
soon after coronary angioplasty. *Circulation* 1991; 84: 2307–12.

63 Fishell TA, Bausack KN, McDonald TV.
Evidence for altered epicardial coronary
artery autoregulation as a cause of distal
coronary vasoconstriction after successful percutaneous transluminal coronary
angioplasty. *J Clin Invest* 1990; 86: 575.

64 Uren NG, Crake T, Lefroy DC, da Silva
R, Davies GJ, Maseri A. Delayed recovery of coronary resistive vessel function
after coronary angioplasty. *J Am Coll
Cardiol* 1993; 21: 612–21.

65 Uren NG, Crake T, Lefroy DC, Davies
GJ, Maseri A. Altered resistive vessel
function after coronary angioplasty is
not due to reduced production of nitric
oxide. *Cardiovasc Res* 1996; 32:
1108–14.

66 Uren NG, Marraccini P, Gistri R, de Silva
R, Camici PG. Altered coronary vasodilator reserve and metabolism in myocardium subtended by normal arteries
in patients with coronary artery disease.
J Am Coll Cardiol 1993; 22: 650–58.

67 Uren NG, Crake T, Tousoulis D, Seydoux
C, Davies GJ, Maseri A. Impairment of
the myocardial blood flow response to
cold pressor in collateral-dependent
myocardium with positron emission
tomography. *Heart* 1997; 78: 61–7.

68 Pupita G, Maseri A, Kaski JC *et al.* Myocardial ischaemia caused by distal coronary artery constriction in stable
angina pectoris. *N Engl J Med* 1990;
323: 514–20.

69 Figueras J, Singh BN, Ganz W, Charuzi Y,
Swan HJC. Mechanism of rest and
nocturnal angina: observations during
continuous haemodynamic and
electrocardiographic monitoring. *Circulation* 1979; 59: 955–68.

70 Uthuralt N, Davies GJ, Parodi O, Beni-
civelli W, Maseri A. Comparative study
of myocardial ischaemia during rest and
on exertion using thallium-201 scintigraphy. *Am J Cardiol* 1981; 48: 410–17.

71 Cotter G, Faibel H, Barash P *et al.* High-
dose nitrates in the immediate management of unstable angina: optimal dosage,
route of administration, and therapeutic
goals. *Am J Emerg Med* 1998; 16:
219–24.

72 Figueras J, Lidon R, Cortadellas J. Rebound myocardial ischaemia following
abrupt interruption of intravenous nitroglycerine infusion in patients with myocardial infarction at rest. *Eur Heart J*
1991; 12: 405–11.

73 Fleckenstein A. *Calcium Antagonism in
Heart and Smooth Muscle.* New York:
John Wiley, 1983

74 Mehta J, Conti CR. Verapamil therapy
for unstable angina pectoris: review of

double-blind placebo-controlled randomized clinical trials. *Am J Cardiol* 1982; 50: 919–22.

75 Gerstenblith G, Ouyang P, Achuff SC *et al*. Nifedipine in unstable angina: a double-blind, randomized trial. *N Engl J Med* 1982; 306: 885–9.

76 Theroux P, Taeymans Y, Morissette D, Bosch X, Pelletier GB, Waters DD. A randomized study comparing propranolol and diltiazem in the treatment of unstable angina *J Am Coll Cardiol* 1985; 5: 717–22.

77 Gobel EJ, van Gilst WH, de Kam PJ, Napel MG, Molhoek GP, Lie KI. Long-term follow-up after early intervention with intravenous diltiazem or intravenous nitroglycerin for unstable angina pectoris. *Eur Heart J* 1998; 19: 1208–13.

78 Held PH, Yusuf S, Furberg CD. Calcium channel blockers in acute myocardial infarction and unstable angina: an overview. *BMJ* 1989; 299: 1187.

79 Frampton J, Buckley MM, Fitton A. Nicorandil. A review of its pharmacology and therapeutic efficacy in angina pectoris. *Drugs* 1992; 44: 625–55.

80 Patel DJ, Purcell HJ, Fox KM. Cardioprotection by opening of the K (ATP) channel in unstable angina. Is this a clinical manifestation of myocardial preconditioning? Results of a randomized study with nicorandil: CESAR 2 Investigation. *Eur Heart J* 1999; 20: 51–7.

81 Davies GJ, Chierchia S, Maseri A. Prevention of myocardial infarction by very early treatment with intracoronary streptokinase. Some clinical observations. *N Engl J Med* 1984; 384: 1488–92.

82 Maseri A, Severi S, Marzullo P. Role of coronary arterial spasm in sudden coronary ischaemic death. *Ann NY Acad Sci* 1982; 382: 204–17.

83 Cipriano PR, Koch FH, Rosenthal SJ, Schroeder JS. Clinical course of patients following the demonstration of coronary artery spasm by angiography. *Am Heart J* 1981; 101: 127–34.

84 Williams MJ, Restieaux NJ, Low CJ. Myocardial infarction in young people with normal coronary arteries. *Heart* 1998; 79: 191–4.

85 Legrand V, Dehege M, Henrard L, Boland J, Kulbertus H. Patients with myocardial infarction and normal coronary arteriogram. *Chest* 1982; 82: 678–85.

86 Lange RA, Reid M, Tzesch D *et al*. Non-atheromatous ischaemic heart disease following withdrawal from chronic industrial nitroglycerin exposure. *Circulation* 1972; 46: 666–78.

87 Lange RA, Cigarroa RG, Yancy CW *et al*. Cocaine-induced coronary artery vasoconstriction. *N Engl J Med* 1989; 321: 1557–62.

88 Hung DZ, Deng JF. Acute myocardial infarction temporally related to betel nut chewing. *Vet Hum Toxicol* 1998; 40: 25–8.

89 Parmar MS, Luque-Coqui AF. Killer dreams. *Can J Cardiol* 1998; 11: 1389–91.

90 Imai Y, Nobuoka S, Nagashima J *et al*. Acute myocardial infarction induced by alternating exposure to heat in a sauna and rapid cooling in cold water. *Cardiology* 1998; 90: 299–301.

91 Lewis HDJ, Davis JW, Archibald DG *et al*. Protective effects of aspirin against acute myocardial infarction and death in men with unstable angina. Results of a Veterans Administration Cooperative Study. *N Engl J Med* 1983; 309: 396–403.

92 Cairns JA, Gent M, Singer J *et al*. Aspirin, sulfinpyrazone, or both in unstable angina. Results of a Canadian multicentre trial. *N Engl J Med* 1985; 313: 1369–75.

93 Theroux P, Waters D, Qiu S *et al*. Aspirin versus heparin to prevent myocardial infarction during the acute phase of unstable angina. *Circulation* 1993; 88: 2045–8.

94 FRISC investigators. Low-molecular-weight heparin during instability in coronary artery disease, Fragmin during Instability in Coronary Artery Disease study group. *Lancet* 1996; 347: 561–8.

95 Fibrinolytic Therapy Trialists' (FTT) Collaborative Group. Indications for fibrinolytic therapy in suspected acute myocardial infarction: collaborative overview of early mortality and major morbidity results from all randomised trials of more than 1000 patients. *Lancet* 1994; 343: 311–22.

96 TIMI IIIb investigators. Effects of tissue plasminogen activator and a comparison of early invasive and conservative strategies in unstable angina and non Q-wave myocardial infarction. Results of the

TIMI IIIB. Trial. Thrombolysis Myocardial Ischemia. *Circulation* 1994; 89: 1545–56.

97 Sharma GV, Deupree RH, Khuri SF *et al.* Coronary bypass surgery improves survival in high-risk unstable angina. Results of a Veterans Administration Co-operative study with an 8-year follow-up. Veterans Administration Unstable Angina Cooperative Study Group. *Circulation* 1991; 84: III260–7.

98 FRISC II, investigators. Invasive compared with non-invasive treatment in unstable coronary artery disease: FRISC II prospective randomised multicentre study. *Lancet* 1999; 354: 708–15.

99 Stone GW, Grines CL, Browne KF *et al.* Predictors of in-hospital and 6-month outcome after acute myocardial infarction in the reperfusion era: the Primary Angioplasty in Myocardial Infarction (PAMI) trial. *J Am Coll Cardiol* 1995; 25: 370–7.

100 Stone GW, Brodie BR, Griffin JJ *et al.* PAMI stent pilot. *J Intervent Cardiol* 1999; 12: 101–7.

101 Lubsen J. Medical management of unstable angina. What have we learned from the randomized trials? *Circulation* 1990; 82: II82–4.

102 The ISIS-4 investigators. ISIS-4: a randomised factorial trial. Assessing early oral captopril, oral mononitrate, and intravenous magnesium sulphate in 58 050 patients with suspected acute myocardial infarction. *Lancet* 1995; 345: 669–85.

5: What is known about the genetics of acute coronary syndromes?

Nilesh J. Samani and Ravi Singh

'The disease may occur in three generations, . . . a father and four children, . . . father and son, . . . brothers, . . . and brother and sister'

William Osler
addressing the Royal College of Physicians of London, 1910.

Although a familial aggregation of coronary artery disease (CAD) has long been appreciated [1], until recently tools were not available to identify the specific genetic components responsible. Therefore, historically, a 'positive' family history has been viewed, by physician and patient alike, as a 'non-modifiable' coronary risk factor, like age and sex. However, progress in molecular biology has dramatically altered this perspective in the last decade. The ability to elucidate the role of variation in potentially relevant genes has fuelled a plethora of research into the genetics of CAD, a situation that shows no sign of abating. Several exciting observations have already been made that provide valuable insights regarding how genetic factors may act to increase the risk of acute coronary syndromes. However, many remain to be confirmed, and conflicting data have raised important issues regarding study design and interpretation. The ultimate hope that genetic characterization may help to improve prevention and treatment, particularly for specific individual subjects, remains to be realized. The aim of this chapter is to provide an overview of where things stand and to consider the challenges and opportunities that lie ahead.

To what extent are acute coronary syndromes genetically determined?

One of the first substantive studies to document a familial aggregation of acute coronary syndromes was that of Rose *et al.* in 1964 [2]. In 717 first-degree relatives of either probands aged 40–70 with myocardial infarction (MI) or controls without MI, they found that the risk of fatal MI or sudden death at any age was increased 2.3-fold in the families of probands with MI. Since then numerous other retrospective studies [3–11] have reached a generally similar conclusion, with the relative risk in first-degree relatives of subjects with MI ranging from around 1.5- to 8-fold higher, compared with subjects without MI (Table 5.1). More recently, prospective studies in which the development of acute CAD phenotypes (fatal or non-fatal MI or sudden death) has been examined in subjects in relation to their family history [12–19] have yielded consistent results (Table 5.2). The relative risks described are similar to, and in some studies higher than, those attributed to other common risk factors such as smoking and hypertension.

Some of the familial risk of CAD could be attributable to familial aggregation of other risk factors for CAD known to have a genetic component themselves, such as hypertension, hypercholesterolaemia and diabetes. Although some of the early studies listed in Tables 5.1 and 5.2 did not take other risk factors into account, recent studies have done so, and it has been established that at least a proportion of the familial risk of acute coronary syndromes appears to be independent of classical risk factors. As with most other risk factors, the familial risk is more obvious the more premature the disease (Tables 5.1 and 5.2).

The demonstration of an increased familial risk, even independent of classical risk factors, does not, of course, by itself prove genetic causation. The effect could be due to a 'shared' adverse environment among members of an affected family, especially in view of the strong impact of socio-economic factors on CAD prevalence. Nonetheless, some elegant studies provide compelling evidence that there is a significant genetic contribution to acute coronary syndromes. Sorensen *et al.* [20] followed up 960 Danish adoptees placed at an early age (> 90% by 2 years of age) with their adopted parents to assess genetic and environmental influences on premature death. A premature death was classed as one occurring in a subject between 16 and 58 years of age. The death of a biological parent before the age of 50 was associated with a relative risk of death in the adoptees of 5 for cardiovascular and cerebrovascular disease. The same classification with respect to adopted parents was associated with a relative risk of 3. Similarly, Marenberg *et al.* [21] followed up 10 502 pairs of Swedish twins for 26 years with respect to susceptibility to death from coronary heart disease. In men the relative hazard of death from coronary heart disease when one's twin died before the age of 55 years, compared with the hazard when one's twin did not die before 55, was 8 for monozygotic twins and 4 for dizygotic twins. Among the women, when one's twin died before the age of 65 years the relative hazard was 15 for monozygotic and 3 for dizygotic.

It has recently been hypothesized that an adverse intrauterine 'environment', perhaps resulting from nutritional deficiencies in the mother, may have a significant impact on the development of chronic adult-onset diseases, including CAD, in the offspring [22]. This hypothesis has fuelled the

Table 5.1 Familial aggregation of acute coronary syndromes: retrospective case-control trials.

Study	No. of cases: controls	Proband description	Number of first degree family members studied	End point in family member	Relative risk of end-point for first degree relatives of cases
Rose 1964 [2]*	75 : 75	MI Age 40–70 Males/Females	717	Fatal MI or sudden death (all ages)`	2.3
Slack 1966 [3]*	217 : 209	Angina/ MI Age <60 males <70 females	1107	Fatal MI or sudden death All ages Premature (<54 males, <64 females)	2.6 4.8
Rissanen 1977 [4]*	106 : 94	Angina (no MI) Age 27–55 Males only	793	Premature (>65) fatal MI or sudden death in —fathers —mothers Premature (<65) MI in siblings	5.0 1.0 8.2
ten Kate 1982 [5]	194 : 94	Non-fatal MI Age 30-59	639	MI (all ages) Males only	2.0
Shea 1984 [6]	145 : 145	Angiographic coronary heart disease +/– MI Age 30–60 Males/females	927	MI (all ages) Cardiac death (all ages)	2.8 (×3.5 MI proband) 2.1 (×3.2 MI proband)

Continued

Table 5.1 *Continued*

Study	No. of cases: controls	Proband description	Number of first degree family members studied	End point in family member	Relative risk of end-point for first degree relatives of cases
Hamsten 1987[7]	223:57	Non-fatal MI Age <45 Males only	399	Fatal/non fatal MI (age 20–60)	4.0
Roncaglioni 1992[8]	85:85	Non-fatal MI All ages Males/females	916	MI (all ages)	2.0
Cirruzzi 1997[9]	916:1106	Non-fatal MI All ages Males/females	916	MI (all ages)	2.2
Freidlander 1998[10]	235:374	Primary cardiac arrest —no previous cardiac history Age 25–74 Males/females	235	MI (all ages) Primary cardiac arrest	1.5 1.6
Pohjola-Sintonen* 1998[11]	707:130	MI (all ages) Age 29–59 Males/females	2658	Angina/MI/sudden death (all ages)	2.0

* Not adjusted for other risk factors.

Table 5.2 Familial aggregation of acute coronary syndromes: prospective trials.

Study	Study population	Mean years of follow up	Definition of family history	Phenotype in cases	Number of events	Relative risk of developing phenotype in presence of positive family history
Gillum 1978 [12]*	8852 Age 15–29 Men only	22	First degree relative with CHD	MI / sudden death	88	2.4
Cambien 1980 [13]	7186 Age 43–54 Men only	6.5	1. Paternal history of MI/sudden death 2. Maternal history of MI/sudden death	Angina/MI/sudden death	258	1.6 1.0
Snowden 1982 [14]	5127 Age 30–62 Men only	26	CHD in older brother	MI / sudden death	68	1.5
Barrett-Conner 1984 [15]	1774 Age 40–79 Men only	9	First degree relative with MI	Fatal MI / sudden death	87	1.6
Colditz 1986 [16]	117 156 Age 30–55 Women only	9	Parental history of MI <60	Non-fatal MI	132	2.8
Phillips 1988 [17]	7735 Age 40–59 Men only	6	1. Paternal death from heart disease 2. Maternal death from heart disease	MI / sudden death	336	2.1 3.1
Jousilahti 1996 [18]	15620 Age 30–59 Men/Women	12	Parental history of angina/MI <60	MI / sudden death	295	1.6 (in men) 1.9 (in women)
Jouven 1999 [19]	7746 Age 43–52 Men only	23	Paternal history of sudden death	Sudden death	118	1.8

* Not adjusted for other risk factors.

nature–nurture debate and raised questions about whether any unaccounted for familial aggregation should be viewed as being indicative of genetic influences. It is, of course, equally possible that any genetic determinants of CAD could act at a very early age and indeed *in utero*. Ultimately, the separation of genetic compared with environmental effects is very difficult when based on results of observational studies alone. Proof of significant genetic influences requires direct demonstration of causal associations of DNA variants and disease. In this context, it is appropriate to emphasize that the general level of increased risk associated with a positive family history, found in the studies described in Tables 5.1 and 5.2, should not be construed as establishing an upper level of increased risk that may occur with a particular genetic factor. Especially in a favourable environment, the relative risk it causes could be much greater, but of course affecting only a fraction of the population.

Candidate genes that may influence risk of occurrence of an acute coronary syndrome

The search for genetic factors predisposing to acute coronary syndromes has, to date, been guided largely by current understanding of the underlying pathophysiology. Thus, the main targets have been genes that code for molecules involved in lipid homeostasis, blood coagulation, platelet function and vessel-wall biology (as processes related to plaque stability and rupture are better defined)[23]. The most common approach used has been to see whether a variant in a particular gene (a polymorphism) is present more (or less) commonly in affected subjects (usually of MI) compared with non-affected controls (case-control study). The implication is that, if this is the case, either the polymorphism itself, or another polymorphism with which it is in linkage disequilibrium, has a consequence that influences the risk of MI. Polymorphisms in genes in each of the above categories have now been associated, in one or more studies, with risk of MI (Table 5.3), and the list continues to grow rapidly. A selective review of some of the main polymorphisms identified follows:

Lipid factors

Hundreds of polymorphisms have now been reported in genes encoding apolipoproteins, lipolytic enzymes, and lipoprotein levels, and many have been shown to impact on levels of various atherogenic plasma lipids [24]. Not surprisingly, given that coronary atherosclerosis provides the substrate for acute coronary syndromes, some of the polymorphisms have been associated with increased risk of MI, although in most cases the associations are relatively weak and inconsistent [25–29] (see below). Recent studies have investigated genes involved in lipid metabolism in the vascular wall. In particular, variation in the gene for paroxonase, an high density lipoprotein (HDL)

Table 5.3 Candidate gene polymorphisms associated with risk of myocardial infarction.

Gene	Polymorphism	Possible functional effect
Lipid factors		
Apolipoprotein A-IV	Exon 3 Q369H	↓HDL, ↑TG
Apolipoprotein B	Exon 1ins/del/	↑apo B
	Exon 26 codon 2488 (Xba 1)	
Apolipoprotein E	E2/E3/E4	↑LDL
Lipoprotein lipase	Intron 3 (Hind III)	↑apo C-III, ↓HDL
Paroxanase	Exon 6 Q192R	↓HDL, ↑oxidation of LDL
Clotting factors		
Fibrinogen	Promoter G-455A	↑Fibrinogen level
Factor V	Exon 10 R506Q	↑Factor V resistance to inactivation
Prothrombin	3′UTR G20210A	↑Prothrombin level
Factor VII	Intron 7 R353Q VNTR	↑Factor VII level
Thrombomodulin	G127A/C1418T	?
Platelet factors		
Glycoprotein IIIa	Exon 3 T1565C	↑Fibrogen binding
Glycoprotein Ia	C807T/G873A	↑Collogen receptor density
Fibrinolytic factors		
Plasminogen activator inhibitor-1	Promoter -675 4G/5G	↑PAI-1
Tissue plasminogen activator	Intron 12 inserion/deletion	?
Vessel wall factors		
Angiotensin converting enzyme	Intron 16 insertion/deletion	↑ACE activity
Angiotensinogen	Exon 2 M235T	Angiotensinogen
Angiotensin II subtype 1 receptor	Exon 5 C1166A	?
Endothelial nitric oxide synthase	Intron 4 VNTR/exon 7 Glu298Asp	↓NO production
Methylenetetrahydroxylase reductase	C677T	↑Homocysteine level

HDL, high density lipoprotein; TG, triglyceride; LDL, low density lipoprotein; PAI-1, plasminogen activator inhibitor-1; ACE, angiotensin converting enzyme; NO, nitric oxide.

linked enzyme that may exert its effect by removing lipid-peroxidation products, has been associated with coronary artery disease, especially in subjects with diabetes, in whom oxidative stress may be particularly prevalent [30–32]. However, an increased risk of acute coronary syndromes has not been observed (see below). On the other hand, a polymorphism in the gene for cholesterol ester transfer protein has been reported to be associated with a higher HDL level and reduced risk of MI, but, interestingly, only in subjects taking moderate amounts of alcohol [33], perhaps illustrating a gene–environment interaction and providing a novel insight into the enigmatic cardioprotective effect of moderate alcohol intake.

Clotting factors

Increased plasma fibrinogen has been recognized as a risk factor for acute coronary syndromes for many years [34]. There is considerable inter-individual variation in plasma fibrinogen level, and at least part of the variation is genetically determined. A polymorphism in the upstream region of the beta-fibrinogen gene (G-455 A) has been evaluated extensively and found to interact with smoking and the level of physical activity in determining plasma fibrinogen level [35]. In some [36,37] but not all [38,39] studies, it has been implicated in influencing the risk of MI. Functional polymorphisms in a number of other coagulation cascade genes (prothrombin, factor V and factor VII) have been defined [40–42] and consistently implicated as important risk factors for venous thrombosis [43]. Some, but again not all, studies have shown an association of the prothrombin and factor V polymorphisms with MI [44–47]. An effect of these polymorphisms on MI risk has been seen most convincingly in young female subjects where thrombosis may be a more major contributor to the development of the event [44], or when other risk factors have also been present [45]. However, the contrast to the ease with which the polymorphisms have been implicated in the pathophysiology of deep venous thrombosis emphasizes inherent differences in the pathophysiology of venous and arterial thrombosis. For Factor VII, one study has recently reported two polymorphisms in the gene associated with lower plasma Factor VII levels, protecting against MI [48]. However, the beneficial effect has been disputed [49]. Two polymorphisms in the gene for thrombomodulin, an endothelial-cell-surface receptor that, on binding thrombin, activates the protein-C-anti-coagulant cascade, have been associated with risk of MI [50,51]. In addition to confirmation of the findings, functional correlates of these polymorphisms need to be identified.

Platelet factors

The recognized importance of platelets in the pathogenesis of arterial thrombosis has led to a search for platelet-related polymorphisms that may influence MI risk. Thus, the report by Weiss *et al.* in 1996 [52] that a relatively common polymorphism in the gene for glycoprotein (GP) IIIa, which in combination with GPIIb constitutes the platelet fibrinogen receptor, was associated with a 2- to 3.6-fold increase in risk for coronary thrombosis caused considerable excitement. The polymorphism, which is responsible for the platelet PlA2 antigen, may increase fibrinogen binding [53]. In a subsequent study, the polymorphism was reported to also increase the risk of in-stent thrombosis following coronary stenting, lending credence to a pathophysiologic role [54]. However, several studies have failed to replicate the association of the GPIIIa polymorphism with MI [55–57] and its importance remains uncertain. Two linked polymorphisms in the gene for GP1a, a component of the platelet collagen receptor, have been reported recently to increase the risk of MI by 3.0-fold overall and possibly 25-fold in smokers [58]. The polymorphisms themselves appear to be silent, but may be linked to a functional mutation that increases receptor density on the platelet surface [59].

Fibrinolytic factors

Interest has focused also on genes coding for proteins involved in fibrinolysis, because of epidemiological associations of plasma levels of tissue-plasmino-gen activator (TPA), and particularly its naturally occurring inhibitor, plas-minogen-activator inhibitor-1 (PAI-1), with risk of acute coronary syndromes [60]. Particular interest has focused on a promoter region polymorphism in the PAI-1 gene (4G/5G), which influences PAI-I expression and plasma levels, with higher levels in those with the 4G allele [35]. Two studies have reported an approximate 2-fold increase in MI risk associated with the 4G allele [61,62]. However, several studies have not observed such an association [63–65]. An *alu* repeat insertion (I)/deletion (D) polymorphism in intron h of the tissue plasminogen-activator gene has also been reported to influence the risk of MI (increased risk of 2.2-fold in II vs. DD genotypes), although the study found no effect of the I allele on plasma TPA level or activity [66].

Vessel-wall factors

In this category, most attention to date has focused on the insertion/deletion polymorphism in intron 16 of the angiotensin-converting-enzyme (ACE) gene. Unlike its counterpart in the TPA gene, the ACE I/D polymorphism is as-sociated with a marked effect on plasma and tissue ACE level, with those with the DD genotype having twice the level of those with the II genotype [67,68]. The mechanism underlying this effect remains to be defined, but is likely to in-volve a linked polymorphism rather than the I/D polymorphism itself. In any case, this interesting observation assumed much greater significance in 1992 when Cambien *et al.* [69] reported an increased risk of MI in individuals carry-ing the DD genotype, especially in those thought to be at low risk on the basis of body mass index and plasma apolipoprotein B level. Since then many stud-ies have focused on the role of the ACE I/D polymorphism in CAD as well as a variety of other disorders. Meta-analysis suggests that, at best, the polymor-phism has probably only a modest effect (around 25% increase) in the risk of MI [70]. However, the importance of the paper by Cambien *et al.* [69] cannot be overemphasized, because, for the first time, it really revealed the prospect to a large number of clinical researchers that it may be possible to identify spe-cific (non-lipid) genetic factors which predispose to MI risk, and laid the foun-dation for much of the work which has followed during this decade. Other polymorphisms in genes of the renin–angiotensin cascade have also been linked to the risk of MI, specifically, a coding region polymorphism in the gene for angiotensinogen [71] (which influences plasma angiotensinogen level and has also been linked to hypertension [72]), and a non-coding polymorphism in the 3′ end of the gene for angiotensin II type-1 receptor, the effect of which was seen only in the presence of the ACE DD genotype [73]. The evidence of the involvement of either of these genes is weak and needs more support.

Two different polymorphisms in the endothelial nitric oxide synthase gene have been associated with a risk of MI. Wang *et al.* [74] reported a highly significant association of a variable number tandem repeat polymorphism in intron 4 of the gene with both severity of angiographic coronary disease and risk of MI (1.8-fold increase in aa genotype). Interestingly, this association was restricted to current and ex-smokers, suggesting an important gene–environment interaction. Subsequently, they reported that the deleterious allele (allele a) was also associated with a lower plasma nitric oxide level [75], implying a possible diminution in the vasodilatory and vaso-protective effects of nitric oxide in those carrying the genotype that might be further aggravated by smoking. A separate polymorphism, Glu298Asp, whose functional effect remains to be determined, has also more recently been associated with risk of MI in a Japanese population [76].

An elevated plasma level of homocysteine is associated with premature atherosclerosis [77]. Mechanisms related mainly to the vessel wall, including effects on endothelial function, smooth muscle cell proliferation and lipid oxidation, have been proposed [77] to explain the association. Homocysteine metabolism is enzymatically regulated, with important involvement of nutritionally derived co-factors including folate and vitamin B_{12}, as well as by genetic factors. Recently a common mutation (C677T) in the gene for a key enzyme, methylene tetrahydrofolate reductase (MTHFR), has been shown to reduce the activity of the gene and increase homocysteine levels [78]. Several studies have investigated the role of the polymorphism as a risk factor for MI [79–82]. Although an effect of the polymorphism on plasma homocysteine level has been observed consistently [77,79,81], most studies have not been able to demonstrate that the mutation increases MI risk [79–81]. In one, however, an increased risk was seen in young male subjects in the presence of other risk factors [82].

A perspective on the current status of genetic factors in acute coronary syndromes

The main dilemma currently facing the field of CAD genetics is the lack of consistency of findings among studies. For virtually all the polymorphisms studied to date, a consistent association with MI has not been found. In a pathophysiologically complex, and genetically heterogeneous, disorder such as MI, one would not expect results of all studies to agree, but the discordance of findings has hampered progress and application of the results. Several factors may account for the marked variability. This sections discusses some of the key issues that need to be considered.

A not uncommon scenario has been an initial report, often in quite small cohorts reporting a strong association, followed by results of other studies, often larger, that do not replicate the finding, interspersed with an occasional further positive study. The possibility of an artefactual association related to small numbers is, of course, not peculiar to genetic studies. Publication bias is an important concern, and more stringent criteria for reporting association studies have been recommended recently [83]. However, it is difficult to dismiss all, or even most, discordance of findings on this basis alone and several other issues need to be considered.

An important aspect concerns the polymorphism being assessed. Often, as alluded to in the previous section, such a polymorphism is not itself the functionally important variant, but rather it acts as a marker for another polymorphism with which it is in linkage disequilibrium. Both the frequency of the marker polymorphism as well as its linkage disequilibrium with the functional polymorphism may vary from population to population, particularly in relation to ethnicity. This has two important consequences for case–control studies [84,85]. First, any unrecognized differences in the population structures of the case and control cohorts may cause a spurious difference in the frequency of the marker allele between cases and controls not related to the disorder. Conversely, failure to reproduce an association of a polymorphism in a particular population may reflect simply a lack of linkage disequilibrium between it and the functional variant that was present in the original population.

The sensitivity of case–control studies to population stratification has led to the development of other methods. One currently in vogue is the transmission disequilibrium test (TDT), which examines whether there is preferential transmission of a putative disease-associated variant from parents to an affected offspring, in a series of such trios [85]. Analyses for such intra-familial association avoids the pitfalls of population stratification. However, such approaches are difficult to apply to a late-onset disorder such as MI, and good studies of this sort pertinent to coronary risk have yet to emerge.

Other issues relate to the phenotype [86]. In a sense, acute coronary syndromes, and in particular MI, have several positive attributes as a phenotype for study. Apart from the clear clinical importance, there are well-defined criteria for diagnosis. Furthermore, in most cases, the time of onset can be determined very precisely allowing any age-dependency of genetic effect (as is the case for many other risk factors) to be examined. Likewise, controls who have not suffered an event by a particular age can usually be identified accurately. However, there is an important downside, namely the unavoidable loss of subjects through fatality when recruitment is based on an incident event. This is the case, even if recruitment is done at the time of admission to a coronary care unit, because more than 50% of deaths from acute MI occur before subjects reach a hospital. An examination of the timing of recruitment of cases in genetic studies of MI shows marked variation; indeed, in the landmark study of Cambien *et al.* [69] cases were not recruited until 3–6 months after an event. This delay and variation could become of paramount importance if a relevant genetic factor unknowingly also influences survival after MI.

Potential confounding, attributable to survival bias, is of course a major reason why findings from prospective studies carry extra weight. However, even for them, one needs to be careful. Some, for example the American Physicians Study [56,64,87], are based on a highly selected group of male subjects with a distinct pattern of life-style risk factors that may markedly modify the effects of specific genetic factors. Recent studies based on broader populations such as the Copenhagen City Heart Study [39,88] provide powerful observations.

An issue that has caused some confusion relates to the complementary effort, in many cases, to link polymorphisms to other coronary phenotypes, and notably the presence/severity of coronary atherosclerosis, as judged by coronary angiography. This phenotype has its own advantages and disadvantages [86]. However, in the context of the current discussion, the important point is that, although coronary atheroma provides the substrate for acute coronary syndromes, the association between the two is less than perfect. It is well recognized that an acute coronary event is as likely to occur as a result of disruption of an angiographically minor plaque as from obstruction of a severe stenosis [89]. Thus, depending on its specific role in the pathophysiology of coronary disease, a genetic factor may be associated more strongly, or indeed only, with one of the two phenotypes. This may explain, in part, the inconsistent findings reported with regard to some polymorphisms, for example some of the lipid polymorphisms and the thermolabile variant of MTHFR, which show stronger associations with atherosclerosis than with acute coronary syndromes.

Finally, a crucial issue is that of gene–environment and gene–gene interactions. Tantalizing evidence points to the importance of both. A lack of a necessary environmental factor, or an appropriate genetic background, could completely mask an effect of a particular polymorphism, and this scenario could explain some of the discordance among findings. One of the problems with genetic studies to date has been that many have sprung from projects with other objectives (a blood sample for DNA analysis is easy to collect!) and have not been designed to allow examination of specific interactions. The subject is difficult to tackle, as, by their nature, many interactions are likely to be obscure until they are identified. However, there is a need for studies to be planned whose primary focus is genetics and in which phenotyping is conducted expressly to allow such interactions to be sought.

Conclusions and future directions

Only a decade ago, there was still uncertainty as to whether it would ever be possible to identify individual genetic factors that could alter the susceptibility to a complex polygenic disorder such as MI. Accordingly the results obtained so far, despite their somewhat inconclusive nature, represent a triumph for the application of molecular techniques. Progress in characterizing the human genome [90] and in defining variation in candidate cardiovascular genes [91,92] is occurring at a remarkably fast pace. At the same time, the ease with which multiplex, large-scale genotyping can be carried out is improving rapidly [93]. Thus, technological issues are unlikely to be a long-term problem. What is required is clinical ingenuity in asking the right questions and designing studies to answer them. Possible questions related to acute coronary syndromes include not only those concerned with risk (the majority of the work so far), but also those addressing whether genetic factors contribute to the undoubted inter-individual response to both acute (e.g. thrombolytic) and chronic (beta-blockers, aspirin, ACE inhibitors) therapy following MI and consequently prognosis. The findings could improve not only risk stratification but also allow therapy to be tailored much more effectively to each individual. The potential is vast. Although important challenges remain to be overcome, the way in which acute coronary syndromes are classified, investigated and managed will almost certainly be very different in the next decade as a consequence of a more robust understanding of their genetic basis.

Acknowledgements

Dr Singh is supported by a British Cardiac Society Fellowship and a British Heart Foundation project grant.

References

1 Osler W. The Lumleian lectures on angina pectoris I-II. *Lancet* 1910; 1: 697–702.
2 Rose G. Familial pattern of ischaemic heart disease. *Br J Prev Soc Med* 1964; 18: 75–80.
3 Slack J, Evans KA. The increased risk of death from ischaemic heart disease in first degree relatives of 121 men and 96 women with ischaemic heart disease. *J Med Genet* 1966; 3: 239–57.

4 Rissanen AM, Nikkila EA. (Editorial.) Coronary heart disease and its risk factors in families of young men with angina pectoris and in controls. *Br Heart J* 1977; 39: 875–83.
5 ten Kate LP, Bowman H, Daiger SP, Motulsky AG. Familial aggregation of coronary heart disease and its relation to known genetic risk factors. *Circulation* 1982; 50: 945–53.

6 Shea S, Ottman R, Gabrieli C, Stein Z, Nichols A. Family history as an independent risk factor for coronary artery disease. *J Am Coll Cardiol* 1984; 4: 793–801.

7 Hamsten A, de Faire U. Risk factors for coronary artery disease in families of young men with myocardial infarction. *Am J Cardiol* 1987; 59: 14–19.

8 Roncaglioni MC, Santoro L, D'Avanzo B *et al.* Role of family history in patients with myocardial infarction. An Italian case-control study. GISSI-EFRIM Investigators. *Circulation* 1992; 85: 2065–72.

9 Ciruzzi M, Schargrodsky H, Rozlosnik J *et al.* Frequency of family history of acute myocardial infarction in patients with acute myocardial infarction. Argentine FRICAS (Factores de Riesgo Coronario en America del Sur) Investigators. *Am J Cardiol* 1997; 80: 122–7.

10 Freidlander Y, Siscovick DS, Weinmann S *et al.* Family history as a risk factor for primary cardiac arrest. *Circulation* 1998; 97: 155–60.

11 Pohjola-Sintonen S, Rissanen A, Liskola P, Luomanmaki K. Family history as a risk factor of coronary heart disease in patients under 60 years of age. *Eur Heart J* 1998; 19: 235–9.

12 Gillum RF, Paffenbarger RS. Chronic disease in former college students. *Am J Epidemiol* 1978; 108: 289–98.

13 Cambien F, Richard JL. Ducimetiere P. Etude des Antecedents Familiaux de Cardiopathies Ischemiques et D'hypertension Arterielle en Liaison avec la Prevalence des Facteurs de Risque et L'incidence des Cardiopathies Ischemiques. *Rev Epidemiol Sante Publique* 1980; 28: 21–37.

14 Snowden CB, McNamara PM, Garrison RJ, Feinleib M, Kannel WB, Epstein FH. Predicting coronary heart disease in siblings — a multivariate assessment. *Am J Epidemiol* 1982; 115: 217–22.

15 Barrett-Connor E, Khaw KT. Family history of heart attack as an independent predictor of death due to cardiovascular disease. *Circulation* 1984; 69: 1065–9.

16 Colditz GA, Stampfer MJ, Willett WC. A prospective study of parental history of myocardial infarction and coronary heart disease in women. *Am J Epidemiol* 1986; 123: 48–58.

17 Phillips AN, Shaper AG, Pocock SJ, Walker M. Parental death from heart disease and the risk of heart attack. *Eur Heart J* 1988; 9: 243–51.

18 Jousilahti P, Puska P, Vartiainen E, Pekkanen J, Tuomilehto J. Parental history of premature coronary heart disease: an independent risk factor of myocardial infarction. *J Clin Epidemiol* 1996; 49: 497–503.

19 Jouven X, Desnos M, Guerot C, Ducimetiere P. Predicting sudden death in the population: the Paris Prospective Study I. *Circulation* 1999; 99: 1978–83.

20 Sorensen TI, Neilsen GG, Andersen PK, Teasdale TW. Genetic and environmental influences on premature death in adult adoptees. *N Engl J Med* 1988; 318: 727–32.

21 Marenberg ME, Risch N, Berkman LF, Floderus B, de Faire U. Genetic susceptibility to death from coronary heart disease in a study of twins. *N Engl J Med* 1994; 330: 1041–6.

22 Barker D. Fetal origins of cardiovascular disease. *Ann Med* 1999; 31 (Suppl. 1): 3–6.

23 Libby P. Molecular basis of the acute coronary syndromes. *Circulation* 1995; 91: 2844–50.

24 Dammerman M. Genetic basis of lipoprotein disorders. *Circulation* 1995; 91: 505–12.

25 Rewers M, Kamboth MI, Hoag S, Shetterly SM, Ferrell RE, Hamman RF. ApoA-IV polymorphism associated with myocardial infarction in obese NIDDM patients. The San Luis Valley Diabetes Study. *Diabetes* 1999; 43: 1485–9.

26 Gardemann A, Ohly D, Fink M *et al.* Association of the insertion / deletion gene polymorphism of the apolipoprotein B signal peptide with myocardial infarction. *Atherosclerosis* 1998; 141: 167–75.

27 Bohn M, Bakken A, Erikssen J, Berg K. XbaI polymorphism in DNA at the apolipoprotein B locus is associated with myocardial infarction (MI). *Clin Genet* 1993; 44: 241–8.

28 Nakai K, Fusazaki T, Zhang T *et al.* Polymorphism of the apolipoprotein E and angiotensin I converting enzyme genes in Japanese patients with myocardial infarction. *Coron Artery Dis* 1998; 9: 329–34.

29 Jemaa R, Fumeron F, Poirier O *et al.* Lipoprotein lipase gene polymorphisms: associations with myocardial infarction and lipoprotein levels, the ECTIM study.

Etude Cas Temoin sur l'Infarctus du Myocarde. *J Lipid Res* 1995; 36: 2141–6.

30 Ruiz J, Blanche H, James RW *et al.* Gln-Arg 192 polymorphism of paroxonase and coronary heart disease in type 2 diabetes. *Lancet* 1995; 346: 869–72.

31 Serrato M, Marian AJ. A variant of human paroxonase / arylesterase (HUMPONA) gene is a risk factor for coronary artery disease. *J Clin Invest* 1995; 96: 3005–8.

32 Pfohl M, Kock M, Enderle MD *et al.* Paroxonase 192 Gln/Arg gene polymorphism, coronary heart disease, and myocardial infarction in type 2 diabetes. *Diabetes* 1999; 48: 623–7.

33 Fumeron F, Betoulle D, Luc G *et al.* Alcohol intake modulates the effect of a polymorphism of the Cholesterol Ester Transfer Protein Gene on plasma high density lipoprotein and the risk of myocardial infarction. *J Clin Invest* 1995; 96: 1664–71.

34 Thompson SG, Kienast J, Pyke SDM, Haverkate F, van de Loo JCW. Haemostatic factors and the risk of MI or sudden death in patients with angina pectoris. *N Engl J Med* 1995; 332: 635–41.

35 Humphries SE, Panahloo A, Montgomery HE, Green F, Yudkin J. Gene–environment interaction in the determination of levels of haemostatic variables involved in thrombosis and fibrinolysis. *Thromb Haemost* 1997; 78: 457–61.

36 Yu Q, Safavi F, Roberts R, Marian AJ. A variant of beta fibrinogen is a genetic risk factor for coronary artery disease and myocardial infarction. *J Invest Med* 1996; 44: 154–9.

37 Zito F, Di Castelnuovo A, Amore C, D'Orazio A, Donati MB, Iacoviello L. Bcl1 polymorphism in the beta-chain gene is associated with the risk of familial myocardial infarction by increasing plasma fibrinogen levels: a case-control study in a sample of GISSI-2 patients. *Arteriosclerosis Thromb Vasc Biol* 1997; 17: 3489–94.

38 Bahague I, Poirei O, Nicaud V *et al.* Beta fibrinogen gene polymorphisms are associated with plasma fibrinogen and coronary artery disease in patients with myocardial infarction (The ECTIM Study). *Circulation* 1996; 93: 440–9.

39 Tybjaerg Hansen A, Agerholm-Larsen B, Humphries SE, Abidgaard S, Schnohr P, Nordestgaard BG. A common mutation (G-433 A) in the beta-fibrinogen promoter is an independent predictor of plasma fibrinogen, but not of ischaemic heart disease: a study of 9127 individuals on the Copenhagen City Heart Study. *J Clin Invest* 1997; 99: 3034–9.

40 Poort SR, Rosendaal FR, Reitsma PH, Bertina RM. A common genetic variation in the 3'-untranslated region of the prothrombin gene is associated with elevated plasma prothrombin levels and an increase in venous thrombosis. *Blood* 1996; 88: 3698–703.

41 Bertina RM, Koeleman BPC, Koster T *et al.* Mutation in blood coagulation factor V associated with resistance to activated protein C. *Nature* 1999; 369: 64–7.

42 Di Castelnuovo A, D'Orazio A, Amore C *et al.* Genetic modulation of coagulation factor VII plasma levels: Contribution of different polymorphisms and gender related effects. *Thromb Haemost* 1998; 80: 592–7.

43 Rosendaal FR. Venous thrombosis: a multicausal disease. *Lancet* 1999; 373: 1167–73.

44 Rosendaal FR, Siscovick DS, Schwartz SM *et al.* Factor V Leiden (resistance to activated protein C) increases the risk of myocardial infarction in young women. *Blood* 1997; 89: 2817–21.

45 Doggen CJ, Cats VM, Bertina RM, Rosendaal FR. Increase risk of myocardial infarction associated with factor V Leiden or prothrombin variant (20210G to A). *Circulation* 1998; 97: 1037–41.

46 Gardemann A, Arsic T, Katz N, Tillmanns H, Hehrlein FW, Haberbosch W. The factor II and factor V G1691A gene transitions and coronary heart disease. *Thromb Haemost* 1999; 81: 208–13.

47 Croft SA, Daly ME, Steeds RP, Channer KS, Samani NJ, Hampton KK. The prothrombin 20210A allele and its association with myocardial infarction. *Thromb Haemost* 1999; 81: 861–4.

48 Iacoviello L, Di Castelnuovo A, de Knijff P *et al.* Polymorphisms in the coagulation factor VII gene and the risk of myocardial infarction. *N Engl J Med* 1999; 338: 79–85.

49 Doggen CJ, Manger CV, Bertina RM, Reitsma PH, Vandenbroucke JP, Rosendaal FR. A genetic propensity to high factor VII is not associated with the

risk of myocardial infarction in men. *Thromb Haemost* 1998; 80: 281–5.

50 Doggen CJ, Kunz G, Rosendaal FR *et al.* A mutation in the thrombomodulin gene, 127G to A coding for Ala25Thr, and the risk of myocardial infarction in men. *Thromb Haemost* 1998; 80: 743–8.

51 Norlund L, Holm J, Zoller B, Ohlin AK. A common thrombomodulin amino acid dimorphism is associated with myocardial infarction. *Thromb Haemost* 1997; 77: 248–51.

52 Weiss EJ, Bray PF, Taybach M *et al.* A polymorphism of a platelet glycoprotein receptor as an inherited risk factor for coronary thrombosis. *N Engl J Med* 1996; 334: 1090–4.

53 Goodall AH, Curzen N, Panesar M *et al.* Increased binding of fibrinogen to glycoprotein IIIa-Proline positive platelets in patients with cardiovascular disease. *Eur Heart J* 1999; 20: 742–7.

54 Laule M, Cascorbi I, Stangl V *et al.* A1/A2 polymorphism of glycoprotein IIIa and association with excess procedural risk for coronary catheter interventions: a case-controlled study. *Lancet* 1999; 353: 708–12.

55 Samani NJ, Lodwick D. Glycoprotein IIIa polymorphism and risk of myocardial infarction. *Cardiovasc Res* 1997; 33: 693–7.

56 Ridker PM, Hennekens CH, Schmitz C, Stampfer MJ, Lindpaintner K. PLAI/A2 polymorphism of platelet glycoprotein IIIa and risks of myocardial infarction, stroke, and venous thrombosis. *Lancet* 1997; 349: 385–58.

57 Gardemann A, Humme J, Stricker J *et al.* Association of the platelet glycoprotein IIIa PlA1/A2 gene polymorphism to coronary artery disease but not to nonfatal myocardial infarction in low risk patients. *Thromb Haemost* 1998; 80: 214–17.

58 Moshfegh K, Wuillemin WA, Redondo M *et al.* Association of two silent polymorphisms of platelet glycoprotein Ia/IIa receptor with risk of myocardial infarction: a case-control study. *Lancet* 1999; 353: 351–4.

59 Kunicki TJ, Kritzic M, Annis DS, Nugent DJ. Hereditary variations in platelet integrin alpha-2 beta-1 density is associated with two silent polymorphisms in the alpha-2 gene coding sequence. *Blood* 1997; 89: 1939–43.

60 Dawson S, Henney A. The status of PAI-1 as a risk factor for arterial and thrombotic disease: a review. *Atherosclerosis* 1992; 95: 195–217.

61 Eriksson P, Kallin B, van't Hooft FM, Bavenholm P, Hampten A. Allele specific increase in basal transcription of the plasminogen-activator inhibitor 1 gene is associated with myocardial infarction. *Proc Natl Acad Sci USA* 1995; 92: 1851–5.

62 Ossei-Gerning N, Mansfield MW, Stickland MH, Wilson IJ, Grant PJ. Plasminogen activator inhibitor-1 promoter 4G/5G genotype and plasma levels in relation to a history of myocardial infarction in patients characterized by coronary angiography. *Arteriosclerosis Thromb Vasc Biol* 1997; 17: 33–7.

63 Ye S, Green FR, Scarabin PY *et al.* The 4G/5G genetic polymorphism in the promoter of the plasminogen activator inhibitor-1 (PAI-1) gene is associated with differences in plasma PAI-1 activity but not with risk of myocardial infarction in the ECTIM study. Etude CasTemoins de l'nfarctus du Mycocarde. *Thromb Haemost* 1995; 74: 837–41.

64 Ridker PM, Hennekens CH, Lindpaintner K, Stampfer MJ, Miletich JP. Arterial and venous thrombosis is not associated with the 4G/5G polymorphism in the promoter of the plasminogen activator inhibitor gene in a large cohort of US men. *Circulation* 1997; 95: 59–62.

65 Iacoviello L, Burzotta F, Di Castelnuovo A, Zito F, Marchioli R, Donati MB. The 4G/5G polymorphism of PAI-1 promoter gene and the risk of myocardial infarction: a meta-analysis [letter]. *Thromb Haemost* 1998; 80: 1029–30.

66 van der Bom JG, de Knijff P, Haverkate F *et al.* Tissue plasminogen activator and risk of myocardial infarction. The Rotterdam Study. *Circulation* 1997; 95: 2623–7.

67 Rigat B, Hubert C, Alhenc-Gelas F, Cambien F, Corval P, Soubrier F. An insertion/deletion polymorphism in the angiotensin 1-converting enzyme gene accounting for half of the variance of serum enzyme levels. *J Clin Invest* 1990; 86: 1343–6.

68 Danser AHJ, Schalekamp MADH, Bax WA *et al.* Angiotensin-converting enzyme in the human heart: effect of the insertion/deletion polymorphism. *Circulation* 1995; 92: 1387–8.

69 Cambien F, Poirer O, Lecerf L et al. Deletion polymorphism in the gene for angiotensin-converting enzyme is a potent risk factor for myocardial infarction. Nature 1992; 359: 641–4.

70 Samani NJ, Thompson JR, O'Toole L, Channer K, Woods K. A meta-analysis of the association of the deletion allele of the angiotensin-converting enzyme gene with myocardial infarction. Circulation 1996; 94: 708–12.

71 Katsuya T, Koike G, Yee TW. Association of angiotensinogen gene T235 variant with increase risk of coronary heart disease. Lancet 1995; 344: 1600–7.

72 Jeunemaitre X, Soubrier F, Kotelevtsev YV et al. Molecular basis of human hypertension: role of angiotensinogen. Cell 1992; 71: 169–84.

73 Tiret L, Bonnardeaux A, Poirier O et al. Synergistic effects of angiotensin-converting enzyme and angiotensin-II type 1 receptor gene polymorphisms on risk of myocardial infarction. Lancet 1994; 344: 910–13.

74 Wang XL, Sim AS, Badenhop RF, McCredie KM, Wilcken DE. A smoking-dependent risk of coronary artery disease associated with a polymorphism of the endothelial nitric oxide synthase gene. Nature Med 1996; 2: 41–5.

75 Wang XL, Mahaney MC, Sim AS et al. Genetic contribution of the endothelial constitutive nitric oxide synthetase gene to plasma nitric oxide levels. Arterioscler Thromb Vasc Biol 1997; 17: 3147–53.

76 Hibi K, Ishigami T, Tamura K et al. Endothelial nitric oxide synthase gene polymorphism and acute myocardial infarction. Hypertension 1998; 32: 521–6.

77 Mayer Y, Jacobson DW, Robinson K. Homocysteine and coronary atherosclerosis. J Am Coll Cardiol 1996; 27: 517–27.

78 Frosst P, Blom HG, Milos R et al. A candidate genetic risk factor for vascular disease: a common mutation in methylenetetrahydrofolate reductase. Nature Genet 1995; 10: 111–13.

79 Ma J, Stampfer MJ, Hennekens CH et al. Methylenetetrahydrofolate reductase polymorphism, plasma folate, homocysteine, and risk of myocardial infarction in US physicians. Circulation 1996; 94: 2410–16.

80 Adams A, Smith PD, Martin D, Thompson D, Lodwick D, Samani NJ. Genetic analysis of thermolabile methylenetetrahydrofolate reductase as a risk factor for myocardial infarction. Q J Med 1996; 89: 437–44.

81 Schwartz SM, Siscovich DS, Malinow R et al. Myocardial infarction in young women in relation to plasma total homocysteine, folate, and a common variant in the methylenetetrahydroflate reductase gene. Circulation 1997; 96: 412–7.

82 Inbal A, Friemark D, Modan B et al. Synergistic effects of prothrombotic polymorphisms and atherogenic factors on the risk of myocardial infarction in young males. Blood 1999; 93: 2186–90.

83 Editorial. Freely associating. Nature Genet 1999; 22: 1–2.

84 Lander ES, Schork NJ. Genetic dissection of complex traits. Science 1994; 265: 2037–48.

85 Risch N, Merikangas K. The future of genetic studies of complex human diseases. Science 1996; 273: 1516–17.

86 Samani NJ. Molecular genetics of coronary artery disease: measuring the phenotype. Clin Sci 1998; 95: 645–6.

87 Lindpaintner K, Pfeffer MA, Kreutz R et al. A prospective evaluation of an angiotensin-converting enzyme gene polymorphism and the risk of ischaemic heart disease. N Engl J Med 1995; 332: 706–11.

88 Agerholm-Larsen B, Nordestgaard BG, Steffensen R, Sorensen TI, Jensen G, Tybjaerg-Hansen A. ACE gene polymorphism: ischaemic heart disease and longevity in 10150 individuals. A case-referent and retrospective cohort study based on the Copenhagen City Heart Study. Circulation 1997; 95: 2258–367.

89 Little WC, Constantinescu M, Applegate RJ et al. Can coronary angiography predict the site of a subsequent myocardial infarction in patients with mild-to-moderate coronary artery disease. Circulation 1988; 78: 1157–66.

90 Collins FH. Medical and societal consequences of the human genome project (The Shattuck Lecture). N Engl J Med 1999; 341: 28–38.

91 Cargill M, Altshuler D, Ireland J et al. Characterization of single-nucleotide polymorphisms in coding regions of human genes. Nature Genet 1999; 22: 231–8.

92 Cambien F, Poirer O, Nicaud V *et al.*
Sequence diversity in 36 candidate genes
for cardiovascular disorders. *Am J Hum
Genet* 1999; 65: 183–91.

93 Lipshatz RJ, Fodor SP, Gingeas TR,
Lakhart DJ. High density synthetic
oligonucleotide assays. *Nature Genet*
1999; 21: 20–4.

Part 2: Diagnosis

6: What is the role of advanced electrocardiology?

Mitchell W. Krucoff and Mikael Dellborg

Background and definitions

Over the last 15 years it has become evident that for patients with coronary heart disease, episodes of ischaemia, either silent or painful, carry important prognostic implications. From the earliest Holter studies and onward [1] it has become clear that particularly for patients suffering acute coronary syndromes (unstable angina and acute myocardial infarction, AMI), continuous ST-segment monitoring provides uniquely valuable, non-invasive, quantitative information to support both early diagnosis and ongoing assessment of response to therapy.

The development of less costly and more efficient microprocessors as well as the development of improved signal processing firmware and software has made multilead, real-time, continuous ST monitoring technically feasible for clinical use [2,3]. In concert with the fidelity and signal processing capabilities of these current devices, clinical judgement with regard to patient selection and software that supports identification of artefact, ectopic or aberrant cardiac cycles in an effective user interface are key elements to the optimal integration of this new technology into clinical practice. Consensus practice standards for use primarily within the American health-care system of continuous 12-lead electrocardiography (ECG) have recently been published [4]. Finally, clinical studies must continue to contribute to the depth and breadth of knowledge about the influence of real-time and/or retrospective ST-segment data on patient management and clinical outcome [5–8].

Historically the discovery of ST-segment deviation during continuous Holter recordings dates back to the very first report of Norman Jeffery Holter in *Science* in 1961. Although Holter speculated that some of these changes might be the result of myocardial ischaemia, subsequent work showed that the record-playback systems themselves introduced low frequency and phase shift artefact capable of producing measurable ST-segment displacement. In addition, ST-segment changes were observed with postural change, hyperventilation, left ventricular hypertrophy, changes in potassium concentration and use of digoxin, all in the absence of coronary artery disease or myocardial ischaemia. Instrument fidelity across the entire record-playback loop was addressed in the early 1980s on both AM and FM systems [9]. In the 1990s integrated circuit devices that digitize the ECG signal early in the recording process have eliminated these particular sources of artefact in ST recordings.

Even with recording of excellent fidelity, non-ischaemic causes of ST-segment change are relatively common in patients who have normal coronary arteries. However, well characterized ST-segment shifts in patients who are highly likely to have coronary artery disease and who have normal atrioventricular conduction patterns at rest have been shown to be *both* sensitive and specific for myocardial ischaemia [10,11]. Thus, it is clear that the optimal application of this technology in its modern form is not as a screening tool to detect coronary disease out of large populations *per se*, but as a tool to measure the activity of highly suspicious clinical presentations or known coronary disease and its response to directed therapy.

With the use of such a Bayesian approach to patient selection, there is now a large and consistent literature showing that ST-segment changes with or without angina not only represent ischaemia, but also carry prognostic information [12–14]. Caution must be exercised, however, over the consequences of aggressive treatment of all detectable ischaemia, as more is unknown than known at this time. As with dysrhythmia monitoring, where cardiologists learned that effectively treating premature ventricular contraction led to increased rather than decreased mortality, the effect of aggressive treatment of ischaemic epsiodes on clinical outcomes must be carefully studied. To date available data suggest that at least two classes of patients may benefit: patients with minimal symptoms but ongoing ST-segment activity on Holter who are revascularized have better outcomes than those who are not; and patients with ST-segment elevation myocardial infarction who are treated earlier and in whom sustained infarct artery patency is achieved earlier have better outcomes than those who do not reach such reperfusion goals [15,16].

Several kinds of device are currently available for multilead continuous ST-segment monitoring. Much of our knowledge comes from older studies using 1- or 2-lead Holter in retrospective settings. Although Holter is a well established, widely available technology, few Holter centres actually attend to the detailed patient selection, skin preparation, lead location and signal calibration features that are necessary to obtain accurate ST-segment measurements with Holter. In addition, the retrospective nature of Holter technologies implicitly limits use in acute settings where real-time information is critical to optimal patient management. With the rapid progress of technologies in this area, including smaller components with greater storage capacities, real-time integrated circuit Holter systems are likely to emerge in the new millenium.

Technical considerations

12-lead ECG

A growing number of ECG and monitoring manufacturers have developed continuous 12-lead ECG monitoring devices. Published reports using continuous 12-lead monitoring have emerged mostly from applications in patients undergoing angioplasty, in patients treated for ST-segment elevation infarction, and, more recently, in patients with chest pain syndromes, unstable angina and non-Q-wave infarction. The vast majority of studies have been done with a portable continuous 12-lead ECG system (ST100, Mortara Instrument, Milwaukee, USA). To minimize artefact, limb leads are placed on the torso lead positions, with a notable effect on QRS axis but very little effect on ST deviation measures [17]. Depending on software and memory structure, systems may differ on how many ECGs can be stored and how frequently they are assessed. In a widely used portable system [2] an ECG is acquired and immediately compared to the patient's baseline ECG every 20 s. If new ST deviation is detected or progresses over four serial acquisitions—i.e. new ST deviation either persists or worsens over a >60 s period—a real-time alarm can sound, and hard-copy ECGs representing both the baseline and the new offending ECG are printed out in a comparison format at the bedside. In the absence of new ST deviation, ECGs are archived in the device's memory according to a manually programmed interval, for instance every 5–10 min. Trends of ST level vs. time for individual leads, lead groups and summated ST deviation are all accessible at the bedside and/or at a central review station.

Continuous vectorcardiography

With the use of 8 leads placed according to Frank [18], a continuous 3-lead ECG, X, Y and Z is recorded. The vast majority of studies have been done with the MIDA Continuous Vectorcardiographic System (Ortivus, Täby, Sweden). After filtering and rejection of ectopic beats, incoming beats are averaged over 30–120-s periods and each such average is stored. Comparison is made with the first 2 min of recording, i.e. the reference. Changes are displayed as trends over time where summarized ST parameters such as ST vector magnitude (ST-VM) and differential QRS parameters such as QRS vector difference (QRS-VD) are displayed [3]. The ST-VM is the summarized deviation of the ST-segment for lead X, Y and Z, added quadratically, i.e. thereby equalizing ST elevation and ST depression. Many reports are based on ST-VM data measured at J+20 ms, whereas others are based on measurements at J+60 ms. The former will lessen the influence of T-wave changes, particularly at higher heart rates, while the latter is more in agreement with standard procedures used during exercise testing, other 12-lead ECG monitor reports and Holter recording. However, the difference between measuring at J + 20 ms vs. J + 60 ms has in clinical trials been minor [19]. The QRS-VD is a differential measurement, comparing the current mean QRS-complex to the initial (the 'reference') QRS-complex. The area of difference between the two is calculated and presented as a trend curve over time. Whereas QRS changes clearly occur with episodes of myocardial ischaemia and infarction, the clinical usefulness is limited by the low specificity of QRS changes, particularly with changes in body position. However, many patients when placed in the left lateral position will exhibit substantial changes in both ST and QRS parameters [20]. The software permits use of variations of the Dower transformation of the vectorcardiogram (VCG) to a transformed 12-lead ECG [21]. However, this 12-lead ECG carries important differences as compared with standard 12-lead ECG, particularly regarding QRS morphology, but to a very small extent regarding ST-segment changes [22].

Which devices should be used?

It is now well appreciated that acute coronary syndromes are highly dynamic clinical and pathophysiological entities. Occasional static ECGs may undersample important information, either to correlate with patient symptoms or to raise alerts when ischaemia is not accompanied by patient symptoms. Thus any device with real-time capability and reasonably modern signal fidelity that provides continuous ECG monitoring will yield important information beyond that encountered in routine practice.

A second basic principle of application is the familiarity of the clinical users with the device and the information it yields. Some devices include automated dysrhythmia detection algorithms that identify ventricular and aberrant beats in order to eliminate them from ST-segment measurements. Users must be aware that the sensitivity and specificity of such 'automatic' beat identification programs are highly variable. Other devices measure ST deviation on all ECG acquisitions, leaving the clinician to determine whether newly detected ST deviation results from ischaemic changes or from a change in conduction or rhythm. Whereas QRS monitoring can be performed only with continuous vectorcardiography, this concept has scientific interest. Interesting observations and possibilities for QRS monitoring have included assessment of patency in patients with less pronounced ST elevation [7] and diagnosis of AMI in patients with bundle-branch block [23]. However, at present, there is no substantial clinically meaningful benefit that can be obtained by adding QRS monitoring to ST-segment monitoring.

A third very important issue in selecting an ST monitoring system is the noise levels of the signal. ST-segment measurements are very susceptible to movement and other 50–60 Hz artefact. Manufacturers differ in the extent to which their often proprietary signal processing elements modulate signal/noise. A substantial part of noise reduction, however, originates in the bedside staff familiarity and competence with the systems in use. Artefacts caused by changes in body position remain a problem for ST as well as QRS monitoring [20,24,25].

If one does not have access to multilead monitoring systems in a coronary care unit (CCU), monitoring 'worst lead', i.e. the lead that shows the most dramatic ST change on the admission standard 12-lead ECG, will clearly provide important information. 'Worst lead' monitoring can be of sufficient use for monitoring during thrombolytic treatment to assess reperfusion and/or reocclusion. It is more problematic in the unstable angina patients where ST changes may be more variable and it is more difficult to prospectively identify the lead where the largest changes will occur [26].

In addition to selections across different device formats, it should be recognized that across publications different measurement points, measurement leads and cut-off values are reported in the evaluation of the information obtained from monitoring. It is therefore important not only to use similar technology but also similar methods of data analysis when results of monitoring are related to reported studies. When study-derived algorithms are applied for clinical use, it is important to tailor the decisions to the technology used and to the data available from rigorous studies.

What is gained by multilead monitoring as compared to standard dysrhythmia monitoring?

Ischaemia, unlike dysrhythmias, can cause local deviation. It has been clearly shown that the more leads monitored, the more ischaemic episode changes are likely to be recognized [26,27]. Precordial mapping with 32, 64 or 128 leads provides more information but is impractical for clinical care and patient comfort. Widespread use and acceptance by CCU nurses and patients of the 8–10 leads used in standard 12-lead and continuous vectorcardiographic monitoring, make the system suitable for use in critically ill patients. With such tools high quality data can be obtained in multicentre studies [28,29]. Most importantly, when standard 1–3 lead monitoring of lead V1 and limb leads for determination of dysrhythmia are used, ischaemic events may be missed completely. Vectorcardiography and 12-lead ECG provide a much more robust monitoring approach for the detection of ischaemia.

Which patients should be monitored?

ST-segment elevation infarction

In ST elevation infarction both continuous ST monitoring with 12-lead ECG and vectorcardiography have been studied extensively as non invasive markers of the quality and stability of reperfusion [6,7,30]. These techniques provide important prognostic information and information regarding infarct size [14,31,32]. Clinically they are suitable for real-time identification of patients with failed reperfusion after thrombolytic therapy, who may be candidates for rescue angioplasty or other additional therapy as well as for triage of patients into high- or low-risk categories. It is important to realize, however, that optimal therapeutic choices in high-risk patients are still largely based on clinical judgement. The presence of criteria that is high risk, such as persistent ST elevation or ST re-elevation after transient ST recovery, does not mean that any or every available therapeutic option will lower that risk profile. Thus, although continuous ST-segment monitoring is useful for ongoing risk stratification and assessment of response to therapy, its integration into the clinical care of patients with ST elevation infarction must be individualized by the decision making of the clinician.

Unstable angina/non-Q-wave infarction

In non-ST elevation and unstable angina ST-segment monitoring clearly can be used to identify patients at increased risk [1,33,34]. This prognostic information is additive to that obtained from a careful clinical history, standard 12-lead ECG, as well as biochemical monitoring such as serial troponin-T measurements [12,35,36]. There are data to suggest that treatments that limit the number of silent or symptomatic ST episodes will also have a beneficial effect on patient outcome [28,37]. However, no clinical trials have yet used ST-segment monitoring as a real-time basis for intervention. ST-

Fig. 6.1 Mr E.M. was a 59-year-old male who presented with accelerated angina. Cardiac catheterization revealed a 95% mid-right-coronary stenosis. Angioplasty of the site was performed and a coronary stent was placed due to sub-optimal angioplasty results. Transient inferior ST-segment monitor (A), reversing completely with balloon deflation. A reasonable angiographic result was obtained, and the patient was taken back to the CCU. The following morning ST-segment monitor alarms (B) drew attention to new inferior ST-segment elevation in a pattern identical to the 'fingerprint' recorded during angioplasty. These changes were not reversed with medical therapies. As the catheterization laboratory was being prepared the patient began to experience chest pain, became hypotensive and hypoxic. He was intubated and taken urgently to the catheterization laboratory where an intra-aortic balloon pump was placed. The right coronary artery was found to be occluded. Re-dilatation and deployment of a second coronary stent resulted in excellent angiographic flow. The ECG quickly normalized and the patient rapidly stabilized. He subsequently rehabilitated and was discharged uneventfully.

Above: Three-dimensional graphic depiction of ST-segment level (Y-axis) plotted for each of the standard 12 ECG leads (X-axis) over time (Z-axis).

Middle: Two-dimensional graphic summated ST deviation (Y-axis) over time (X-axis) showing markers (A = ST deviation during PCI, B = ST deviation during abrupt closure).

Below: Standard analogue 12-lead ECG waveforms from time A, showing minor inferior ST elevation during PCI and from time B, showing more marked ST elevation in identical precordial 'fingerprint' pattern during abrupt closure.

Modified from Crater *et al. Critical Care Nurse* 2000; 20: 93–9. Reprinted with permission.

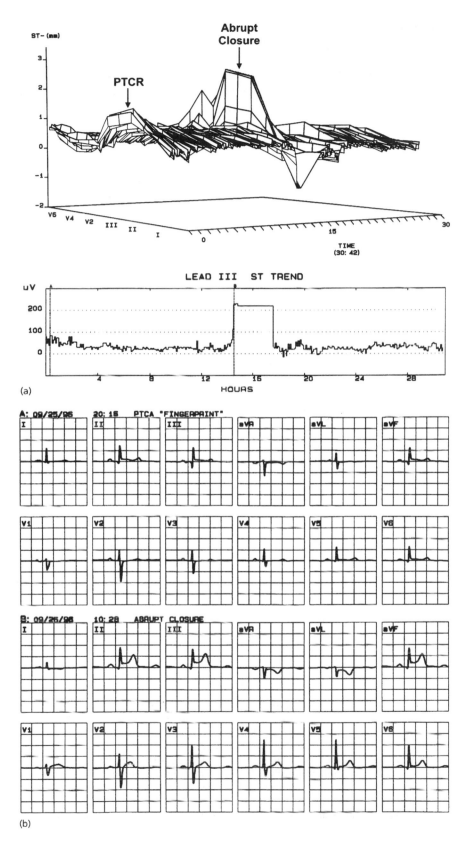

(a)

(b)

segment monitoring is a powerful tool to identify high risk and as such may be used to assign intensive care vs. regular ward beds facilities and/or to otherwise more appropriately distribute interventional resources when supply is limited.

Post-angioplasty

Sudden reocclusions and complications after routine angioplasty are relatively uncommon but may be disastrous and unexpected. Multilead ST-segment monitoring is clearly valuable after high-risk angioplasty [38]. Patterns of ST deviation over multiple leads may be acquired during the balloon occlusion at a known coronary site for an individual patient like an occlusion 'fingerprint' [39,40]. Recurrence of this same pattern then becomes a highly sensitive and specific marker of abrupt closure of the percutaneous transluminal coronary revascularization (PTCR) site (see Fig. 6.1). Such unequivocal ST-segment changes frequently precede clinically recognizable patient symptoms. This 'early warning' may allow the catheterization laboratory to assemble earlier or otherwise promote earlier, more effective therapy to be given.

Chest pain units

Multilead ST-segment monitoring has also been used in chest pain units for early diagnosis of ischaemia and infarction [41–43]. It is not infrequent for patients who experience chest pain at home to be pain free by the time they arrive

---

Fig. 6.2 D.H. was a 70-year-old white man who was found pulseless and in ventricular fibrillation after a low-impact motor vehicle accident. Pulse and a narrow complex rhythm were restored in the field after 9 countershocks. He was intubated and unresponsive with decerebrate posturing on transfer to the CCU. He suffered episodes of intermittent hypotension. Echocardiogram showed preserved left ventricular function with an ejection fraction of 50%. Initial ECG was unremarkable for acute changes. Continuous 12-lead ECG monitoring was initiated, and several hours later a 30-minute episode of ST segment depression of 2 mm in V_2, 1 mm in V_3, and down-sloping of the J point in leads V_4 and V_5 were observed. Chest pain could not be evaluated. On the second day of admission a similar ST segment depression event occurred. On the third day of admission, ST segment depressions of 2 mm in V_2, >5 mm in V_3 and V_4, >4 mm in V_5. This ischaemic event did not reverse after several hours and the patient was taken as an emergency to the coronary procedure unit where a 100% occluded left circumflex coronary artery was revascularized with percutaneous transluminal coronary angioplasty. D.H. was extubated and neurological deficits resolved and he was discharged in good condition. A pre-discharge echocardiogram showed an EF of 50% and no significant regional wall motion defects.

Above: Three-dimensional graphic depiction of ST-segment level (Y-axis) plotted for each of the standard 12 ECG leads (X-axis) over time (Z-axis).

Middle: Two-dimensional graphic of summated ST deviation (Y-axis) over time (X-axis) showing markers (A = baseline ST levels, B = ST depression during an episode of ischaemia).

Below: Standard analogue 12-lead ECG waveforms from time ! at baseline and during time B ischaemic episode.

Modified from Crater *et al. Critical Care Nurse* 2000; 20: 93–9. Reprinted with permission.

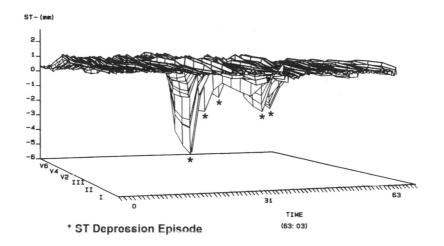

* ST Depression Episode

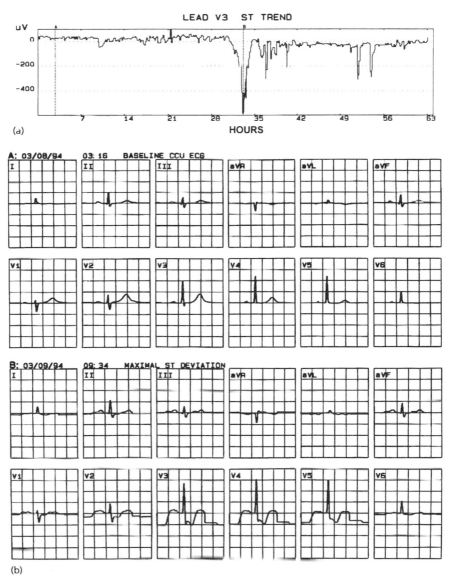

(a)

(b)

in the emergency department. Such patients may have non-diagnostic ECGs on arrival either because the pain was not cardiac pain to begin with, or because the ischaemia that caused the pain has abated. Continuous ECG monitoring may document unequivocal episodes of ischaemia in the absence of symptoms (see Fig. 6.2) or may capture ECG changes at the time of recurrent symptoms, assisting in more timely and definitive diagnosis. As with ischaemia monitoring in general, it is important to understand Bayesian probabilities. Continuous monitoring of patients who are very unlikely to have ischaemic heart disease, such as young females or adolescent males with chest pains, will yield significantly more non-specific ST deviation. Monitoring patients with multiple risk factors for coronary disease or patients who have known coronary disease who present with chest pain will detect transient episodes of ST deviation that are more specific for ischaemia. Combined with focused clinical attention, rapid serum marker assays and sometimes more advanced tools such as echocardiography, the chest pain unit application of continuous ST-segment monitoring represents one of the most exciting new areas of application for these devices.

Perioperative ischaemia

Patients with cardiac risk factors or known coronary artery disease who undergo non-cardiac surgery may suffer postoperative ischaemia, infarction or death as a result of perioperative stressors with alarming frequency. Such patients undergoing non-cardiac vascular surgery suffer ischaemic episodes in about 20% of cases [44]. These patients are at higher risk for myocardial infarction and death; however, work to show that real-time detection of and therapy for ST episodes can improve these outcomes will require focused clinical trials.

Bundle-branch block/pacemaker

In patients with suspected acute coronary artery disease and bundle-branch block or pacemaker ST-segment deviations, monitoring has been assessed by the use of continuous 12-lead technique and continuous vectorcardiography [23,45]. Small changes in heart rate and body position create such marked changes on the surface ECG that ST-segment monitoring by and large is not yet clinically useful in these patients.

What questions can be answered by continuous monitoring?

Reperfusion therapy: early risk stratification

Continuously monitored ST-segment recovery provides what is perhaps the most reliable predictor of the quality and stability of coronary reperfusion in patients with ST elevation myocardial infarction treated with fibrinolytic agents. As a non-invasive, widely available, relatively inexpensive device for clinical use, continuous ST-segment monitoring is ideally suited to the acute care of these high-risk patients. Integration of ST-segment monitoring data with clinical assessment, rapid-turnaround biochemical assays and arrythmia monitoring may further increase risk stratification accuracy at the bedside.

In comparison with the 'gold standard', acute angiogram, the relative information content of invasive and non-invasive markers must be understood as complementary rather than compared as 'accurate' or 'inaccurate' surrogates of myocardial salvage through interruption of infarction. The angiogram is an anatomical examination of the epicardial vessel patency, documented over a short 'snap shot' window of time. Continuous ST-segment monitoring is a continuous quantification of a physiological nature, reflecting the ongoing and dynamic response of myocardial cells to the presence or absence of nutritive blood flow [46]. Recently, the appreciation of the importance of understanding reperfusion at the cellular level in humans has increased the awareness that a more physiological marker such as early ST recovery may in fact be a better prognostic marker than a 90-min angiogram [47]. Although reperfusion is often considered to be a dichotomous event, it is actually a continuous variable with highly dynamic properties. Cyclic flow changes in the infarct artery have been reported in 30–50% of patients treated with reperfusion therapy. These ongoing changes are clearly reflected as the peaks and troughs observed on continuous ST-segment monitoring [31,48,49] (see also the case recorded in Fig. 6.3).

In clinical use, continuous real-time assessment of ST-segment activity may be of special assistance in patients who are intubated or obtunded and who are unable to feel or communicate the experience of chest pain *per se*. Even in the awake patient, however, reocclusion following reperfusion may not cause chest pain, as the nociceptive system within the 'stunned' myocardium's distribution may remain dysfunctional for weeks. On the other hand, such reocclusion generally does generate significant ST-segment elevation on ECG and very adversely affects clinical outcomes [50].

Serial static ECGs have been reported to have prognostic significance in patients treated with thrombolytics for ST elevation infarction [51–53]. While it is intuitively obvious that repeated static standard 12-lead ECGs have greater information content than would a single ECG, the undersampling error intrinsic to serial static ECGs over the course of a dynamic event such as an infarction is corrected by continuous monitoring [54].

Recurrent ischaemia after reperfusion

Recurrent ischaemia occurring late during a hospital stay is a risk factor for subsequent cardiac morbidity and mortality. Recurrent ischaemia may

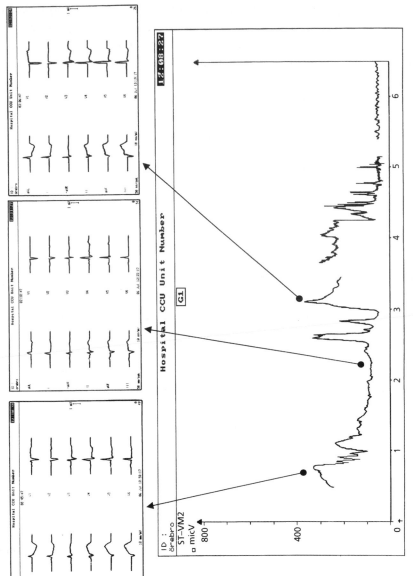

Fig. 6.3 A 57-year-old man was admitted with chest pain and anterior ST-segment elevation. He was treated with 100 mg alteplase over 90 min. Continuous ST-segment monitoring revealed high-grade ST recovery of 65% at 90 min. After 2 h 30 min he began having episodes of ST-VM change, indicating reocclusion with rapid spontaneous reperfusion. After 3 h monitoring he experienced a sustained reocclusion with concomitant chest pain. Illustrative 12-lead ECGs are shown, indicating severe inferior ischaemia. The patient was transferred to the catheterization laboratory where angiography revealed an occluded right coronary artery. An angioplasty with stent placement was performed and subsequent recovery was uneventful.

represent ischaemia from outside the infarct zone, for instance in patients with multivessel coronary disease whose non-infarct myocardial segments are overcompensating for the compromised function of the 'stunned' infarct area. Until recently it has not been clear what the incidence or importance is of early (during the initial 24 h) recurrent ischaemia. The experience from the GUSTO-I ischaemia monitoring substudy clearly indicates that early recurrent ischaemia is a strong prognostic factor [14]. While occasional episodes of recurrent ST-segment deviation seem to carry little adverse risk, repeated episodes identified a subgroup of patients with a substantial risk in the short- and long-term. By continuous ST-segment monitoring we can thus identify a subgroup of patients towards whom further research may be directed regarding early intervention or addition of potent medical therapies.

Chest pain

Improved definition of patient risk categories with continuous ST-segment monitoring in the chest pain unit includes a spectrum of applications. In moderate- to low-risk patients, continuous ST-segment monitoring enhances the basis for decisions to discharge the patient home or to admit the patient to hospital. In moderate- to high-risk patients, ST-segment monitoring may support the decision on whether to admit the patient to a ward bed or to an intensive care bed, on whether to anticoagulate and on whether a patient is a candidate for antiplatelet therapies such as IIb/IIIa inhibitors, etc. ST-segment monitoring may also be very helpful in the early identification of a patient who presents with chest pain and ST-segment depression to sudden, progressive ST elevation infarction.

Risk stratification in unstable coronary syndromes

Both for short-term and long-term risk stratification continuous ST-segment monitoring is very powerful. The prognostic value exceeds that of the admission ECG and various clinical characteristics including recurrent pain. The prognostic value is additive to that from biochemical markers such as troponin-T. In situations of restricted access to coronary interventions or even restricted number of hospital beds, ST-segment monitoring may be helpful in supporting selection of patients for early intervention or early discharge. However, it must be pointed out that there are no formal controlled trials that support the use of only ST-segment monitoring for this kind of triage.

The cases shown in Figs 6.4 and 6.5 demonstrate the occurrence of several episodes of asymptomatic ST-segment change, presented as ST-vector magnitude change in two patients with acute unstable angina. Available data indi-

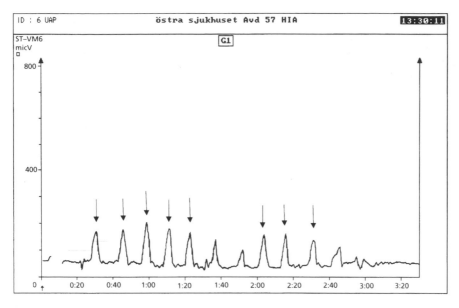

Fig. 6.4 A patient with unstable angina. During the first 4 h of monitoring the patient was asymptomatic but had 8 episodes of recurrent ST change, illustrated as reversible increases of >50 µV of the summarized ST vector magnitude, i.e. the ST-VM. The largest episode was just above 200 µV. The patient stabilized on aspirin, LMW heparin and i.v. nitrates; subsequent angiography revealed triple vessel disease. In a health-care system with limited access to coronary angiography ST monitoring can be utilized in this way for proper selection of patients for early angiography/revascularization.

cate that the mere occurrence of ST-VM episodes indicates an increased early and late risk [12,28]. The number of episodes and, more importantly, the magnitude of the largest episode, indicate further increased risk [55].

Summary and conclusion

Continuous ST-segment monitoring either by continuous 12-lead ECG or continuous vectorcardiography provides reliable information regarding ST changes in patients with ongoing myocardial ischaemia with or without concurrent chest pain. ST-segment monitoring enables the clinician to continuously follow the dynamic changes that characterize unstable angina and acute myocardial infarction syndromes. It provides important information for risk stratification in unstable coronary syndromes and helps in differentiating between extra-cardiac chest pain and acute coronary disease. Futher evolution in semiautomatic evaluation software, body position detectors and ongoing clinical trials will further enhance the utility of this very important clinical tool.

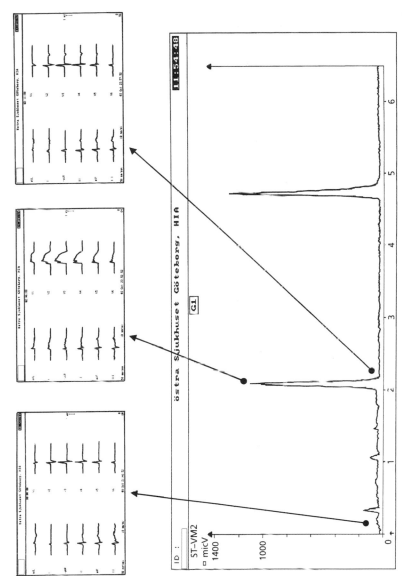

Fig. 6.5 A patient was admitted with chest pain. On admission the patient was free of pain and was treated with aspirin, low molecular weight (LMW) heparin and i.v. nitrates. Standard 12-lead ECG revealed only flat T-waves in anterior leads. Over the next 6 h the patient was pain free but had two very large episodes of ST-VM change corresponding to 3–4 mm ST-segment elevation in anterior leads. Angiography later the same day revealed high-grade proximal stenosis of the left anterior descending coronary artery which was dilated and stented.

References

1 Johnson S, Mauritson D, Winniford M *et al.* Continuous electro-cardiographic monitoring in patients with unstable angina pectoris: Identification of high-risk subgroups with severe coronary disease, variant angina and/or impaired early prognosis. *Am Heart J* 1982; 103 (1): 4–12.

2 Krucoff M, Wagner N, Pope J *et al.* The portable programmable microprocessor-driven real-time 12-lead electrocardiographic monitor: a preliminary report of a new device for the noninvasive detection of successful reperfusion or silent coronary reocclusion. *Am J Cardiol* 1990; 65: 143–8.

3 Dellborg M, Riha M, Swedberg K. Dynamic QRS and ST-segment changes in myocardial infarction monitored by continuous on-line vectorcardiography. *J Electrocardiol* 1990; 23 (Suppl.): 11–19.

4 Drew BJ, Krucoff MW. Multilead ST-segment monitoring in patients with acute coronary syndromes: a consensus statement for healthcare professionals. ST-Segment Monitoring Practice Guideline International Working Group. *Am J Crit Care* 1999; 8 (6): 372–86.

5 Krucoff M, Jackson Y, Kehoe M, Kent K. Quantitative and qualitative ST segment monitoring during and after percutaneous transluminal coronary angioplasty. *Circulation* 1990; 81 (Suppl. IV): IV20–6.

6 Krucoff M, Croll M, Pope J *et al.* Continuous 12-lead ST-segment recovery analysis in the TAMI 7 study: performance of a noninvasive method for real-time detection of failed myocardial reperfusion. *Circulation* 1993; 88 (2): 437–46.

7 Dellborg M, Steg PG, Simoons M *et al.* Vectorcardiographic monitoring to assess early vessel patency after reperfusion therapy for acute myocardial infarction. *Eur Heart J* 1995; 16: 21–9.

8 Andersen K, Eriksson P, Dellborg M. Ischaemia detected by continuous on-line vectorcardiographic monitoring predicts unfavourable outcome in patients admitted with probable unstable coronary disease. *Coron Artery Dis* 1996; 7 (10): 753–60.

9 Holter NJ. The development of Holter electrocardiography. *Clin Eng* 1980; 8 (6): 65–7.

10 Deanfield JE, Shea M, Ribiero P *et al.* Transient ST-segment depression as a marker of myocardial ischemia during daily life. *Am J Cardiol* 1984; 54 (10): 1195–200.

11 Chierchia S, Lazzori M, Freedman B, Brunelli C, Maseri A. Impairment of myocardial perfusion and function during painless myocardial ischemia. *J Am Coll Cardiol* 1983; 1: 924–30.

12 Andersen K, Eriksson P, Dellborg M. Non-invasive risk stratification within 48 h of hospital admission in patients with unstable coronary disease. *Eur Heart J* 1997; 18 (5): 780–8.

13 Langer A, Minkowitz J, Dorian P *et al.* Pathophysiology and prognostic significance of holter-detected ST segment depression after myocardial infarction. *J Am Coll Cardiol* 1992; 20 (6): 1313–37.

14 Langer A, Krucoff MW, Klootwijk P *et al.* Prognostic significance of ST segment shift early after resolution of ST elevation in patients with myocardial infarction treated with thrombolytic therapy: the GUSTO-I ST Segment Monitoring Substudy. *J Am Coll Cardiol* 1998; 31 (4): 783–9.

15 Mulcahy D, Keegan J, Phadke K *et al.* Effects of coronary artery bypass surgery and angioplasty on the total ischemic burden: a study of exercise testing and ambulatory ST segment monitoring. *Am Heart J* 1992; 123 (3): 597–603.

16 Corbalan R, Prieto JC, Chavez E, Nazzal C, Cumsille F, Krucoff M. Bedside markers of coronary artery patency and short-term prognosis of patients with acute myocardial infarction and thrombolysis. *Am Heart J* 1999; 138 (3, Part 1): 533–9.

17 Krucoff MW, Loeffler KA, Haisty WK Jr. *et al.* Simultaneous ST-segment measurements using standard and monitoring-compatible torso limb lead placements at rest and during coronary occlusion. *Am J Cardiol* 1994; 74 (10): 997–1001.

18 Frank E. An accurate, clinically practical system for spatial vectorcardiography. *Circulation* 1956; 13: 737–44.

19 Dellborg M, Malmberg K, Ryden L, Svensson AM, Swedberg K. Dynamic on-line vectorcardiography improves and simplifies in-hospital ischemia monitoring of patients with unstable angina. *J Am Coll Cardiol* 1995; 26 (6): 1501–7.

20 Norgaard BL, Rasmussen BM, Dellborg M, Thygesen K. Temporal and positional variability of the ST segment during continuous vectorcardiography monitoring in healthy subjects. *J Electrocardiol* 1999; 32 (2): 149–58.

21 Dower GE. The ECGD: a derivation of the ECG from VCG leads. *J Electrocardiol* 1984; 17 (2): 189–91.

22 Dower GE, Machado HB. XYZ data interpreted by a 12-lead computer program using the derived electrocardiogram. *J Electrocardiol* 1979; 12 (3): 249–61.

23 Eriksson P, Andersen K, Swedberg K, Dellborg M. Vectorcardiographic monitoring of patients with acute myocardial infarction and chronic bundle branch block. *Eur Heart J* 1997; 18 (8): 1288–95.

24 Bergman K, Stevenson W, Tillisch J, Stevenson L. Effect of body position on the diagnostic accuracy of the electrocardiogram. *Am Heart J* 1989; 117: 204–7.

25 Adams M, Drew B. Body position effects on the ECG. Implication for ischemia monitoring. *J Electrocardiol* 1997; 30: 285–91.

26 Klootwijk P, Meij S, von Es GA *et al.* Comparison of usefulness of computer assisted continuous 48-h 3-lead with 12-lead ECG ischaemia monitoring for detection and quantitation of ischaemia in patients with unstable angina. *Eur Heart J* 1997; 18 (6): 931–40.

27 Krucoff MW. Poor performance of lead V5 in single- and dual-channel ST-segment monitoring during coronary occlusion. *J Electrocardiol* 1988; 21 (Suppl.): S30–4.

28 Andersen K, Dellborg M. Heparin is more effective than inogatran, a low-molecular weight thrombin inhibitor in suppressing ischemia and recurrent angina in unstable coronary disease. Thrombin Inhibition Myocardial Ischemia (TRIM) Study Group. *Am J Cardiol* 1998; 81 (8): 939–44.

29 Langer A, Krucoff M, Klootwijk P *et al.* Noninvasive assessment of speed and stability of infarct-related artery reperfusion: Results of the GUSTO ST segment monitoring study. *J Am Coll Cardiol* 1995; 25 (7): 1552–7.

30 Klootwijk P, Langer A, Meij S *et al.* Noninvasive prediction of reperfusion and coronary artery patency by continuous ST segment monitoring in the GUSTO-I trial. *Eur Heart J* 1996; 17: 689–98.

31 Dellborg M, Riha M, Swedberg K. Dynamic QRS-complex and ST-segment monitoring in acute myocardial infarction during recombinant tissue-type plasminogen activator therapy. The TEAHAT Study Group. *Am J Cardiol* 1991; 67 (5): 343–9.

32 Dellborg M, Herlitz J, Risenfors M, Swedberg K. Electrocardiographic assessment of infarct size: comparison between QRS scoring of 12-lead electrocardiography and dynamic vectorcardiography. *Int J Cardiol* 1993; 40 (2): 167–72.

33 Langer A, Freeman M, Armstrong P. ST segment shift in unstable angina: Pathophysiology and association with coronary anatomy and hospital outcome. *J Am Coll Cardiol* 1989; 13 (7): 1495–502.

34 Patel D, Holdright D, Knight C *et al.* Early continuous ST segment monitoring in unstable angina: prognostic value additional to the clinical characteristics and the admission electrocardiogram. *Heart* 1996; 75: 222–8.

35 Holmvang L, Andersen K, Dellborg M *et al.* Relative contributions of a single-admission 12-lead electrocardiogram and early 24-hour continuous electrocardiographic monitoring for early risk stratification in patients with unstable coronary artery disease. *Am J Cardiol* 1999; 83 (5): 667–74.

36 Norgaard BL, Andersen K, Dellborg M, Abrahamsson P, Ravkilde J, Thygesen K. Admission risk assessment by cardiac troponin T in unstable coronary artery disease: additional prognostic information from continuous ST segment monitoring. TRIM study group. Thrombin Inhibition in Myocardial Ischemia. *J Am Coll Cardiol* 1999; 33 (6): 1519–27.

37 Klootwijk P, Meij S, Melkert R, Lenderink T, Simoons ML. Reduction of recurrent ischemia with abciximab during continuous ECG-ischemia monitoring in patients with unstable angina refractory to standard treatment (CAPTURE). *Circulation* 1998; 98 (14): 1358–64.

38 Krucoff M. Identification of high-risk patients with silent myocardial ischemia after percutaneous transluminal coronary angioplasty by multilead monitoring. *Am J Cardiol* 1988; 61: 29F–34F.

39 Krucoff M, Parente A, Bottner R *et al.* Stability of multilead ST-segment 'fingerprints' over time after percutaneous

transluminal coronary angioplasty and its usefulness in detecting reocclusion. *Am J Cardiol* 1988; 61: 1232–7.

40 Bush H, Ferguson J, Angelini P, Willerson J. Twelve-lead electrocardiographic evaluation of ischemia during percutaneous transluminal coronary angioplasty and its correlation with acute reocclusion. *Am Heart J* 1991; 121 (6): 1591–9.

41 Gustafsson G, Dellborg M, Lindahl B, Wallentin L. Dynamic vectorcardiography for early diagnosis of acute myocardial infarction compared with 12-lead electrocardiogram. BIOMACS Study Group. *Coron Artery Dis* 1996; 7 (12): 871–6.

42 Lundin P, Eriksson S, Erhardt L, Strandberg L-E, Rehnqvist N. Continuous vectorcardiography in patients with chest pain indicative of acute ischemic heart disease. *Cardiology* 1992; 81: 145–56.

43 Fesmire FM, Smith EE. Continuous 12-lead electrocardiograph monitoring in the emergency department. *Am J Emerg Med* 1993; 11 (1): 54–60.

44 Mangano DT, Browner WS, Hollenberg M, London MJ, Tubau JF, Tateo IM. Association of perioperative myocardial ischemia with cardiac morbidity and mortality in men undergoing noncardiac surgery. The Study of Perioperative Ischemia Research Group [see comments]. *N Engl J Med* 1990; 323 (26): 1781–8.

45 Stark K, Krucoff M, Schryver B, Kent K. Quantification of ST-segment changes during coronary angioplasty in patients with left bundle branch block. *Am J Cardiol* 1991; 67: 1219–22.

46 Hackett D, Davies G, Chierchia S, Maseri A. Intermittent coronary occlusion in acute myocardial infarction. Value of combined thrombolytic and vasodilator therapy. *N Engl J Med* 1987; 317 (17): 1055–9.

47 Ito H, Okamura A, Iwakura K *et al.* Myocardial perfusion patterns related to thrombolysis in myocardial infarction perfusion grades after coronary angioplasty in patients with acute anterior wall myocardial infarction. *Circulation* 1996; 93 (11): 1993–9.

48 Kwon K, Freedman B, Wilcox I *et al.* The unstable ST segment early after thrombolysis for acute infarction and its usefulness as a marker of recurrent coronary occlusion. *Am J Cardiol* 1991; 67 (2): 109–15.

49 Krucoff M, Croll M, Pope J *et al.* Continuously updated 12-lead ST-segment recovery analysis for myocardial infarct artery patency assessment and its correlation with multiple simultaneous early angiographic observations. *Am J Cardiol* 1993; 71: 145–51.

50 Ohman M, Califf R, Topol E *et al.* Consequences of reocclusion after successful reperfusion therapy in acute myocardial infarction. *Circulation* 1990; 82 (3): 781–91.

51 Barbash G, Roth A, Hod H *et al.* Rapid resolution of ST elevation and prediction of clinical outcome in patients undergoing thrombolysis with alteplase (recombinant tissue-type plasminogen activator): results of the Israeli Study of Early Intervention in Myocardial Infarction. *Br Heart J* 1990; 64: 241–7.

52 Schröder R, Dissmann R, Brüggemann T *et al.* Extent of early segment elevation resolution; A simple but strong predictor of outcome in patients with acute myocardial infarction. *J Am Coll Cardiol* 1994; 24 (2): 384–91.

53 Mauri F, Maggioni A, Franzosi M *et al.* A simple electrocardiographic predictor of the outcome of patients with acute myocardial infarction treated with thrombolytic agent. A gruppo Italiano per lo studio della Sopravvivenza nell'Infarto Miocardico (GISSI-2)—Derived Analysis. *J Am Coll Cardiol* 1994; 24: 600–7.

54 Veldkamp RF, Green CL, Wilkins ML *et al.* Comparison of continuous ST-segment recovery analysis with methods using static electrocardiograms for noninvasive patency assessment during acute myocardial infarction. Thrombolysis and Angioplasty in Myocardial Infarction (TAMI) 7 Study Group. *Am J Cardiol* 1994; 73 (15): 1069–74.

55 Abrahamsson P, Andersen K, Eriksson P, Dellborg M. Prognostic value of maximum ST-vector magnitude during the first 24 h of vectorcardiographic monitoring in patients with unstable angina pectoris. *Eur Heart J* 1999; 20 (16): 1166–74.

7: Biochemical tests in suspected acute coronary syndromes: which test when?

Paul O. Collinson and Peter J. Stubbs

The rationale for biochemical diagnostic tests

The electrocardiogram (ECG) remains the most important first diagnostic test in the management of patients who present with suspected acute coronary syndromes (ACS), although the diagnostic accuracy of the ECG is only 55–75% [1–4]. In an audit of patients presenting to a typical district general hospital (DGH) only 10% of the patients presented with characteristic ECG changes (Fig. 7.1). Thus, biochemical criteria are needed to confirm or exclude a diagnosis of acute myocardial infarction (AMI) for 90% of patients who present with suspected ACS. The ECG helps in identifying patients who are candidates for interventions such as thrombolysis, but it does not provide a definitive diagnostic test for AMI [5,6].

Currently available biochemical markers in routine clinical use

Biochemical tests for diagnosis of myocardial damage can be divided into cytosolic catalytic proteins and structural proteins (Table 7.1). The original World Health Organization (WHO) criteria for the diagnosis of AMI include the use of cardiac enzymes [7,8] with measured values exceeding twice the upper reference limit. The WHO criteria do not prescribe which enzymes should be used, or the sampling frequency. The *de facto* standard has been measurement of creatine kinase (CK) and its MB isoenzyme (CK-MB). Measurement of CK-MB was first performed by electrophoresis. This has been replaced by measurement of CK-MB activity and latterly by measurement of CK-MB mass.

The range of tests offered by individual laboratories varies from country to country. Despite clinical studies and rigorous statistical analysis which have shown that CK-MB is the best of the current enzymes [9–11] and CK-MB mass to be the best test [12–14], routine measurement of CK-MB mass is not performed in all laboratories. The routine clinical practice in many UK hospitals is the measurement of 'daily cardiac enzymes', often a combination of CK,

Table 7.1 Typical figures for currently available markers to indicate timing for optimal diagnostic accuracy.

Marker	Time to reach maximum sensitivity		Sensitivity	Specificity
	Onset of symptoms	From admission		
Cytosolic				
Myoglobin	4	2	90	80
CK	24	18	90	90
CK-MB activity	20	16	95	95
CK-MB mass	16	12	100	100
Delta myoglobin	3	1	100	80
Delta CK	6	4	100	90
Delta CK-MB	6	4	100	95
Structural				
cTnT	16	12	100	100
cTnI	16	12	100	100

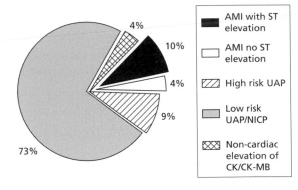

Legend:
- AMI with ST elevation
- AMI no ST elevation
- High risk UAP
- Low risk UAP/NICP
- Non-cardiac elevation of CK/CK-MB

4%, 10%, 4%, 9%, 73%

Fig. 7.1 Final diagnosis of patients admitted with suspected acute coronary syndromes. NICP, Non-ischaemic chest pain; UAP, unstable angina pectoris.

aspartate transaminase and lactate dehydrogenase. This approach is of little value to the clinician and often does not contribute to patient management. In centres where CK-MB tests are offered, only the activity measurement may be available and then only when total CK is elevated. This approach is fundamentally flawed since CK-MB, especially CK-MB mass, is more sensitive than CK alone [12–14]. Initial measurement of CK followed by measurement of CK-MB only if total CK is elevated will fail to detect MI in 5% of patients in whom it could be detected by CK-MB measurement [15,16]. The use of CK-MB/CK ratio to distinguish between cardiac and non-cardiac elevations of CK is unreliable [17].

A more proactive approach is required. The existing biochemical tests can be used more efficiently. Diagnosis can be achieved reliably within 12 h from admission by serial measurement of myoglobin, CK or CK-MB [18–22]. The use of rate of change of these markers, delta values, allows very early, accurate diagnostic categorization of patients with suspected ACS into those with or without AMI within as little as 2–4 h from admission [23–25]. The advent of real-time immunoassay means the laboratory is now able to provide a 24-hour, 7-day-a-week service precisely and accurately measuring CK-MB mass.

Immunoassays for the cardiac structural proteins, cardiac troponin T (cTnT) and cardiac troponin I (cTnI) provide detection of a marker that is completely specific for cardiac damage [17]. In situations in which there is substantial elevation of CK such as arduous physical training, marathon running or endurance cycling, there is no elevation of cTnT or cTnI [17,26–29]. It has been shown recently that even when only minor elevation of cTnT or cTnI occur following extreme endurance competition, cardiac dysfunction is evident [30]. Conversely, there is no rise in cTnT or cTnI after DC cardioversion [31–33].

Measurement of cTnT and cTnI appears to be 100% sensitive for the diagnosis of AMI. The specificity of both markers in non-AMI populations with unstable angina has been reported to be less than 100% [34–37]. This result arises because of reliance on CK-MB mass as the 'gold standard' against which all other tests are evaluated. The classification of patients positive for AMI becomes circular. AMI is diagnosed when CK-MB mass is elevated, making CK-MB mass measurement by definition 100% sensitive and specific. Cardiac TnT has not been detected in the serum of anyone in a large normal population. In patients with a final diagnosis of unstable angina, detectable cTnT and cTnI in the serum predicts risk of cardiac death and recurrent cardiac events [38–45]. Risk is proportional to the degree of both cTnT [40] and cTnI elevation [43]. This explains the apparent reduction in specificity of the cardiac troponins. Measurement of cTnT and cTnI detects small degrees of myocardial necrosis not detected by conventional markers. In this respect, it has been noted that small elevations of CK-MB do occur in patients with suspected ACS and that these are associated with a poor prognosis. Histologically, microinfarcts due to plugging of small arteries by platelet aggregates have been demonstrated. These platelet microemboli arise due to platelet aggregation on a ruptured unstable plaque which then break off and lodge distally [46,47]. The presence of cTnT and cTnI in the serum is often indicative of an active unstable plaque.

In patients with unstable angina pectoris (UAP), cTnT and cTnI can be combined with other diagnostic modalities. In patients admitted without ST segment elevation, measurement of cTnT on admission and at 12–24 h from admission allows separation into high-, intermediate- and low-risk categories (Fig. 7.2) [48]. Both admission and peak cTnT values can be combined with ECG category (ST depression, T wave inversion, normal ECG or uncodeable ECG) to allow further prognostic risk stratification [40,49]. Measurement of

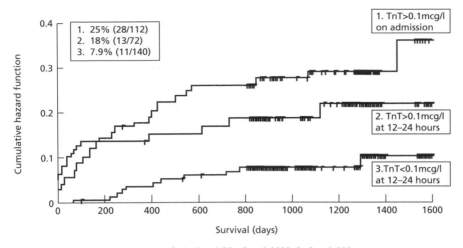

Fig. 7.2 Cardiac death as first event according to timing of Troponin T measurement and concentration in patients admitted with chest pain without ST-segment elevation—survival curves in patients presenting without ST-segment elevation according to presence of cTnT ≤0.1 μg/l on admission or 12–24 h from admission. (Adapted from Collinson, P.O. *European Heart J* 1998; 19: (supplement N) N16–24.

cTnT can be combined with the stress ECG [50] and ST segment monitoring [51,52]. Patients with undetectable cTnT and a negative stress test are at very low risk. In patients admitted with ST segment elevation, measurement of cTnT provides additional prognostic information [49,53]. An elevated cTnT on admission correlates with failure to achieve TIMI 3 flow [54] but does not correlate with time of onset of symptoms [55].

cTnT measurements can be used to guide the need for therapy in patients with unstable angina. Revascularization in patients with unstable angina who have elevated cTnT values leads to a reduction of cardiac events [41]. Measurement of cTnT can be used to identify patients with a reduced ejection fraction in whom ACE inhibitors will be beneficial [56]. Because detectable cTnT and cTnI in the serum is often indicative of platelet aggregation and platelet emboli *in vivo*, drugs inhibiting thrombosis may be maximally effective in patients with elevated values. The response to low molecular weight heparin [57] and to inhibitors of the glycoprotein IIb/IIIa receptor is better in patients in whom cTnT can be detected [58,59]. Measurement of cTnT can therefore be used to guide therapy.

A scheme delineating the current utility of the available tests is shown in Table 7.1. Although time from onset of symptoms is often quoted in the literature, in routine clinical practice its estimation is unreliable because of several factors including perception of symptoms by the patient, denial of illness and true silent infarction [60–62]. We have found that even when a detailed history is taken, including time of occurrence of worst chest pain, in 30% of patients the reported duration of symptoms does not correspond to the time of onset of the acute event. Hence, the only accurately recorded time that can be relied upon is the time of admission.

In formulating a policy for the use of cardiac markers a number of questions must be addressed. Typically biochemical testing is only used primarily or exclusively to rule in or rule out AMI. However:

> The challenge is not always simply to rule in or rule out myocardial infarction, but rather to distinguish patients with acutely unstable coronary lesions from those with either stable coronary disease or none.   Eagle. N Engl J Med 1991; 325: 1250

Hence the requirements for a cardiac marker strategy must take into account its value with respect to the following.

1 Confirming the diagnosis of AMI — 'rule in diagnosis' — maximal sensitivity.
2 Excluding AMI as a cause of suspected acute coronary syndromes (ACS) — 'rule-out' diagnosis — maximal specificity.
3 Allowing prognostic risk stratification.
4 Identifying patients who will respond to interventions.

It is no longer acceptable solely to divide patients into those with AMI or those without AMI with the use of the conventional WHO criteria. Ischaemic heart disease entails a spectrum of pathophysiology with full-thickness transmural Q-wave AMI representing one extreme through stable angina induced by exercise with a flow-limiting stenosis to asymptomatic coronary atheroma at the other. Seventy per cent of cardiac events occur in patients without a flow-limiting stenosis. Clinical studies have shown that cardiac troponin measurements can predict to outcome, which is important in an era of cost containment and evidence-based medicine. The ability to detect prognostically significant myocardial damage means that it is necessary to reconsider current diagnostic criteria incorporating both new laboratory methods and therapeutic approaches. The measurement of cardiac troponin can reveal the presence of unsuspected myocardial damage. Several methods are available for cTnI determinations. Results are not necessarily the same with each. The lack of standardization of cTnI methods from different manufacturers and problems relating to differing epitope recognition and epitope stability have led to confusion [63–65].

Strategies for clinical decision making in patients with suspected ACS incorporating biochemical testing

An integrated clinical decision-making strategy for management of chest pain and suspected ACS is required. It entails the use of the initial clinical and ECG findings together with admission values of cardiac markers to assign patients into risk categories (Fig. 7.3a). Thereafter, the strategy followed will depend on the risk group. Results with the three modalities, clinical findings, ECG results and measurement of biochemical markers are additive and inclusive, not exclusive. The initial clinical assessment and ECG are required to assign the appropriate prior probability of disease. Thereafter, an appropriate test strategy is aimed at using the sensitivity and specificity of the markers appropriately.

The interaction of test sensitivity and specificity with the prior probability of disease is extremely important and is summarized in Table 7.2. In the coronary care unit (CCU) setting when the prior probability of ischaemic heart disease (IHD) is high most tests will perform well. The importance then is to have a high sensitivity to detect myocardial damage. In the Emergency Department (ED) setting the prior probability is lower. Thus, the lower specificity of CK and CK-MB mass will result in an appreciable number of false positives. These problems can be overcome by measurement of cTnT or cTnI. The prior probability of disease can be used to advantage when designing a test strategy, as will be discussed later. One disadvantage of cardiac troponin measurement is related to persistent elevations. This means that timing of the onset of infarction can be difficult unless multiple samples are taken. For this reason the use of a second marker with a different temporal profile is desirable. The choice here is between myoglobin, CK or CK-MB. In reality, CK is readily available and has a low cost. It would therefore seem sensible to use this. In conclusion, strategies for using biochemical markers for elevation of patients with acute chest pain should be based on the following criteria.

1 The clinical efficiency of the tests.
2 The use to which the information will be put.
3 The probability of disease.

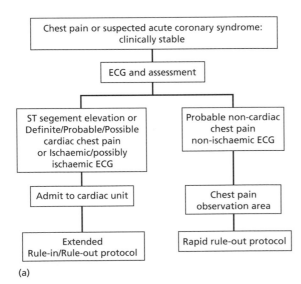

(a)

Fig. 7.3 (a) Initial diagnostic categorization. (b) Extended rule-in/rule-out prognostic risk stratification protocol for patients admitted with a high probability of ischaemic heart disease. (c) Rapid rule-out protocol—patients considered at low risk for ACS scheduled for discharge from the ED.

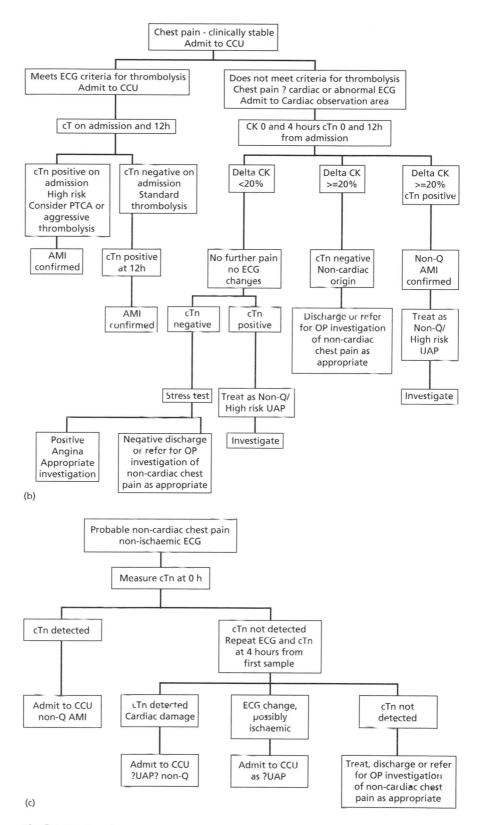

Fig. 7.3 *Continued.*

Table 7.2 Categorization of patients by risk group.

Selection criteria	Incidence of AMI	Prevalence of IHD	Strategy

ECG–ST segment elevation	95–99%	99%	Opening the artery
			  Thrombolysis
			  PTCA
			Rule in AMI

Non-specific ECG change Clinical suspicion	20%	50%	Rule out AMI Rule in IHD
No ECG changes Atypical clinical features	5%	10%	Rule out AMI Rule out IHD

AMI, acute myocardial infarction; ECG, electrocardiogram; IHD, ischaemic heart disease; PTCA, percutaneous transluminal coronary angioplasty.

Marker	Admission	4 hours	12 hours
Cardiac troponin	x	x	x
CK/CK-MB	x	x	x

Table 7.3 Sampling times for markers in patients admitted with suspected ACS.

An attractive sampling strategy is summarized in Table 7.3. The actual strategy used within any given institution will be constrained by the organization of and resources for patient care, which may influence the template. The algorithms shown have been developed and are in general use in a typical UK DGH (community hospital) and were developed to provide a cost-effective modification.

Integrated chest pain management including biochemical markers

Initial categorization will be into patients at high and low risk of IHD (Fig. 7.3a). Thereafter, management will be by an extended rule-out protocol (Fig. 7.3b) or a rapid rule-out protocol (Fig. 7.3c).

Extended protocols for patients admitted with a high probability of IHD (Fig. 7.3b)

Patients presenting with a definite diagnosis of AMI

These patients will present with ST segment elevation, with or without the presence of new Q-waves. In such patients the probability of AMI is 95–99%.

The role of biochemical testing is to confirm the diagnosis of AMI for the purpose of audit and to quantify the effect of damage. This can be achieved by a single troponin measurement 12–24 h from admission. Measurement of cTnT at this time point correlates with the extent of damage and can be used to predict the subsequent ejection fraction. A secondary role for cardiac markers may be to determine whether reperfusion has occurred. The rate of change of concentrations of markers such as myoglobin may be particularly helpful [66]. Whether monitoring ST segment change alone is sufficient has not been determined. Measurement of cTnT on admission can be used for prognostic risk stratification in patients admitted with ST segment elevation. It is likely that in this group aggressive revascularization therapy will be needed. Hence a policy of admission and 12-h cTn measurement should be sufficient.

Patients admitted to hospital with a suspected diagnosis of ACS

Most patients admitted to hospital with suspected ACS do not have AMI. Most are either low-risk patients with IHD or have non-cardiac causes of chest pain. The objectives in this group are as follows.

1 *To identify patients at low risk of subsequent cardiac events for early stepdown care and evaluation.*

Measurement of both cTnT and cTnI provides prognostically useful risk stratification criteria. The literature on cTnT is extensive, compared to cTnI. The measurement of cTnT can therefore be combined with the admission ECG, ECG monitoring and stress ECG to identify low-risk patients. Patients with no cTnT detectable at 12–24 h can be followed in a stepdown unit. Patients with no ECG changes, no detectable cTnT and a negative stress test can be rapidly discharged. Subsequent follow up will depend on clinical judgement. For patients presenting with a single episode of chest pain and without a history of previous IHD, further cardiac outpatient follow up is unlikely to be beneficial. The combination of a short time window marker (CK or CK-MB) with cTn (cardiac troponin) measurement is sufficient. This strategy has the potential for very rapid (within 24 h) risk stratification with potential for major cost savings [67,68].

2 *To identify those at high risk who require evaluation.*

The presence of detectable cTnT indicates patients who may benefit from early revascularization and treatment with low molecular weight heparin and a glycoprotein IIb/IIIa antagonist. In those in whom cTnT is not detectable at 12–24 h, such therapy can be discontinued with further evaluation as outlined above. In patients admitted with ACS, 100% sensitivity is achieved only 12 h after admission; hence, a sample should be taken on admission and at least 12 h later for cTn measurement.

The combined strategy of assaying CK or CK-MB plus a troponin allows

Table 7.4 Diagnostic classification in patients with IHD presenting with ACS combining current and new markers.

ECG	CK/CK-MB	Cardiac	Diagnostic category troponin
ST-segment elevation	Exceeds upper discriminant	Positive	AMI (classical Q-wave AMI)
No ST-segment elevation	Exceeds upper discriminant	Positive	AMI (non-Q-wave AMI)
No ST-segment elevation	Does not exceed upper discriminant	Positive	UAP with myocardial necrosis
No ST-segment elevation	Does not exceed upper discriminant	Negative	UAP without myocardial necrosis

The discriminant for CK or CK-MB can be the upper reference limit, twice the upper reference limit or a significant delta value. The choice will alter the number of patients in the borderline classified as AMI rather than UAP with myocardial necrosis.
The discriminant for cardiac troponin is the upper reference limit for the assay.

Table 7.5 Diagnostic classification based on new markers and ECG.

ECG	CK/CK-MB	Cardiac troponin	Diagnostic category
ST-segment elevation	Exceeds upper discriminant	Positive	AMI
No ST-segment elevation	Does not exceed upper discriminant	Positive	ACS with myocardial necrosis
No ST-segment elevation	Does not exceed upper discriminant	Negative	ACS without myocardial necrosis

timing of occurrence of events and permits diagnostic classification that can be related to existing guidelines whilst incorporating the value of cardiac troponin measurement (Table 7.4). Abnormal cTn measurements have been defined differently for UAP and for AMI [69,70]. Using diagnostic criteria based on CK-MB mass by WHO criteria, Gerhardt showed that 9% of patients with a final diagnosis of AMI had cTnT values within the UAP discriminant band [71]. The distinction between non-Q-wave AMI and cTn positive unstable angina may be arbitrary. The distinction between non-Q-wave AMI and cTn positive UAP may not alter treatment (Table 7.5), but whether such patients should be referred to as having sustained 'AMI' remains a matter of discussion.

Rapid rule-out protocol—patients considered at low risk for ACS scheduled for discharge from emergency facilities (Fig. 7.3c)

The incidence of missed AMI has been estimated to be 11.8% in an audit of patients discharged from an ED [72]. The figure usually quoted is 6–8% of all ED discharges [73,74]. Strategies to reduce the incidence of missed AMI have included the use of serial measurements of cardiac markers and the use of delta values. Protocols have been developed utilizing serial measurements over short time frames (4–9 h) followed by stress testing or radionucleide imaging. More recently the use of cardiac troponins has been studied.

Results of measurement of cTnT and cTnI at the point of care (POCT, point of care testing) have been shown to be equivalent to those obtained in laboratory testing and can be used in the ED [75]. Follow up of patients discharged from the ED in whom cTnT and cTnI are not detected 4 h from admission (≥6 h from onset of chest pain) has shown an event rate of <1%. This is consistent with our experience. In patients identified on the basis of clinical and ECG criteria to be at low risk of IHD (prevalence ≤5%) a strategy of measurement of cardiac troponin on admission and 4 h from admission will allow early discharge or appropriate study or follow up. It must be remembered that this will not detect 100% of all patients, but the risk of subsequent cardiac events in patients without ECG change, negative cTn and atypical symptoms is extremely low. Subsequent stress testing or radionucleide imaging can identify those at risk.

Detection of the cytosolic and cardiac structural proteins often reflects the consequence of plaque rupture. It may be possible by measurement of markers of platelet activation such as p-selectin to identify even earlier consequences of plaque rupture.

References

1 McQueen M, Holder D, El-Maraghi N. Assessment of the accuracy of serial electrocardiography in the diagnosis of acute myocardial infarction. *Am Heart J* 1983; 105: 258–61.

2 Zarling EJ, Sexton H, Milnor P. Failure to diagnose acute myocardial infarction. *JAMA* 1983; 250: 1177–81.

3 Brush JE, Brand DA, Acampora A, Chalmer B, Wackers FJ. Use of the admission electrocardiogram to predict in-hospital complications of acute myocardial infarction. *N Engl J Med* 1985; 312: 1137–41.

4 Yusuf S, Pearson M, Sterry H *et al*. The entry ECG in the early diagnosis and prognostic stratification of patients with suspected acute myocardial infarction. *Eur Heart J* 1984; 5: 690–6.

5 Fibrinolytic Therapy Trialists Collaborative Group. Indications for fibrinolytic therapy in suspected acute myocardial infarction: collaborative overview of early mortality and major morbidity results from all randomised trials of more than 1000 patients. *Lancet* 1994; 343: 311–22.

6 Effects of tissue plasminogen activator

and a comparison of early invasive and conservative strategies in unstable angina and non Q-wave myocardial infarction. Results of the TIMI IIIBTrial. Thrombolysis Myocardial Ischemia *Circulation* 1994; 89: 1545–56.

7 WHO Working group on establishment of ischaemic heart disease registers. Report of fifth working group. Copenhagen. World Health Organisation. *WHO Eur* 1972; 821 (5).

8 Task Force on Standardisation of Clinical Nomenclature. *Circulation* 1979; 59: 607–9.

9 Lee TH, Goldman L. Serum enzyme assays in the diagnosis of acute myocardial infarction. *Ann Int Med* 1986; 105: 221–33.

10 Werner M, Brooks SH, Mohrbacher RJ, Wasserman AG. Diagnostic performance of enzymes in the discrimination of myocardial infarction. *Clin Chem* 1982; 28: 1297–302.

11 Leung FY, Galbraith LV, Jablonsky G, Henderson AR. Re-evaluation of the diagnostic utility of serum total creatine kinase and creatine kinase-2 in myocardial infarction. *Clin Chem* 1989; 35: 1435–40.

12 Mair J, Artner-Dworzak E, Dienstl A *et al.*
Early detection of acute myocardial infarction by measurement of mass concentration of creatine kinase-MB. *Am J
Cardiol* 1991; 68: 1545–50.

13 Collinson PO, Rosalki SB, Kuwana T *et al.*
Early diagnosis of acute myocardial in-
farction by CK-MB mass measurements.
Ann Clin Biochem 1992; 29: 43–7.

14 Gerhardt W, Katus H, Ravkilde J *et al.* S-
Troponin T in suspected ischaemic
myocardial injury compared with mass
and catalytic concentrations of S-creatine
kinase isoenzyme B. *Clin Chem* 1991;
37: 1405–11.

15 Heller GV, Blaustein AS, Wei JY. Implications of increased myocardial isoenzyme
level in the presence of normal serum creatine kinase activity. *Am J Cardiol* 1983;
51: 24–7.

16 Clyne CA, Medeiros LJ, Marton KI. The
prognostic significance of immuno-
radiomeric CK-MB (IRMA) diagnosis
of myocardial infarction in patients
with a low total CK and elevated MB
isoenzymes. *Am Heart J* 1989; 118:
901–6.

17 Collinson PO, Chandler HA, Stubbs PJ,
Moseley DS, Lewis D, Simmons MD. Cardiac troponin T and CK-MB concentration in the differential diagnosis of
elevated creatine kinase following arduous physical training. *Ann Clin Biochem*
1995; 32: 450–3.

18 Collinson PO, Rosalki SB, Flather M,
Wolman R, Evans T. Early diagnosis of
myocardial infarction by timed sequential
enzyme measurements. *Ann Clin Biochem*
1988; 25: 376–82.

19 Gibler WB, Runyon JP, Levy RC *et al.* A
rapid diagnostic and treatment centre for
patients with chest pain in the emergency
department. *Ann Emerg Med* 1995; 25:
1–8.

20 Brogan GX Jr, Friedman S, McCuskey C *et
al.* Evaluation of a new rapid quantitative
immunoassay for serum myoglobin versus
CK-MB for ruling out acute myocardial
infarction in the emergency department.
Ann Emerg Med 1994; 24: 665–71.

21 Lindahl B, Venge P, Wallentin L. Early
diagnosis and exclusion of acute myocardial infarction using biochemical monitoring. *Coron Artery Dis* 1995; 6: 321–8.

22 Gibler WB, Young GP, Hedges JR for the
Emergency Medicine Cardiac Research

Group. Early detection of acute myocardial infarction in patients presenting with
chest pain and non-diagnostic ECGs:
serial CKMB sampling in the emergency
department. *Ann Emerg Med* 1990; 19:
1359–66.

23 Collinson PO, Stubbs PJ. 4 hour 'rule-in'
diagnosis of acute myocardial infarction
for early risk stratification by creatine
kinase increment (CK change). *Ann Clin
Biochem* 1996; 33: 308–13.

24 Mair J, Smidt J, Lechleiter P, Dienstl F,
Puschendorf B. Rapid accurate diagnosis
of acute myocardial infarction in patients
with non-traumatic chest pain within 1
hour of admission. *Coron Artery Dis*
1995; 6: 539–45.

25 Young GP, Gibler WB, Hedges JR *et al.* for
the EMREG II study group. Serial creatine
kinase-MB results are a sensitive indicator
of acute myocardial infarction in chest
pain patients with non-diagnostic electrocardiograms: The second emergency
medicine cardiac research group study.
Acad Emerg Med 1997; 4: 869–77.

26 Artner-Dworzak E, Mair J, Seibt I, Koller
A, Haid C, Puschendorf B. Cardiac tro-
ponin T identifies unspecific increases of
CK-MB after physical exercise (letter).
Clin Chem 1990; 36: 1853.

27 Mair J, Wohlfarter T, Koller A, Mayer M,
Artner-Dworzak E, Puschendorf B. Serum
troponin T after extraordinary endurance
exercise (letter). *Lancet* 1992; 340: 1048.

28 Adams JE, Bodor GS, Davila-Roman VG
et al. Cardiac troponin I, a marker with
high specificity for cardiac injury. *Circulation* 1993; 88: 101–6.

29 Muller-Bardorff M, Hallermayer K,
Schroder A *et al.* Improved troponin T
ELISA specific for cardiac troponin T isoform: assay development and analytical
and clinical validation. *Clin Chem* 1997;
43: 458–66.

30 Rifai N, Douglas PS, O'Toole M, Rimm E,
Ginsburg GS. Cardiac troponin T and I,
electrocardiographic wall motion analyses, and ejection fractions in athletes par-
ticipating in the Hawaii Ironman
Triathlon. *Am J Cardiol* 1999; 83:
1085–9.

31 Garre L, Alvarez A, Rubio M *et al.* Use of
cardiac troponin T rapid assay in the diagnosis of a myocardial injury secondary to
electrical cardioversion. *Clin Cardiol*
1997; 20: 619–21.

32 Bonnefoy E, Chevalier P, Kirkorian G, Guidolet J, Marchand A, Touboul P. Cardiac troponin I does not increase after cardioversion. *Chest* 1997; 111: 15–18.

33 Rao ACR, Naeem N, John C, Collinson PO, Canepa-Anson R, Joseph SPDC. Cardioversion does not cause cardiac damage: evidence from cardiac troponin T estimation. *Heart* 1998; 80: 229–30.

34 Mair J, Artner-Dworzak E, Lechleitner P, Smidt J, Wagener I, Dienstl F *et al*. Cardiac Troponin T in diagnosis of acute myocardial infarction. *Clin Chem* 1991; 37: 845–52.

35 Collinson PO, Moseley D, Stubbs PJ, Carter GD. Troponin T for the differential diagnosis of ischaemic myocardial damage. *Ann Clin Biochem* 1993; 30: 11–16.

36 Wu AHB, Valdes R, Apple FS, Gornet I, Stone MA, Mayfield-Stokes S *et al*. Cardiac troponin T immunoassay for diagnosis of acute myocardial infarction. *Clin Chem* 1994; 40: 900–7.

37 Baum H, Braun S, Gerhardt W *et al*. Multicenter evaluation of a second-generation assay for cardiac troponin T. *Clin Chem* 1997; 43: 1877–84.

38 Hamm CW, Ravkilde J, Gerhardt W *et al*. The prognostic value of serum Troponin T in unstable angina. *N Engl J Med* 1992; 327: 146–50.

39 Ravkilde J, Horder M, Gerhardt W *et al*. The predictive value of cardiac Troponin T in serum of patients suspected of acute myocardial infarction. *Scand J Clin Invest* 1993; 53: 677–85.

40 Lindahl B, Venge P, Wallentin L. Relation between troponin T and the risk of subsequent cardiac events in unstable coronary artery disease. *Circulation* 1996; 93: 1651–7.

41 Stubbs P, Collinson P, Moseley D, Greenwood T, Noble M. Prospective study of the role of cardiac troponin T in patients admitted with unstable angina. *BMJ* 1996; 313: 262–4.

42 Wu AHB, Lane PL. Meta-analysis in clinical chemistry: Validation of cardiac troponin T as a marker for ischaemic heart disease. *Clin Chem* 1995; 41 (B): 1228–33.

43 Antman EM, Tanasijevic MJ, Thompson B *et al*. Cardiac specific troponin I levels to predict the risk of mortality in patients with acute coronary syndromes. *N Engl J Med* 1996; 335: 1342–9.

44 Galvani M, Ottani F, Ferrini D *et al*. Prognostic influence of elevated values of cardiac troponin I in patients with unstable angina. *Circulation* 1997; 95: 2053–9.

45 Panteghini M, Bonora R, Pagani F. Rapid and specific immunoassay for cardiac troponin I in the diagnosis of myocardial damage. *Int J Clin Lab Res* 1997; 27: 60–4.

46 Falk E. Unstable angina with fatal outcome: dynamic coronary thrombosis leading to infarction and/or sudden death. Autopsy evidence of recurrent mural thrombosis with peripheral embolization culminating in total vascular occlusion. *Circulation* 1985; 71: 699–708.

47 Davies MJ, Thomas AC, Knapman PA, Hangartner JR. Intramyocardial platelet aggregation in patients with unstable angina suffering sudden ischemic cardiac death. *Circulation* 1986; 73: 418–27.

48 Collinson PO. Troponin T or Troponin I or CK-MB (or none?). *Eur Heart J* 1998; 19 (Suppl. N): N16–24.

49 Ohman ME, Armstrong PW, Christenson RH *et al*. Cardiac troponin T levels for risk stratification in acute myocardial ischaemia. *N Engl J Med* 1996; 335: 1333–41.

50 Lindahl B, Andren B, Ohlsson J, Venge P, Wallentin L. Risk stratification in unstable coronary artery disease. Additive value of troponin T determinations and predischarge exercise tests. FRISK Study Group *Eur Heart J* 1997; 18: 762–70.

51 Hudson MP, White HD, Anderson RD *et al*. Bedside risk stratification using both troponin T and ST-segment resolution in acute myocardial infarction: a GUSTO II sub-study. *Circulation* 1999; 98 (Suppl.) 1–493.

52 Jernberg T, Isaksson A, Lindahl B, Wallentin L. Prognostic importance of troponin T and continuous 12 lead ischaemia monitoring with the ST-guard system. *Circulation* 1999; 98 (Suppl.) 1–424.

53 Stubbs P, Collinson P, Moseley D, Greenwood T, Noble M. Prognostic significance of admission troponin T concentrations in patients with myocardial infarction. *Circulation* 1996; 94: 1291–7.

54 Ramanathan K, Stewart JT, Theroux P, French JK, White HD. Admission Troponin T level may predict 90 minute TIMI III flow after thrombolysis. *Circulation* 1997; 96 (Suppl.): 1–270.

55 Ohman EM, Armstrong PW, Weaver WD *et al*. Prognostic value of a whole blood qualitative Troponin T testing in patients with acute myocardial infarction in the GUSTO-III trial. *Circulation* 1997; 96 (Suppl.): 1–216.

56 Rao AC, Collinson PO, Canepa-Anson R, Joseph SP. Troponin T measurement after myocardial infarction can identify left ventricular ejection of less than 40%. *Heart* 1998; 80: 223–5.

57 Lindahl B, Venge P, Wallentin L. Troponin T identifies patients with unstable coronary artery disease who benefit from long-term antithrombotic protection. Fragmin in Unstable Coronary Artery Disease (FRISC) Study Group. *J Am Coll Cardiol* 1997; 29: 43–8.

58 Hamm CW, Heeschen C, Goldman B *et al*. Benefit of acbciximab in patients with refractory unstable angina in relation to serum troponin T levels. *N Engl J Med* 1999; 340: 1623–9.

59 Heeschen C, Hamm CW, Goldman B, Deu A, Langenbrink L, White HD. Troponin concentrations for stratification of patients with acute coronary syndromes in relation to therapeutic efficacy of tirofiban. *Lancet* 1999; 354: 1757–62.

60 Barsky AJ, Hochstrasser B, Coles NA, Zisfein J, O'Donnell C, Eagle KA. Silent myocardial ischaemia. Is the person or the event silent? *JAMA* 1990; 264: 1132–5.

61 Hofgren C, Karlson BJ, Herlitz J. Prodromal symptoms in subsets of patients hopitalised for suspected acute myocardial infarction. *Heart Lung* 1995; 24: 3–10.

62 Ruston A, Clayton J, Calnan M. Patients' actions during their cardiac event: qualitative study exploring differences and modifiable factors. *BMJ* 1998; 316: 1060–5.

63 Wu AH, Feng YJ, Moore R *et al*. Characterization of cardiac troponin subunit release into serum after acute myocardial infarction and comparison of assays for troponin T and I. American Association for Clinical Chemistry Subcommittee on cTnI Standardisation. *Clin Chem* 1998; 44: 1198–208.

64 Katrukha AG, Bereznikova AV, Filatov VL *et al*. Degradation of cardiac troponin I. implication for reliable immunodetection. *Clin Chem* 1998; 44: 2433–40.

65 Apple FS. Clinical and analytical standardisation issues confronting cardiac troponin I. *Clin Chem* 1999; 45: 18–20.

66 Apple FS. Biochemical markers of thrombolytic success. *Scand J Clin Lab Invest* 1999; 59 (Suppl. 230): 60–6.

67 Collinson PO. Cost economics of new cardiac markers—CK-MB and cardiac troponins. In: Kaski CJ, Holt D, eds. *Myocardial Damage: Early Detection by Novel Biochemical Markers*. The Netherlands: Kluwer Academic Publishers B. V., 1998: 173–87.

68 Collinson PO. The need for point of care testing evidence-based appraisal. *Scand J Clin Lab Invest* 1999; 59 (Suppl. 230): 67–73.

69 Wu AHB, Apple FS, Gibler WB, Jesse RL, Warshaw MM, Valdes R. National Academy of Clinical Biochemistry Standards of Laboratory Practice: Recommendations for the use of cardiac markers in Coronary Artery Diseases. *Clin Chem* 1999; 45: 1104–21.

70 Panteghini M, Apple FS, Christenson RH *et al*. Recommendations on use of biochemical markers of cardiac damage in acute coronary syndromes. *Scand J Clin Lab Invest* 1999; 59 (Suppl. 230): 103–12.

71 Gerhardt W, Ljungdahl NG. Can troponin T replace CK-MB mass as 'gold standard' for Acute Myocardial Infarction ('AMI')? *Scand J Clin Lab Invest* 1999; 59 (Suppl. 230): 83–9.

72 Emerson PA, Russel NJ, Wyatt J *et al*. An audit of doctors' management of patients with chest pain in the accident and emergency department. *Q J Med* 1989; 70: 213–20.

73 Lee TH. Clinical characteristics and natural history of patients sent home from the emergency room. *Am J Cardiol* 1987; 60: 220–4.

74 McCarthy BD, Beshansky JR. Missed diagnosis of acute myocardial infarction in the emergency department: Results from a multicentre study. *Ann Emerg Med* 1993; 22: 579–82.

75 Hamm CW, Goldmann BU, Heeschen C, Kreymann G, Berger J, Meinertz T. Emergency room triage of patients with acute chest pain by means of rapid testing for cardiac troponin T or troponin I. *N Engl J Med* 1997; 337: 1648–53.

8: What is the role of MRI in coronary syndromes?

Penelope R. Sensky and Graham R. Cherryman

Magnetic resonance imaging (MRI) is a rapidly evolving and powerful non-invasive tool for the diagnosis and evaluation of patients with coronary artery disease (CAD). It has great potential to aid clinical decision-making and patient management. Early MRI of the heart was beset by long scanning times and technical difficulties caused by cyclic cardiac motion and respiration. The development of ultrafast imaging techniques and cardiac dedicated hardware has markedly facilitated the implementation and clinical utility of cardiac MRI. Magnetic resonance (MR) scanners with cardiac imaging capability are now available in many centres.

The integrated cardiac MRI examination

A striking advantage of MRI, compared with other diagnostic procedures, is that it has the potential to offer an integrated examination of cardiac anatomy, myocardial function and perfusion, coronary vasculature and myocardial metabolism (Table 8.1). Three-dimensional reconstruction of the heart and great vessels can be achieved with commercially available image post-processing software. The physics of image acquisition are discussed elsewhere [1]. A list of the current MRI techniques available for cardiac imaging, together with their clinical applications, is shown in Table 8.2.

Cardiac anatomy

The high spatial resolution of MRI and the ability to image in any orientation permits finely detailed delineation of cardiac structures and morphology. The epicardial and endocardial borders can be easily defined. Intrinsic tissue contrast can be enhanced with the use of paramagnetic contrast agents. Intra-cardiac and extra-cardiac structures such as masses, thrombi and pericardial abnormalities can be visualized (Fig. 8.1).

Table 8.1 Advantages and disadvantages of cardiac MRI.

Technique	Myocardial perfusion	Myocardial function	Myocardial strain	Coronary vasculature	Myocardial metabolism	Invasive	Ionizing radiation	Spatial resolution
MRI	+	+	+	±	+	−	−	~1 mm
TTE	±	+	−	−	−	−	−	~1–2 mm
SPECT	+	+	−	−	±	−	+	~6–10 mm
PET	+	−	−	−	+	−	+	~5–8 mm
CA	−	+	−	+	−	+	+	~0.5–2 mm

CA, coronary angiography; PET, positron emission tomography; SPECT, single photon emission computed tomography; TTE, transthoracic echocardiography.

Table 8.2 Cardiac applications of MRI techniques.

Clinical application	MRI technique
Cardiac structure/anatomy	ECG-gated spin echo
	Segmented breath-hold cine-GRE
Global and regional ventricular function/ chamber volumes/LV mass	Segmented breath-hold cine-GRE
	Real time imaging
Myocardial perfusion	Contrast-enhanced snapshot FLASH (saturation/ inversion recovery)
	Echo-planar imaging
Aortic disease	Breath-hold MR angiography
	Segmented breath-hold cine-GRE
Coronary artery/aortic flow velocity	Velocity-encoded segmented cine-GRE
Coronary artery imaging	Fat-saturated segmented GRE

FLASH, fast low angle shot; GRE, gradient recalled echo.

Myocardial function

MR images acquired throughout the cardiac cycle facilitate evaluation of regional (Fig. 8.1c,d) and global myocardial function. They can be presented in a cine format and subjected to frame-by-frame analysis for quantitative assessment of myocardial thickening [2]. Repeated short-axis slices, encompassing the entire myocardium, can be stacked to calculate left and right ventricular mass, ejection fraction and cardiac volumes. When measured by MRI, these variables have been shown to be accurate and highly reproducible [3], reflecting precise myocardial border discrimination and whole heart coverage. Thus, the reliance on geometric assumptions required by echocardiography and ventriculography is not needed.

With the use of a localized radiofrequency saturation technique, a tagged grid that deforms with cardiac motion can be superimposed on the image

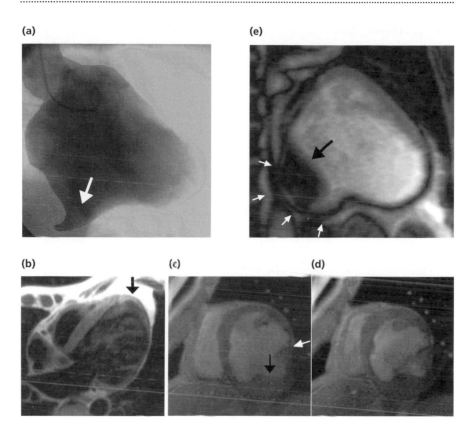

Fig. 8.1 MR images from a patient with a remote inferior infarction. (a) Left ventriculography showed an apparent false aneurysm (arrow). (b) Fat suppression excluded the presence of pericardial blood (arrow). End-diastolic (c) and systolic (d) short axis cine frames showed a thinned lateral wall (white arrow), thickened inferior wall (arrow) and poor systolic function. (e) Contrast enhancement (vertical long axis) revealed a true inferobasal aneurysm (white arrows) containing a large thrombus (black arrow), explaining the angiographic appearance.

(Fig. 8.2a). The nodes of the grid can be used to track the exact in-plane, through-plane and rotational displacement of the ventricle during the cardiac cycle. The information obtained permits correction of any quantitative calculations to account for complicated ventricular movements. Subendocardial and epicardial thickening, myocardial strain and wall stress can be measured based on the extent of grid deformation. The dynamic spatial parameters of the grid nodes can be reconstructed to create 3-D models of the working cardiac pump [4].

Valvular leaflet morphology and motion can be visualized with the use of standard cine sequences. Abnormal valvular jets can be identified by the presence of signal voids in the cardiac chambers (Fig. 8.2d). Velocity-encoded cine sequences facilitate the quantification of valvular and vascular blood flow [5].

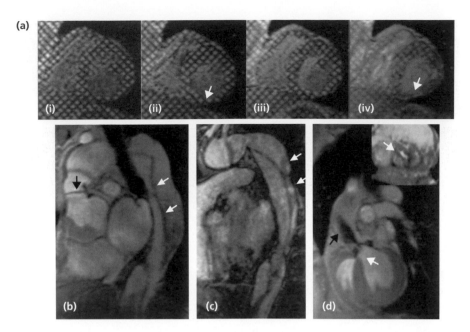

Fig. 8.2 (a) End-diastolic (i, iii) and systolic (ii, iv) tagged cine frames showing resting inferior hypokinesia (ii, arrow) and dobutamine-induced inferior dyskinesia (iv, arrow) in a patient with right coronary artery stenosis. (b) Ascending aortic graft (black arrow) and descending aortic dissection (white arrows). (c) MR angiography of an aortic dissection extending into the descending aorta (arrows). (d) Cine images demonstrating thickened aortic valve leaflets (white arrows) and a high velocity jet (black arrow) in a patient with aortic stenosis.

Myocardial perfusion

The advent of ultrafast subsecond imaging to track the changing MR variables following the first pass of a contrast agent bolus has stimulated the increasing use of MRI to evaluate myocardial perfusion. The contrast media in clinical use (gadolinium chelates) act by shortening the T1 relaxation rate of the myocardium. Although they are not purely intravascular agents, being taken up into the myocardial interstitium, their uptake during the first pass circulation has been shown to be related to blood flow in both animal and human studies [6]. Figure 8.3a shows a typical first pass perfusion sequence. With current scanners, the image quality is sufficient to allow a qualitative assessment of perfusion defects [7]. However, there is considerable interest in using MRI to quantify regional myocardial blood flow. Approaches are complicated by the distribution kinetics of the gadolinium compounds. Semi-quantitative methods for analysing the signal intensity curves have been proposed [8,9]. However, for absolute quantification, complicated mathematical models are mandatory [10,11]. Imaging planes have to be sacrificed to provide optimal temporal resolution to track the first pass circulation of a contrast bolus. Thus,

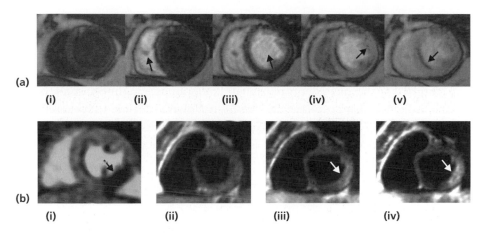

Fig. 8.3 (a) Sequential first pass perfusion images during adenosine infusion from a patient with a severe right coronary artery stenosis. The bolus of gadolinium contrast (arrows) appears first in the right ventricle (RV, ii) and then in the left ventricular cavity (LV, iii). Normally perfused myocardium is enhanced (arrow, iv). An inferoseptal subendocardial perfusion deficit is seen (arrow, v). (b) (i) First pass image demonstrating a full thickness lateral wall infarction. Spin echo images from the same patient pre-contrast (ii), at 15 minutes (iii) and 30 minutes (iv) after a contrast bolus. Note the increasing signal enhancement with time in the area of infarction (white arrows).

a compromise between cardiac coverage and quantitative model requirements has to be reached. Techniques in development, such as echo-planar imaging, may reduce the need for any such concessions. Future improvements in automated edge-detection software for image analysis will improve the practical application of quantitative methods.

Coronary vasculature

Much research is directed towards visualization of the coronary arterial tree [12]. The challenges facing MRI include the high spatial resolution required, the tortuous anatomical course of the coronary vessels and the sensitivity of the images to cardiac and respiratory motion. Recent approaches have incorporated ECG and respiratory gating, saturation pulses to suppress fat from the image, contrast angiography and complex 3-D post-processing programs. Large clinical studies are likely to be justified only when the rapid rate of technical advancement in this area reaches a plateau [13]. Current clinical applications permit evaluation of left main stem disease and the detection of coronary vessel anatomical anomalies. The measurement of flow reserve provides an indirect method for establishment of coronary artery patency. This technique can also be used to assess the internal mammary arteries [14] and aortocoronary bypass grafts [15].

Myocardial metabolism

MR spectroscopy offers a means by which to study the metabolic characteristics of ischaemic myocardium and infarction. Most studies have concentrated on the high-energy phosphate compounds, e.g. the phosphocreatinine:adenosine triphosphate ratio has been shown to decline after exercise in patients with CAD before revascularization but not after corrective surgery [16]. At present, MR spectroscopy is not widely available and remains a research tool.

Application of MRI to coronary artery disease

MRI as a diagnostic tool

As with other investigative tools for the diagnosis of CAD, the accuracy of MRI is augmented by increasing the cardiac workload. In a conventional clinical scanner, there is limited room for the subject to perform physical exercise. Thus pharmacological stress agents are employed.

Myocardial function

Regional wall motion abnormalities are a hallmark of myocardial ischaemia. In patients with clinically significant disease they may be present at rest, ranging from mild hypokinesia with ischaemia to dyskinesia with infarction. Dobutamine is the optimal agent for the precipitation of stress-induced myocardial ischaemia. It increases both myocardial contractility and the rate-pressure product, resulting in an oxygen supply demand mismatch in territories supplied by stenosed coronary vessels. Echocardiographic data have demonstrated the diagnostic and prognostic value of dobutamine stress examinations [17]. Long imaging times and difficulty in ECG-gating during inotrope-induced tachycardias hampered initial work with MRI. However, despite the use of only a modest dose of dobutamine, MRI demonstrates comparable diagnostic sensitivities and specificities compared with those of stress echocardiography and scintigraphy (Table 8.3) [2,17,18]. Modern MR sequences have facilitated the use of optimal stress regimens. Using a high-dose dobutamine–atropine protocol, Nagel *et al.* proved that MRI is superior to dobutamine stress echocardiography for the detection of CAD [20]. MRI had an 86% (98% in patients with three-vessel disease) positive and an 86% negative predictive accuracy for the detection of CAD. In their study, transthoracic echocardiography had a 74% positive and 70% negative diagnostic accuracy. The favourable MRI result appeared to be attributable entirely to the excellence of image quality. The difficulties with suboptimal acoustic

Table 8.3 Investigative methods for the detection of angiographic coronary artery disease.

Modality	Sensitivity	Specificity
Db wall motion MRI [2]	91%	80%
Exercise electrocardiography [18]	64%	30%
Db echocardiography [17]	72–86%	77–95%
Db MIBI-SPECT [18]	95%	71%

CA, coronary angiography; Db, dobutamine; MIBI-SPECT, [99]technetium- single photon emission computed tomography.

windows and subendocardial delineation that plague stress echocardiography were surmounted.

Myocardial perfusion

Disruption of myocardial perfusion is an early phenomenon in the pathophysiology of myocardial ischaemia. Hypoperfusion initially affects the subendocardium. The spatial resolution of the traditional perfusion imaging modalities is insufficient to evaluate the subendocardial layer *per se*. However, MRI is ideal for this purpose. Perfusion imaging is performed optimally with a vasodilating stress agent such as dipyridamole or adenosine. Both agents initiate a four- to five-fold increase in blood flow, enhancing heterogeneity of myocardial perfusion in patients with CAD because of the relative or absolute lack of increased flow distal to coronary obstructive lesions. In our institution, adenosine is the preferred agent because its short half-life is beneficial in terms of limiting patient side-effects and facilitating the remainder of the examination. The longer half-life of dipyridamole can produce prolonged myocardial ischaemia and increase the duration of any adverse events, thus compromising further imaging. If adenosine is contraindicated, dobutamine can be used, but a submaximal vasodilatory effect is obtained [21].

Perfusion MRI has been compared with other modalities (Table 8.4) [8–11]. The computation of regional myocardial perfusion reserve, i.e. the ratio of maximal blood flow during hyperaemia to basal blood flow, may improve the accuracy and clinical application of perfusion imaging [10]. A potential role for perfusion MRI lies in the appreciation of the end-organ effects of coronary atheroma. The functional significance of single and sequential coronary artery lesions and collateral vessel development on myocardial perfusion can be evaluated. In addition, measurement of myocardial perfusion reserve may prove to be a valuable means of assessing patients with angina with angiographically normal coronary arteries [11].

Comparison	Findings
*MRI vs. CA [8]	70% agreement
*MRI vs. SPECT [8]	90% agreement
*MRI vs. CA and SPECT [9]	65% sensitivity, 76% specificity
†MRI MPR vs. CFR [11]	Correlation: $r = 0.8$
†MRI MPRI vs. CA stenosis diameter [10]	Correlation: $r = -0.81$

Table 8.4 MRI stress perfusion studies.

* adenosine; † dipyridamole.
CA, coronary angiography; CFR, coronary flow reserve; MPR(I), myocardial perfusion reserve (index); SPECT, single photon emission computed tomomography.

Differential diagnosis

MRI is useful in assessment of chest pain that cannot be attributed clearly to myocardial ischaemia, e.g. in the detection of pericardial abnormalities, pulmonary emboli and aortic disease. Haemorrhagic pericardial fluid and pericardial fat (Fig. 8.1b) have characteristic signal intensities. The high spatial resolution of MRI allows detailed assessment of pericardial thickening. MRI has the potential to be as accurate as traditionally used techniques for the identification of pulmonary emboli [22]. Breath-hold MR angiography has become the imaging method of choice for the initial and continued assessment of patients with aortic disease [23]. MRI is of particular value in patients with aortic dissection (Figs 8.2b,c). The site and extent of the dissection, true and false lumen anatomy and blood flow can be delineated. In addition, the integrity of the aortic valve and the involvement of the abdominal vasculature, i.e. the coeliac axis and renal arteries, can be readily appreciated. The rapid acquisition of such accurate information delineating anatomical detail is invaluable in the planning of surgical interventions.

MRI in myocardial infarction

Characteristic MR features are present in patients with acute and remote myocardial infarction (MI). In acute infarction, changes in relaxation times caused by myocardial oedema characterize the injured tissue. These changes are seen on T2 imaging and are enhanced by the use of contrast agents [24] (Fig. 8.3b). A perfusion defect can be seen in the immediate period post-infarction. A study of 103 patients 2–6 days after presentation delineated regional hypoperfusion on first pass imaging in 72.5% [25]. Hypoperfusion was more likely to be seen in patients with full-thickness (Q-wave) anterior infarction. Perfusion MRI may have a role in the differentiation between reperfused and non-reperfused infarcts. We have observed a trend towards normality with early treatment with thrombolytic drugs.

Remote MI is depicted by the presence of thinned, akinetic or dyskinetic regions. The spatial extent of the territory of infarction can be assessed together with acquisition of an accurate and reproducible measure of ejection fraction. The clear definition of the epicardial and endocardial borders provided by MRI makes it an ideal tool with which to evaluate the remodelling process following infarction, i.e. the wall thinning in the injured territory and the compensatory hypertrophy in spatially remote regions. The attenuation of this deleterious process, induced by drug therapy, has been demonstrated with MRI in experimental animals [26]. Certainly, the non-invasive nature of MRI makes it eminently suitable for serial assessments after potentially therapeutic strategies in human subjects. In particular, the use of tagging techniques to evaluate wall stress between adjacent zones of infarction and remote territories is likely to play an important role in such applications.

The catastrophic sequelae that can follow MI, such as true and false ventricular aneurysm formation, ventricular thrombi (Fig. 8.1), pericardial effusions, haemopericardium and tamponade with free wall rupture, ventricular septal defects and mitral regurgitation, can be evaluated easily.

Assessment of myocardial hibernation and viability

A rapidly developing use of cardiac MRI is in the detection of myocardial hibernation. Hibernating myocardium is a state of apparently persistent left ventricular contractile dysfunction that is fully reversible with reperfusion [27]. It appears to reflect repeated stunning in tissue with adequate perfusion to maintain viability at rest but inadequate flow reserve to preclude ischaemia with physiological stress. Its identification is vital in the assessment of patients with global or regional myocardial impairment. In comparison with behaviour of myocardial scar tissue, territories consisting predominantly of hibernating tissue show functional improvement following successful revascularization. The recognition of myocardial hibernation is based on the following properties: a recruitable contractile reserve accompanying increased perfusion or transiently increased stimulation, preserved basal metabolic perfusion and preserved cell membrane integrity.

Contractile reserve

A key diagnostic feature of hibernating myocardium is a recruitable contractile reserve following stimulation with low doses of agents with positive inotropic effects. Stress echocardiography is employed traditionally to detect this, but it is both subject and operator dependent. Dobutamine MRI has a

Table 8.5 Comparison of techniques for the assessment of viability.

Modality	Sensitivity	Specificity	Standard parameter
Db MRI [28]	94%	100%	FDG-PET
Db TOE [29]	77%	81%	FDG-PET
Db MRI [30]	89%	94%	LV recovery*
Db echocardiography [31]	94%	80%	LV recovery*
Thallium reinjection scintigraphy [31]	100%	80%	LV recovery*
Thallium redistribution [31]	91%	50%	LV recovery*

* Post-revascularization.
Db, dobutamine; FDG-PET, 18-fluorodeoxyglucose positron emission tomography; TOE, transoesophageal echocardiography.

high specificity and sensitivity for detection of hibernation (Table 8.5) [28–30]. The myocardial edge discrimination available with cine MRI techniques has enabled investigators to assess variables quantitatively. Baer *et al.* found that induced systolic thickening greater than 2 mm predicted left ventricular recovery following revascularization with 89% sensitivity and 94% specificity [30]. Mathematical physiologically based models, predicting the extent of left ventricular recovery after revascularization and the addition of quantitative MRI tagging methods, should increase the potential utility of functional MRI.

Preservation of perfusion

The preservation of sufficient perfusion to sustain myocardial metabolism and cell membrane integrity is clearly vital for cell viability. A hypoenhancement pattern, seen on contrast-enhanced first pass and early pseudoequilibrium imaging, has been shown to be a predictor of poor recovery following acute MI [32]. This sign appears to represent microvascular injury and compression from extracellular oedema, and it is typically seen in the centre of an infarction. Reversible perfusion defects and those limited to the subendocardial region alone may be indicative of hibernation. Biochemical data and evidence from positron emission tomography (PET) studies suggest that a minimum resting blood flow of 0.25–0.3 ml/g/min is required to maintain cell viability [33]. With the use of quantitative MRI techniques, it may be possible to measure not only perfusion under conditions of rest, but also myocardial perfusion reserve.

Cell membrane integrity

The signal intensity enhancement seen with delayed contrast imaging may be a marker of non-viable myocardium. This principle exploits the low molecular weight of MRI contrast media and the resulting free distribution of contrast between the intravascular and extracellular spaces. A breach in cell membrane integrity increases interstitial accumulation of contrast medium and changes the tissue signal characteristics. Measurement of the contrast fractional distribution has been proposed as a means of distinguishing normal from necrotic myocardial tissue. Wendland *et al.* demonstrated an increase in fractional distribution in relation to the severity of graded myocardial injury in experimental animals [34]. Further clinical research is required to determine whether this method can quantify the percentage of non-viable cells within an infarct zone.

Clinical application

Although the identification of myocardial hibernation is important in the assessment of patients after MI, it is of greatest consequence in patients with significant left ventricular dysfunction being considered for revascularization procedures. The coronary artery surgery study (CASS) demonstrated the benefit of surgical revascularization compared with medical therapy in patients with low ejection fractions. However, patients with left ventricular impairment have substantial perioperative morbidity and mortality [35]. Thus, the decision to proceed with a revascularization procedure needs to be based on sound criteria. Information required by the surgeon ideally includes accurate assessment of ejection fraction, the site of regional wall dysfunction, the extent of myocardial hibernation and scar, and the extent and reversibility of regional perfusion abnormalities. Thus, integrated examination of cardiac structure, function and perfusion is likely to be particularly valuable.

We have developed a dual adenosine–dobutamine stress (DADS) MRI protocol that is designed to provide optimal preoperative assessment [36]. Functional imaging is used to measure ejection fraction and assess regional systolic wall thickening at rest and during a two-step low-dose dobutamine infusion. The latter is used to evaluate the presence or absence of contractile reserve in resting dysfunctional segments. The first pass of gadolinium-DTPA at rest and during adenosine infusion provides information relevant to the transmural extent and reversibility of perfusion defects. The MRI findings can be correlated accurately with the angiographically delineated anatomy obtained by superimposing a Green Lane report on a bull's eye display of the MRI data [7] (Fig. 8.4). The protocol can be completed in less than an hour and is safe, well tolerated and provides valuable and comprehensive information.

MRI in coronary artery disease: limitations and safety

Conventional contraindications to MRI also apply to cardiac patients (Table 8.6). Permanent pacemaker systems were originally thought to be an absolute contraindication to MRI. However, there is now evidence to show that certain

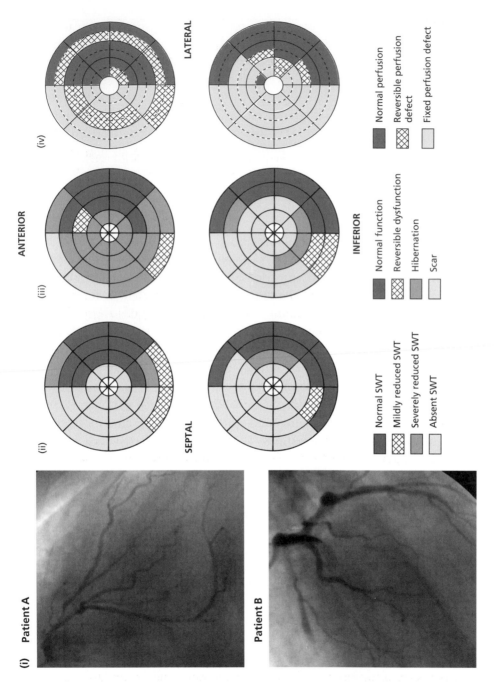

Fig. 8.4 Polar maps displaying regional MRI data from two patients with an anteroseptal MI and angiographic left anterior descending artery occlusion (i). Concentric rings from outside to inside represent the short axis slices: maps (ii) and (iii) basal, papillary and apical; map (iv) basal epicardium (EP) and subendocardium (SE), papillary EP and SE, and apical EP and SE. SE is indicated by a dashed outer border. The shading key is shown below each map. Maps indicate: resting systolic wall thickening (SWT) (ii); regional characterization with low dose dobutamine (iii) and evaluation from rest and adenosine stress perfusion scans (iv). In both patients there is absent anteroseptal thickening at rest. In patient A, significant hibernating myocardium is seen with dobutamine and there is some evidence of perfusion defect reversibility in the area of infarction. The infarction zone in patient B consists predominantly of scar tissue. No reversibility of the defect is seen on perfusion imaging. Revascularization should be considered in Patient A, but is unlikely to be beneficial in patient B.

Table 8.6 Standard contraindications to magnetic resonance imaging.

Metallic implants
Intra-cranial clips
Intra-ocular foreign bodies/implants
Cochlear implants
Shrapnel
Pacemakers *(see text)*/internal cardiac defibrillators
Temporary pacing devices/Swan-Ganz catheters
Dehiscing Starr-Edwards prosthetic valves (1960–1964)
Clinical instability
Contraindications to stress agents (if required)
Contraindications to contrast agents (if required)
Pregnancy/breast-feeding
Severe claustrophobia

pacing units are unaffected by 0.5 Tesla machines [37]. However, a marked temperature rise has been demonstrated in some types of electrodes in higher magnetic fields [38]. Thus, the presence of an implanted pacing system remains a relative contraindication to MRI in the majority of patients. The only valve prostheses contraindicated are Starr-Edwards valves produced between 1960 and 1964, and then only if clinical dehisence is suspected [5]. There have been no reports to suggest that the magnet adversely affects coronary artery stents. Most companies have taken the conservative position that stents should be allowed to endothelialize undisturbed. However, the literature suggests that stents can be scanned early after placement [39]. Safety is an important consideration for patients undergoing stress MRI. An adequate electrocardiogram tracing, blood pressure monitoring and supervision by trained personnel are mandatory. An experienced reader should view scans immediately after acquisition.

MRI as a research tool

MRI has enormous potential as a cardiac research tool. An important factor for clinical studies is that no ionizing radiation is required, ensuring that serial studies are safe. The multiple aspects of ischaemia that can be evaluated during a single examination make MRI an ideal means to study the complex manifestations and pathophysiology of CAD. Perfusion imaging is already being used to assess the value of established and novel revascularization options, such as transmyocardial laser revascularization and gene therapy.

Future directions

Progress in the development of cardiac dedicated scanners, image quality and acquisition speed of imaging sequences over the last few years has been exponential. It has resulted from collaborations between clinicians, researchers, physicists and industry. Numerous clinical studies are in progress. The need for prospective multicentre research has been recognized. As cardiologists and radiologists become more familiar with current MRI techniques and their clinical applications in patients with CAD, integrated cardiac examination by magnetic resonance is likely to become a clinical investigation of choice in the very near future.

References

1 Axel L. Physics and technology of cardiovascular MR imaging. *Cardiol Clin* 1998; 16: 125–33.

2 van Rugge FP, van der Wall EE, Spanjersberg SJ *et al.* Magnetic resonance imaging during dobutamine stress for detection and localization of coronary artery disease. Quantitative wall motion analysis using a modification of the centerline method. *Circulation* 1994; 90: 127–38.

3 Martin ET, Fuisz AR, Pohost GM. Imaging cardiac structure and pump function. *Cardiol Clin* 1998; 16: 135–60.

4 Bundy JM, Lorenz CH. TAGASIST. a post-processing and analysis tools package for tagged Magnetic Resonance Imaging. *Comput Med Imaging Graph* 1997; 21: 225–32.

5 Schmidt M, Crnac J, Dederichs B, Theissen P, Schicha H, Sechtem U. Magnetic resonance imaging in valvular heart disease. *Int J Card Imaging* 1997; 13: 219–31.

6 Wilke N, Simm C, Zhang J *et al.* Contrast-enhanced first pass myocardial perfusion imaging: correlation between myocardial blood flow in dogs at rest and during hyperemia. *Magn Reson Med* 1993; 29: 485–97.

7 Sensky PR, Jivan A, Hudson NM *et al.* Coronary artery disease: combined stress MR imaging protocol–one-stop evaluation of myocardial perfusion and function. *Radiology* 2000; **215**: 608–14.

8 Eichenberger AC, Schuiki E, Kochli VD *et al.* Ischemic heart disease: assessment with gadolinium-enhanced ultrafast MR imaging and dipyridamole stress. *J Magn Reson Imaging* 1994; 4: 425–31.

9 Matheijssen NA, Louwerenburg HW, van Rugge FP *et al.* Comparison of ultrafast dipyridamole magnetic resonance imaging with dipyridamole SestaMIBI SPECT for detection of perfusion abnormalities in patients with one-vessel coronary artery disease: assessment by quantitative model fitting. *Magn Reson Med* 1996; 35: 221–8.

10 Cullen JH, Horsfield MA, Reek CR *et al.* A myocardial perfusion reserve index in humans using first-pass contrast-enhanced magnetic resonance imaging. *J Am Coll Cardiol* 1999; 33: 1386–94.

11 Wilke N, Jerosch-Herold M, Wang Y *et al.* Myocardial perfusion reserve: assessment with multisection, quantitative, first-pass MR imaging. *Radiology* 1997; 204: 373–84.

12 Danias PG, Edelman RR, Manning WJ. Coronary MR angiography. *Cardiol Clin* 1998; 16: 207–25.

13 Duerinckx AJ. Coronary MR angiography. *Radiol Clin North Am* 1999; 37: 273–318.

14 Miller S, Scheule AM, Hahn U *et al.* MR angiography and flow quantification of the internal mammary artery graft after minimally invasive direct coronary artery bypass. *Am J Roentgenol* 1999; 172: 1365–9.

15 Molinari G, Sardenelli F, Zandrino F, Balzan C, Masperone MA. Magnetic resonance assessment of coronary artery bypass grafts. *Rays* 1999; 24: 131–9.

16 Bottomley PA, Weiss RG. Human cardiac spectroscopy. *Magma* 1998; 6: 157–60.

17 Krahwinkel W, Ketteler T, Godke J *et al.* Dobutamine stress echocardiography. *Eur Heart J* 1997; 18 (Suppl. D): D9–15.

18 Senior R, Sridhara BS, Anagnostou E, Handler C, Raftery EB, Lahiri A. Synergistic value of simultaneous stress dobutamine sestamibi single-photon-emission computerized tomography and echocardiography in the detection of coronary artery disease. *Am Heart J* 1994; 128: 713–18.

19 Baer FM, Voth E, Theissen P, Schicha H, Sechtem U. Gradient-echo magnetic resonance imaging during incremental dobutamine infusion for the localization of coronary artery stenoses. *Eur Heart J* 1994; 15: 218–25.

20 Nagel E, Lehmkuhl HB, Bocksch W *et al.* Noninvasive diagnosis of ischemia-induced wall motion abnormalities with the use of high-dose dobutamine stress MRI. Comparison with dobutamine stress echocardiography. *Circulation* 1999; 99: 763–70.

21 Orlandi C. Pharmacology of coronary vasodilation: a brief review. *J Nucl Cardiol* 1996; 3: S27–S30.

22 Bongartz G, Boos M, Scheffler K, Steinbrich W. Pulmonary circulation. *Eur Radiol* 1998; 8: 698–706.

23 Biederman RW, Fuisz AR, Pohost GM. Magnetic resonance angiography. *Curr Opin Cardiol* 1998; 13: 430–7.

24 van der Wall EE, Vliegen HW, de Roos A, Bruschke AV. Magnetic resonance imaging in coronary artery disease. *Circulation* 1995; 92: 2723–39.

25 Cherryman GR, Jivan A, Tranter J *et al.* The prevalence, utility and relationship to first pass regional hypo-enhancement of boundary zone equilibrium phase hyper-enhancement in patients with acute myocardial infarction. *Proceedings of ISMRM* 1999: 24.

26 Zierhut W, Rudin M, Robertson E *et al.* Time course of spirapril-induced structural and functional changes after myocardial infarction in rats followed with magnetic resonance imaging. *J Cardiovasc Pharmacol* 1993; 21: 937–46.

27 Rahimtoola SH. Clinical aspects of hibernating myocardium. *J Mol Cell Cardiol* 1996; 28: 2397–401.

28 Baer FM, Voth E, Schneider CA, Theissen P, Schicha H, Sechtem U. Comparison of low-dose dobutamine-gradient-echo magnetic resonance imaging and positron emission tomography with [18F]fluorodeoxyglucose in patients with chronic coronary artery disease. A functional and morphological approach to the detection of residual myocardial viability. *Circulation* 1995; 91: 1006–15.

29 Baer FM, Voth E, LaRosee K *et al.* Comparison of dobutamine transesophageal echocardiography and dobutamine magnetic resonance imaging for detection of residual myocardial viability. *Am J Cardiol* 1996; 78: 415–19.

30 Baer FM, Theissen P, Schneider CA *et al.* Dobutamine magnetic resonance imaging predicts contractile recovery of chronically dysfunctional myocardium after successful revascularization. *J Am Coll Cardiol* 1998; 31: 1040–8.

31 Haque T, Furukawa T, Takahashi M, Kinoshita M. Identification of hibernating myocardium by dobutamine stress echocardiography: comparison with thallium-201 reinjection imaging. *Am Heart J* 1995; 130: 553–63.

32 Rogers WJ, Kramer CM, Geskin G *et al.* Early contrast-enhanced MRI predicts late functional recovery after reperfused myocardial infarction. *Circulation* 1999; 99: 744–50.

33 Gewirtz H, Fischman AJ, Abraham S, Gilson M, Strauss HW, Alpert NM. Positron emission tomographic measurements of absolute regional myocardial blood flow permits identification of nonviable myocardium in patients with chronic myocardial infarction. *J Am Coll Cardiol* 1994; 23: 851–9.

34 Wendland MF, Saeed M, Arheden H *et al.* Toward necrotic cell fraction measurement by contrast-enhanced MRI of reperfused ischemically injured myocardium. *Acad Radiol* 1998; 5 (Suppl. 1): S42–S44.

35 Alderman EL, Fisher LD, Litwin P *et al.* Results of coronary artery surgery in patients with poor left ventricular function (CASS). *Circulation* 1983; 68: 785–95.

36 Sensky PR, Jivan A, Cherryman GR *et al.* Stress magnetic resonance imaging for the evaluation of hibernating myocardium: a one-stop assessment of regional left ventricular function and perfusion. *Proceedings of ISMRM* 1999: 24.

37 Lauck G, von Smekal A, Wolke S *et al.* Effects of nuclear magnetic resonance imaging on cardiac pacemakers. *Pacing Clin Electrophysiol* 1995; 18: 1549–55.

38 Achenbach S, Moshage W, Diem B, Bieberle T, Schibgilla V, Bachmann K. Effects of magnetic resonance imaging on cardiac pacemakers and electrodes. *Am Heart J* 1997; 134: 467–73.

39 Kramer CM, Rogers WJ, Mankad SV *et al.* Short- and long term safety of magnetic resonance imaging soon after stenting for acute myocardial infarction. *Proceedings of SCMR* 1999: 24.

9: Advance imaging — PET

Paolo G. Camici and Terry J. Spinks

Introduction

Positron emission tomography (PET) offers unrivalled sensitivity and specificity for research to unravel biochemical pathways and pharmacological mechanisms *in vivo* [1]. This is so because of the availability of short-lived isotopes of biological elements and the manner in which their emissions are detected. Cardiological and neurological research with PET has flourished for more than 20 years, but it is only relatively recently that clinical cardiology has begun to benefit. From the physical point of view, scanning the heart presents more challenges than scanning the brain because of greater complexity for correction for photon attenuation and scattered radiation and because of heart and respiratory motion [2–4]. A distinction has been made in the evolution of positron tomography between so-called 2-D and 3-D modes of scanning. These will be explained below and refer essentially to detection 'efficiency'. Higher efficiency (3-D) is not straightforward because of the more rigorous corrections that have to be applied to the data and the much greater volumes of data and processing times required [5–7].

Positron emitting tracers

The success of PET is founded on the properties of the isotopes listed in Table 9.1. Their short half-lives make it possible to administer a tracer dose high enough to obtain useful data, with a radiation burden to the patient that is acceptably low [8]. Production of isotopes with the shortest half-lives has to be carried out in the immediate vicinity of the scanner and necessitates the installation of cyclotron and radiochemistry facilities. However, ^{18}F compounds can be delivered from a relatively remote site of production. The commercial success of PET has been driven by ^{18}F-labelled fluorodeoxyglucose (FDG) which is used to measure glucose metabolism in the brain, heart and tumours. Trapping of FDG in the metabolic pathway gives images of good quality, although only relative, as opposed to absolute, metabolic rates [9]. Many

Table 9.1 Physical characteristics of the most common positron emitting isotopes.

Isotope	Half-life (min)	Position energy (MeV)		Mean range in tissue (mm)	Examples of labelled compounds
		Mean	Maximum		
^{15}O	2.03	0.74	1.74	2.97	$H_2{}^{15}O$—blood flow $^{15}O_2$—oxygen consumption $C^{15}O$—blood volume
^{13}N	10.0	0.49	1.20	1.73	$^{13}NH_3$—blood flow
^{11}C	20.4	0.39	0.97	1.23	^{11}C-HED and ^{11}C-CGP— pre-and postsynaptic autonomic function ^{11}C-MQNB muscarinic receptors
^{18}F	109.8	0.25	0.64	0.61	^{18}F-FDG—metabolism ^{18}F-Fdopa—dopamine storage

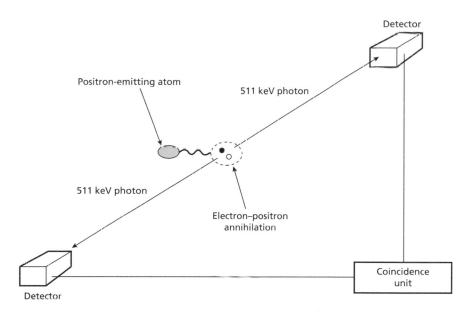

Fig. 9.1 Physics of positron emission, annihilation and coincidence detection.

centres, particularly in the USA, rely on production from a centralized cyclotron and thus avoid the expense of individual facilities. However, research centres aiming to derive most from the power of PET require on-site production of a range of tracers.

Positrons emitted from a tracer injected into the body are not measured directly but indirectly from the photons emitted in opposite directions when the positron annihilates with an electron. This process is illustrated in Fig. 9.1. Detectors placed on either side of the active volume are connected in a so-called coincidence circuit so that if both detectors record an event within a very short interval (**coincidence resolving time** which is about 10^{-8}s), it is assumed that a positron annihilation has taken place. Photons are emitted isotropically from the active volume and so improvement in statistical accuracy, and hence quality of data recorded is directly related to the number of coincidence detector pairs surrounding the body. This number is inevitably dictated by financial constraints, but the volume of the body covered by PET scanners has increased steadily over the years, and at present commercial designs with an axial field-of-view (FOV) up to about 25 cm are available [7,10]. The majority of scanners consist of multiple concentric rings of small detector elements, but other devices consisting of planar gamma-cameras [11] or rotating partial rings [12] are becoming more common. Data acquisition and tomograph design are outlined in more detail in the following sections.

The fundamentals of coincidence detection and photon scattering

Positrons are emitted with a continuous range of energies up to a maximum, characteristic of the particular isotope (Table 9.1). The positron is successively slowed down by Coulomb interaction with atomic electrons and annihilates with an electron when its energy has been reduced to close to zero. Annihilation (Fig. 9.1) results in a pair of photons flying off in opposite directions. They each have an energy of 511 keV (the rest mass energy of the positron and electron that have both disappeared) and their relative 180° direction is a consequence of conservation of momentum (with a small angular spread (~0.3°) around the 'back-to-back' photon paths due to some residual momentum). The distance between emitting atom and the point of annihilation depends on positron energy and, for the respective mean energies, ranges from 0.61 mm to 2.97 mm for the principal isotopes (Table 9.1). This distance, and the photon angular spread, 'blur' the true tracer distribution slightly and lower the resolution of current tomographs from about 4 mm to 5 mm.

The physical limitation imposed by this blurring, however, is relatively minor compared with the consequences of **photon scattering**. For photons of 511 keV travelling through a dense medium such as the body, there is a high probability that they will be scattered by interaction with atomic electrons and undergo change of direction and loss of energy (a negligible proportion give up all their energy in the photoelectric effect). The importance of photon scattering can be explained by considering the fundamental aspects of annihilation coincidence detection illustrated in Fig. 9.2, where a point source A of photons is located between the detectors. Simultaneous detection of photons γ' automatically localizes the annihilation to somewhere on the line joining the two detectors D_1 and D_2. In reality, the 'line' is, of course, a 'tube' of finite width, but it is usually referred to as a **line-of-response (LOR)**. No coincidence counts would be recorded, from annihilations in A, in the adjacent detector pair D_3

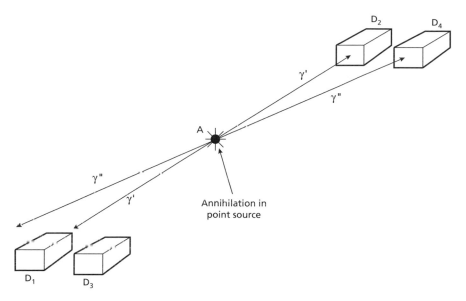

Fig. 9.2 'Electronic collimation' with annihilation coincidence detection.

and D_4. For instance, one of the photon pair γ'' might strike detector D_4 but the other would not strike D_3. The directional information, and hence spatial resolution, thus offered by coincidence detection, known as **electronic collimation**, obviates the need to place lead collimators in front of the detectors. If only single photons were being recorded, the events in detectors D_2 and D_4 would, without collimation, have contained no information regarding where the photons arose. The need for lead collimation in imaging with radioactive isotopes which emit only single photons from the nucleus (the conventional mode in nuclear medicine) unfortunately prevents a large fraction of those photons from reaching the detector. This accounts for a detection efficiency in PET some two orders of magnitude greater [13].

However, this advantage needs to be qualified in the context of photon scattering. If the source is contained within a dense medium (e.g. the body) and one of the photon pair scatters through an angle ϕ (Fig. 9.3, point S) then a coincidence event might be recorded in detectors D_1 and D_4. In order to capture as many photon pairs as possible, many detectors (several thousand in the latest devices) surround the patient and multiple coincidence circuits are set up between them. In this case, the origin of the annihilation would be wrongly assigned to the line (dashed) between D_1 and D_4. Although one photon has lost energy, the types of detectors that are generally employed in PET (described below) have relatively poor ability (energy resolution) to measure precise photon energy. A lower energy threshold is normally applied, but coincidences in which one or both of the photons have scattered still have quite a high

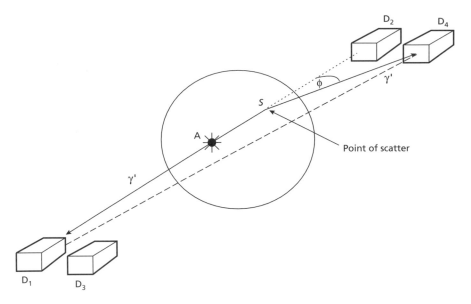

Fig. 9.3 Photon scattering and detection.

probability of being accepted. Contamination of the data by events attributable to scatter lead to poor contrast and inaccurate quantification. A number of correction schemes have been used, based on the spatial or energy characteristics of events [14–16] or on iterative calculation of the distribution of scattered events from raw image data and analytical formulae developed in basic physics [3].

If a photon is scattered it is 'lost' to the original LOR, and the radioactivity measured along that LOR will be in error. This effect is known as **attenuation**. Correction for attenuation is relatively straightforward in PET [17], again because of the mechanism underlying coincidence detection. If the thicknesses of medium on either side of a source is a cm and b cm (Fig. 9.4) then the attenuation factors along the two distances are $\exp\{-\mu a\}$ and $\exp\{-\mu b\}$ where μ is a constant for a given material known as the **linear attenuation coefficient**. The total attenuation along the LOR is the product of these two factors:

$$\exp\{-\mu(a+b)\}$$

which is independent of the position of the source along the LOR. Correction for attenuation is accomplished by placing a radioactive source in the detector field of view and taking measurements with and without the (inactive) patient in position. The source can be in the form of rings, rotating rods or point sources with relatively long-lived activity such as ^{68}Ge or ^{137}Cs [2]. The ratio of counts recorded in the two sets of conditions gives the total attenuation factor needed. Again, contamination from scattered events (lost to one LOR but

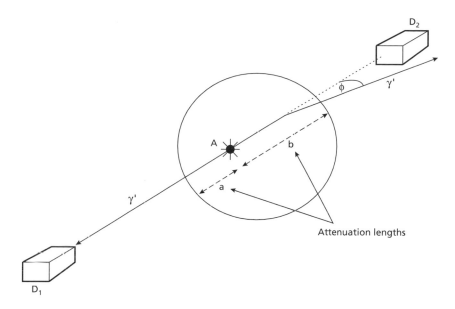

Fig. 9.4 Photon attenuation.

possibly recorded in another) should be corrected. This has been achieved based on a knowledge of source position in the case of rotating rod sources or by 'segmenting' an image of the density map into regions of known attenuation coefficient.

Coincidence detection of two photons, whether they have scattered or not, is referred to as a **true coincidence** (both photons arose from the same annihilation). However, by chance, photons that did not originate from the same annihilation might interact within the time resolution of two detectors connected in coincidence. The result is termed a **random coincidence**. Like scattered events, these would lead to impairment of contrast and quantification if not subtracted [18]. The correction is carried out automatically in modern tomographs and will be discussed more fully below.

The fundamentals of tomograph design

The greater the number of coincidence LORs that pass through the patient, the greater is the efficiency of detection. Thus, greater use is made of the radiation dose given to the patient. The continuing theme of the history of PET instrumentation has been that of improving detection efficiency, while simultaneously improving spatial resolution.

The earliest successful commercial tomographs consisted of a single ring of detectors with thick lead shielding on either side to stop photons arising from outside the plane of the ring (which can yield only random or scattered

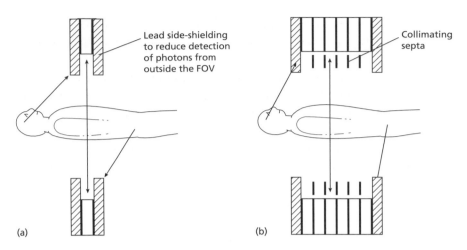

Fig. 9.5 Axial cross-sections of single ring and multiple ring (with septa) tomographs.

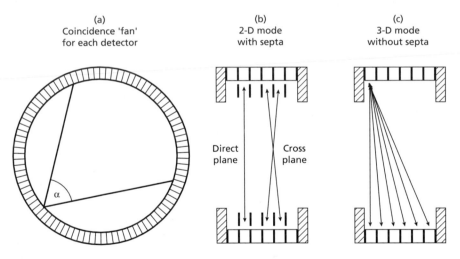

Fig. 9.6 Arrangement of lines-of-response (LORs). (a) Transaxially, between each detector and an opposing 'fan' of detectors; (b) example of interring combinations in 2-D mode (with septa); (c) interring combinations in 3-D (without septa).

coincidences) [19]. Figure 9.5(a) shows an axial cross-section of a single ring scanner. Development of smaller detector elements and the desire for a larger FOV led to the introduction of tomographs with multiple rings of detectors, but concern about the increased random and scattered coincidence rate resulted in the insertion of lead or tungsten annuli, known as **septa**, between the detector rings (Fig. 9.5b) [20]. Data acquisition in such systems is organized as a series of **planes** or **slices** through the patient. This is illustrated in diagrammatic form in Fig. 9.6. Figure 9.6(a) shows the typical arrangement of coincidence LORs, between a given detector element and a number ('fan') of elements on the other side of the detector ring. The angle α of the fan determines the transaxial FOV of the tomograph.

A detector can be in coincidence with detectors in other rings of a multi-ring scanner. Conventionally, the raw data are formatted into matrices known as **sinograms,** each element of which contains the number of events ('counts') recorded in each LOR. Each row of the sinogram represents a one-dimensional view (or **projection**) of the patient at a given angle and the sinogram encompasses all angles around the patient. Sinograms in a modern PET tomograph consist of roughly 50000 elements (LORs) and a single data set can consist of many hundreds of these. The standard process of **image reconstruction** extrapolates or **backprojects** the projection data into the 'image space' (FOV) of the tomograph, as well as applying a spatial frequency filter to remove blurring [21].

For a scanner with septa (Fig. 9.6b) the concept of 'direct' (LORs only within one ring) and 'cross' planes (LORs between adjacent rings) arises. With early multiring devices, the data are organized exactly as shown in Fig. 9.6b. Images are then derived from distinct direct and cross planes through the patient (known as the **2-D mode** of scanning). Each image is treated essentially as a 2-D plane, although, of course, its thickness is finite and determined by (i) detector width; (ii) septa geometry; and (iii) whether the plane is 'direct' or 'cross'.

The trend towards higher spatial resolution with smaller detector width led to thinner septa and the summing of more adjacent ring-to-ring combinations (to maintain efficiency) so that all planes were then effectively cross-planes [22]. However, it became clear that the presence of septa was significantly reducing the detection efficiency of unscattered true events even though it reduced scattered and random events. These concerns prompted the development of the **3-D mode** of data acquisition in PET which is illustrated in Fig. 9.6(c), where coincidence LORs are active between each detector ring and all other rings. The increase in the detection efficiency of true unscattered coincidences is about a factor of 5 between 2-D and 3-D modes, a combination of increase in the number of LORs and removal of shielding by the septa. For practical scanning *in vivo*, this advantage is reduced because of increased random and scattered events, but the improvement in statistical quality is still a factor of 3 even for higher count rate studies [23]. The improvement is measured in terms of **noise-equivalent counts,** that is the effective number of counts recorded when the statistical effect of subtraction of random and scattered events is taken into account.

Automatic subtraction of random events has become standard with commercial tomographs. The technique employed is to measure the number of coincidences occurring in each LOR when signals from one detector pair are 'delayed' relative to those from the other, typically by 128 ns. Coincidences recorded in the delayed channel cannot possibly be true coincidences and so are taken to be an accurate measure for calculation of the rate of random coincidences.

Scanning in 3-D mode has, of course, raised challenges and questions regarding the accuracy of (i) the subtraction of scattered and random events; (ii) detector dead time; and (iii) detector normalization. Although the subtraction of random coincidences is accurate, it does inevitably involve an increase in **statistical noise**. Different methods of smoothing, before subtraction, are being actively investigated [24,25].

Current and future developments in PET

Topics of current and future methodological importance in PET, apart from the data corrections mentioned above, include (i) detector performance and novel data acquisition schemes; (ii) image reconstruction; and (iii) tracer kinetic modelling. Only the first two will be addressed here.

Most PET tomographs today use bismuth germanate (BGO) detectors. This substance has one of the highest densities known for a so-called scintillation crystal and 511 keV photons have a high probability of being stopped in the crystal and giving up their energy. The energy is transformed into visible light (scintillation) that is amplified by a photomultiplier tube (PMT). In practice, an array of BGO detector elements (a **'block'**) is viewed by a smaller number of PMTs and the element struck by a photon is identified based on the ratio of PMT signals [26]. This identification method is similar to that used in a nuclear medicine gamma camera. Some physical characteristics of scintillation crystals used in PET are shown in Table 9.2. Sodium iodide crystals, the standard for gamma cameras and also for many commercial PET scanners, have very high scintillation efficiency but relatively low density and poor photon

Table 9.2 Properties of scintillation detectors.

	Sodium iodide (NaI(Tl))	Bismuth germanate (BGO)	Lutetium orthosilicate (LSO)
Density (g/ml)	3.7	7.1	7.4
Scintillation efficiency (% of NaI(Tl))	100	15	75
Scintillation decay time (ns)	230	300	40
Hygroscopic?	Yes	No	No

stopping power. The high light output gives it good energy resolution, but the density deficiency has led to domination by BGO in most modern PET machines. The introduction of lutetium orthosilicate (LSO), a very dense scintillator with high light output and more rapid response to an interaction, reflected by a short scintillation decay time [27], is predicted to yield advantages because of the associated decrease in electronic **dead time** and rate of random events [6]. The faster a detector can record and process a photon interaction, the more rapidly it can respond to another event. For the detectors *per se*, the single photon event rate or (**singles** rate) is the fundamental determinant of dead time. In some cardiac PET studies 50% or more of the photons impinging on the detectors can be lost (at the peak counting rates) because of dead time, i.e. during intervals in which the detector electronics are 'busy' processing previous events. The far superior timing properties of LSO should greatly lessen dead time and thus capitalize on the injected dose of tracer. Of equal importance is the fact that the timing resolution of an event is much better with LSO. This shortens the coincidence resolving time and hence the ratio of random to true events. Count rate limitations are particularly relevant in cardiac PET in which a large fraction of the injected dose can be in the scanner FOV (blood pool) at one time. At present only a few experimental LSO systems are in existence, but large volume production is being aggressively pursued.

Improvements in timing resolution are relevant not only to detector material but also to the way in which raw data are acquired. Most PET scanners operate in **frame mode** in which many (usually) contiguous time frames are defined before acquisition commences. Frame lengths are selected to accommodate the varying kinetic components at different times after injection. However, especially in 3-D mode with rapidly decaying tracers (such as ^{15}O and ^{11}C), it is more efficient to store each event separately in **list mode** (event-by-event). The reason for this is that a large fraction of LORs contain no events at all. This fraction becomes greater as the isotope decays. Furthermore, list mode acquisition offers the researcher data of the highest possible temporal resolution that can be (i) subsequently **rebinned** into different frame sequences, as desired, for image reconstruction; and (ii) partitioned into different gates on the basis of cardiac and respiratory recorded movements.

Image reconstruction is another focus [28,29]. The standard method of producing an image in PET has been **filtered backprojection,** which is based on frequency filtering and is a convenient technique because of the use of the fast Fourier transform (FFT). However, potentially superior **iterative** methods are now undergoing widespread development [30]. In these, the image is iteratively adjusted to be consistent with the projection (LOR) data to within specified tolerances. Iterative schemes are much more flexible but are also computationally intensive. The well known explosion in computing power is rendering them more practical. Current research pertinent to instrumentation, data acquisition and processing will undoubtedly uncover novel procedures for cardiology. New methods of reconstruction and processing of data are likely to enhance the potential of less expensive partial ring and dual-head gamma cameras.

Applications of PET in cardiology

Current applications of PET imaging in cardiology comprise approaches to the assessment of regional **myocardial blood flow, metabolism and pharmacology.**

Myocardial blood flow

Radionuclide imaging techniques, e.g. the use of thallium-201, have enabled the assessment of nutritive tissue perfusion as opposed to measurements of epicardial coronary flow as measured by either thermodilution [31] or Doppler catheter techniques [32,33]. Before the advent of PET imaging technology, only **directional changes in regional myocardial blood flow** could be assessed by either planar gamma scintigraphy or by single photon emission computed tomography (SPECT) [34]. Quantification of myocardial blood flow with these techniques was impossible because of the physical limitations of the imaging systems and the properties of the tracers available. **PET overcomes the physical limitations of previously available imaging systems** by providing the means for accurate attenuation correction, thus enabling absolute quantification of the concentration of radiolabelled tracer in the organ of interest [35]. As PET technology has advanced and rapid dynamic imaging has become possible, quantification of myocardial blood flow has been achieved following the development of suitable tracer kinetic models.

A number of tracers have been used for measurement of myocardial blood flow by PET, in particular, oxygen-15 labelled water ($H_2{}^{15}O$) [36–39], nitrogen-13 labelled ammonia ($^{13}NH_3$) [40–43], the cationic potassium analogue rubidium-82 (^{82}Rb) [44], carbon-11 and gallium-68 labelled albumin microspheres [45,46]. Currently, $H_2{}^{15}O$ and $^{13}NH_3$ are the tracers most widely used for the quantification of regional myocardial blood flow with PET. Tracer kinetic models for quantification of myocardial blood flow have been validated in animals against the radiolabelled microsphere method over a wide flow range for both $H_2{}^{15}O$ [36–39] and $^{13}NH_3$ [42,43]. The values of myocardial blood flow determined in normal human volunteers studied with both tracers at rest or during pharmacologically induced coronary vasodilatation are similar [36,43]. The use of $H_2{}^{15}O$ for quantification of regional myocardial blood is theoretically superior to the use of $^{13}NH_3$ in that $H_2{}^{15}O$ is a metabolically inert and freely diffusible tracer [47] which exhibits virtually complete myocardial extraction independent of both flow rate [48] and myocardial metabolic state [38]. This makes $H_2^{15}O$ a particularly suitable tracer for measurements of absolute perfusion also under circumstances in which metabolic abnormalities that could affect myocardial trapping of $^{13}NH_3$ [49] may be present. However, the quality of myocardial $^{13}NH_3$ images is superior to that of $H_2^{15}O$ images. Both $H_2^{15}O$ and $^{13}NH_3$ have short physical half lives (2 and 10 min, respectively). Thus, repeat measurements of myocardial blood flow is practical in the same imaging session.

Before the advent of PET, quantitative investigations of regional coronary blood flow in humans were restricted to flow up the epicardial coronary artery. However, the major regulatory site of tissue perfusion is at the level of the arterioles that are not amenable to catheterization. With the development of quantitative myocardial blood flow measurements by PET, it became possible to assess the function of the **coronary microvasculature** by measuring **coronary vasodilator reserve** (CVR), calculated as the ratio of maximal flow after pharmacologically induced coronary vasodilatation to rest flow. CVR is, however, dependent on the coronary perfusion pressure and the extent to which maximal vasodilatation is actually achieved [50]. PET studies in healthy human volunteers have shown that normal CVR in response to a standard intravenous dose of dipyridamole (0.56 mg/kg over 4 min) is approximately 3.5–4.0 [36,43] (Fig. 9.7a and Table 9.3). The data are similar to those reported with the use of the Doppler catheter technique for measuring epicardial coronary flow velocity [51].

Table 9.3 PET measurements of myocardial blood flow in normal subjects.

Author	Tracer	Agent	No. of subjects	Age	MBF_{bas}	MBF_{hyp}	$MBF_{hyp/bas}$
Bergmann et al.	$H_2^{15}O$	Dip	11	25	0.9±0.2	3.6±1.2	4.1±1.2
Geltman et al.	$H_2^{15}O$	Dip	16	25±4	1.2±0.3	4.6±1.6	3.8±1.1
Camici et al.	$^{13}NH_3$	Dip	12	51±8	1.0±0.2	2.7±0.9	2.9±1.0
Sambuceti et al.	$^{13}NH^3$	Dip	14	49±7	1.1±0.3	3.7±0.8	3.6±0.9
Chan et al.	$^{13}NH_3$	Ado	20	35±16	1.1±0.2	4.4±0.9	4.4±1.5
Chan et al.	$^{13}NH_3$	Dip	20	35±16	1.1±0.2	4.3±1.3	4.3±1.9
Araujo et al.	$C^{15}O_2$	Dip	11	26 to 42	0.8±0.1	3.5±1.1	4.2±1.2
Merlet et al.	$H_2^{15}O$	Dip	6	51±5	0.9±0.1	3.5±0.8	4.0±0.7
Muzik et al.	$^{13}NH_3$	Ado	6	26±3	0.8±0.2	3.6+1.0	
Uren et al.	$H_2^{15}O$	Dip/Ado	43	47±20	1.0+0.2	3.2±1.3	3.4±1.3
Radvan et al.	$C^{15}O_2$	Dip	8	27±5	0.8±0.2	3.1+08	3.8±0.8
Czernin et al.	$^{13}NH_3$	Dip	18	31±9	0.8±0.2	3.0±0.8	4.1±0.9
Czernin et al.	$^{13}NH_3$	Dip	22	64±9	0.9±0.3	2.7±0.6	3.0±0.7

Ado, adenosine; Dip, dipyridamole; MBF_{bas}, baseline myocardial blood flow; MBF_{hyp}, hyperaemic myocardial blood flow; $MBF_{hyp/bas}$, coronary flow reserve. Data are mean ± SD. (Adapted from [98].)

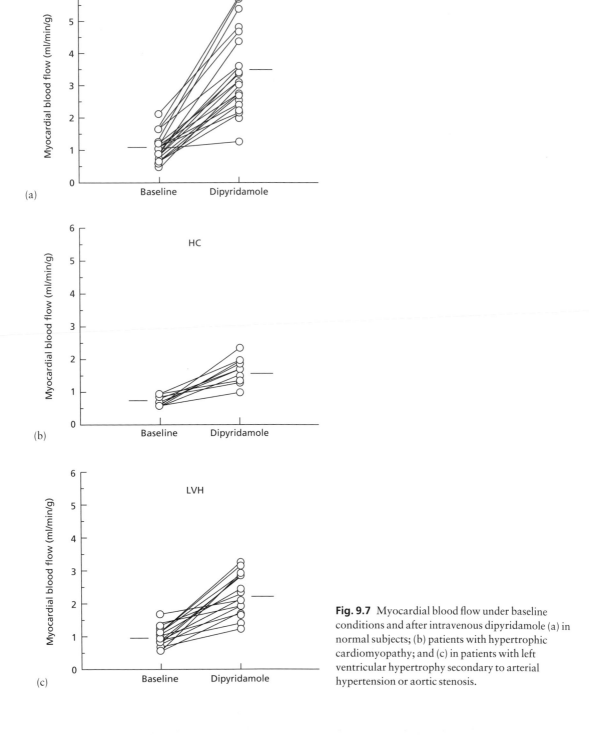

Fig. 9.7 Myocardial blood flow under baseline conditions and after intravenous dipyridamole (a) in normal subjects; (b) patients with hypertrophic cardiomyopathy; and (c) in patients with left ventricular hypertrophy secondary to arterial hypertension or aortic stenosis.

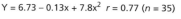

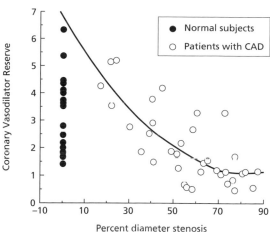

$Y = 6.73 - 0.13x + 7.8x^2$ $r = 0.77$ ($n = 35$)

Fig. 9.8 Coronary vasodilator reserve falls with increasing per cent diameter stenosis and is exhausted for stenoses >80%. Normal controls' values of coronary vasodilator reserve are shown at zero per cent diameter stenosis on the left of the panel.

Use of PET with $H_2{}^{15}O$ has highlighted the effects of age [52,53], sex and alteration in sympathetic tone [54] on myocardial blood flow and CVR. Thus, it has been demonstrated that myocardial blood flow under basal conditions and with hyperaemia remain rather constant up to 60 years of age. Above this age, there is a significant increase in basal flow associated with an increase in systolic blood pressure and a significant reduction in hyperaemic myocardial blood flow and CVR [53].

The measurement of CVR is useful for the assessment of the **functional significance of coronary stenoses** in patients with coronary artery disease [55] (Fig. 9.8). In addition, PET is particularly helpful in those circumstances including the CVR is diffusely (and not regionally) blunted, e.g. in patients with hypertrophic cardiomyopathy or hypertensive heart disease [56] because of a widespread abnormality in the coronary microcirculation (Fig. 9.7b,c). It may aid in the differentiation of pathological from physiological left ventricular hypertrophy [57] and in the exclusion of myocardial ischaemia in patients with chest pain and angiographically normal coronary arteries [58]. The improved spatial resolution of the latest generation of PET cameras affords a realistic prospect of quantification of transmural distribution of myocardial blood flow [59].

Myocardial metabolism

Oxidative metabolism

In the postabsorptive state the normoxic heart relies mainly upon oxidation of free fatty acid (FFA) as its main source of high-energy phosphates, whereas the uptake and oxidation of carbohydrates (glucose, lactate and pyruvate) is low. Conversely, in the fed state, the uptake of carbohydrate is high and accounts for virtually all of the concurrent oxygen uptake [60]. This change is explained in part by the glucose-FFA cycle identified by Randle. An important observation was that the oxidation of glucose by the isolated rat heart was inhibited markedly by concurrent provision of FFA. The factors that regulate myocardial substrate utilization are complex and depend, in addition to substrate concentration, upon the action of different hormones. Insulin, which stimulates myocardial glucose uptake and utilization also inhibits adipose tissue lipolysis, yielding decreased circulating levels of FFA. Catecholamines decrease rather than increase glycolysis in the heart together with a greatly increased uptake and oxidation of FFA. Myocardial utilization of carbohydrates is affected also by cardiac workload, with oxidation of carbohydrates accounting for more than 50% of energy produced during conditions of maximal stress [61]. Glucose utilization is increased under conditions of reduced oxygen supply, in which exogenous glucose uptake and glycogen breakdown are increased, glycolysis is stimulated and ATP production is largely from anaerobic glycolysis with concomitant formation of lactate [60].

In order to measure the flux through this pathway under normoxic and ischaemic conditions, PET imaging has been performed after intravenous administration of the natural free fatty acid palmitate labelled with carbon-11 (^{11}C-palmitate) [62]. Results indicated that the clearance of ^{11}C-palmitate from the myocardium was related to the extent of oxidative metabolism, although absolute quantification of utilization rates was not possible because of the over-complexity of the model required to explain the behaviour of ^{11}C-palmitate in tissue. Interpretation of myocardial uptake and clearance of ^{11}C-palmitate is complicated further by the dependence of these two variables on the prevailing blood flow and dietary state.

Carbon-11 labelled acetate (^{11}C-acetate) has been used as a tracer of tricarboxylic acid cycle activity [63] and as an indirect marker of myocardial oxygen consumption (MVO_2) by PET in experimental animals [64–66] and in humans [67,68]. A number of studies have shown that the rate constant describing the clearance of ^{11}C-acetate from the myocardium correlates well with catheter measurements of oxygen extraction fraction (OEF) from analysis of arteriovenous differences of blood oxygen content with the use of the Fick principle. However, the lack of appropriate models that accurately describe the complex tissue kinetics of ^{11}C-acetate have prevented absolute quantification of MVO_2 with the use of this tracer. Furthermore, measurements of MVO_2 based on its behaviour will be subject to the influence of blood flow and dietary constraints similar to those influencing measurements made with the use of labelled FFA.

A method to quantify MVO_2 after inhalation of oxygen-15 labelled molecular oxygen gas ($^{15}O_2$) has been developed recently [69]. Its accuracy for measurement of myocardial OEF and MVO_2 has been validated over a wide range of values in experimental animal studies [70]. Preliminary studies in human subjects yielded mean OEF and MVO_2 values of 61±8% and 9.4± 1.8 ml/min/100 g, respectively [69], consistent with values previously obtained in invasive catheterization sudies. Use of $^{15}O_2$ is attractive in that it offers a means for quantification of MVO_2 independent of myocardial substrate utilization.

Utilization of glucose

The utilization of exogenous glucose by the myocardium can be assessed with PET with[^{18}F]-2-fluoro-2-deoxyglucose (FDG) as a tracer [71]. FDG is transported into the myocyte by the same trans-sarcolemmal carrier as glucose and phosphorylated to FDG-6-phosphate by the enzyme hexokinase. This is essentially a unidirectional reaction and results in FDG-6-phospate accumulation within the myocardium since glucose-6-phosphatase (the enzyme that hydrolyses FDG-6-phosphate back to free FDG and free phosphate) does not appear to be present in cardiac muscle. Thus, measurement of the myocardial uptake of FDG is proportional to the overall **rate of trans-sarcolemmal transport and hexokinase-phosphorylation of exogenous (circulating) glucose** by heart muscle. Measurement of myocardial FDG uptake by PET, however, does not provide any information about the further intracellular disposal of glucose (i.e. glycogen synthesis, glycolysis or flux through the pentose shunt).

A number of kinetic modelling approaches have been used for the quantification of glucose utilization rates using FDG [72]. Their major limitation is that quantification of glucose metabolism requires the knowledge of **the lumped constant,** a factor that relates the kinetic behaviour of FDG to that of naturally occurring glucose in terms of the relative affinity of each molecule for the trans-sarcolemmal transporter and for hexokinase. Unfortunately, the value of the lumped constant in humans under different physiological and pathophysiological conditions is not known, thus making accurate *in vivo* quantification of myocardial metabolic rates of glucose utilization very difficult. Still, the quantification of the uptake of FDG (particularly if obtained under standardized conditions such as with euglycaemic insulin clamps) allows comparison of absolute values from different individuals and may help to characterize absolute rates of glucose utilization (in FDG units) in normal and pathological myocardium [73].

Application of quantitative FDG uptake for detection of
hibernating myocardium

With the advent of coronary revascularization and thrombolysis, it has become apparent that restoration of blood flow to asynergic myocardial segments may result in improved regional and global left ventricular (LV) function [74,75]. The greatest clinical benefit is seen in those patients with the most severe forms of dysfunction [76]. Initial studies indicated that myocardial ischaemia and infarction could be distinguished by analysis of PET images of the perfusion tracer $^{13}NH_3$ and the glucose analogue FDG acquired after an oral glucose load [77]. Regions that exhibited a concordant reduction in both myocardial blood flow and FDG uptake (**'flow-metabolism match'**) were hypothesized to be infarct and irreversibly injured, whereas regions in which FDG uptake was relatively preserved or increased despite a perfusion defect (**'flow-metabolism mismatch'**) were considered to reflect ischaemic yet viable myocardium. The uptake of FDG by the myocardium, however, depends on many factors such as dietary state, cardiac workload, insulin resistance, sympathetic drive and the presence and severity of ischaemia. These factors may contribute to the regional variability observed with FDG imaging and the concomitant difficulty of data interpretation in the fasted or glucose-loaded state. Therefore, measurement of the uptake of FDG as previously implemented, though indicative of the presence of metabolically active tissue components, may not accurately define the amount of metabolizing viable tissue within the asynergic region.

The recent suggestion that semiquantitative and quantitative analyses of FDG uptake may enhance detection of viable myocardium, required rigorous standardization of conditions [73]. In addition, many patients with coronary artery disease are insulin resistant, i.e. the amount of endogenous insulin released after feeding will not induce maximal stimulation because of partial resistance to the action of the hormone. In many cases, this results in poor FDG image quality after an oral glucose load. To circumvent the problem of insulin resistance, an alternative protocol has been applied recently in PET studies of viability [78]. The protocol is based on the use of the **hyperinsulinaemic euglycaemic clamp**, essentially the simultaneous infusion of insulin and glucose acting on the tissue as a *metabolic challenge* and stimulating maximal FDG uptake. The use of the euglycaemic hyperinsulinaemic glucose clamp provides excellent image quality, demonstrates uniform tracer uptake throughout the heart and enables PET studies to be performed under standardized metabolic conditions. This permits a comparison of the absolute values of the metabolic rate of glucose uptake (μmol/g/min) amongst different subjects and centres (Fig. 9.9).

By using the euglycaemic hyperinsulinaemic glucose clamp in conjunction with regional wall motion information (derived from echocardiography or conventional radionuclide ventriculography), the need for a simultaneous flow tracer is obviated. The images obtained with FDG with the clamp technique are of sufficient quality to reduce the period of image acquisition to approximately 30 min, giving a total scan time of about an hour. Another significant benefit is particular sensitivity in patients with coronary artery disease and poor left ventricular function. With this approach we have studied a large series of patients undergoing different revascularization procedures and have demonstated the good predictive accuracy of PET under different clinical

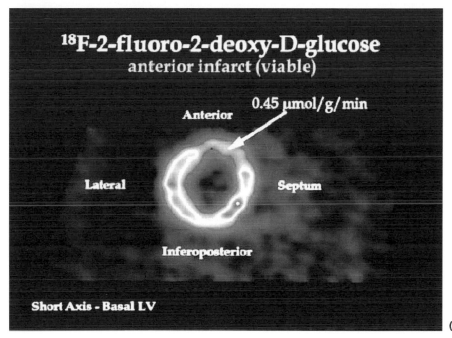

(a)

Fig. 9.9 Myocardial viability in two patients with coronary artery disease and severe chronic left ventricular dysfunction assessed by PET with ^{18}F-labelled fluorodeoxyglucose (FDG) during hyperinsulinaemic euglycaemic clamp. Both patients had previous myocardial infarctions. The scan illustrated in (a) shows that FDG uptake in the previously infarcted anteroseptal segment is 0.45 μmol/min/g, suggesting the presence of viable myocardium. In the scan illustrated in (b), the uptake of FDG in the anterior wall and the interventricular septum is significantly reduced (0.14 μmol/min/g), suggesting absence of viability in this large area. A cut-off point of 0.25 μmol/min/g is routinely used in our laboratory to differentiate between viable and non-viable myocardium. This cut-off value was derived from our database of patients with coronary artery disease and chronic left ventricular dysfunction who underwent FDG-PET and were subsequently revascularized. The proportion of dysfunctional segments that improved following revascularization increased linearly with FDG uptake. To determine the value of FDG uptake above which the best prediction of improvement in functional class of at least one grade could be obtained, a receiver-operator characteristic curve (ROC) was constructed. According to this analysis the optimal operating point on the curve (point of best compromise between sensitivity and specificity) was at the FDG uptake value of 0.25 μmol/min/g.

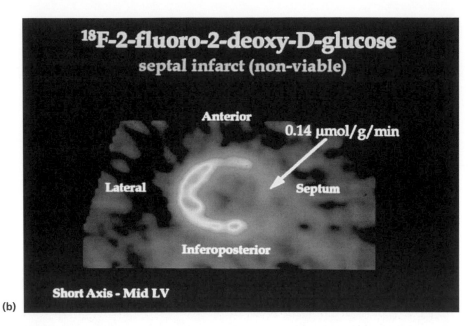

(b)

Fig. 9.9 *Continued.*

conditions. A threshold value for the metabolic rate of glucose of 0.25 μmol/g/min allowed the best prediction of improvement in functional class of at least one grade after revascularization [79].

Myocardial pharmacology

Several beta-blocker drugs have been labelled with carbon-11 to act as radio-ligands for imaging by PET [80]. The most promising is CGP 12177, a non-selective β-adrenoceptor anatagonist that is particularly well suited for PET studies because of its high affinity and low lipophilicity, facilitating character-ization of the functional receptor pool on the cell surface [81]. A graphical method for quantification of **β-adrenoceptor density** (B_{max}, pmol/ml) from the PET data has been developed [82]. The approach requires two injections of ^{11}C-(S)-CGP 12177, one at a high specific activity followed by a second at a lower specific activity. The analytical approach is particularly attractive for clinical studies because it does not require an input function and thus obviates the need for arterial cannulation. Studies in our institution [83] in a group of healthy subjects over a broad range of ages have yielded B_{max} values of 8.4±2.0 pmol/ml, a figure comparable to values obtained in studies of binding *in vitro* [84]. In addition, studies in patients have demonstrated diffuse **downregulation of myocardial β-adrenoceptors** in hypertrophic cardiomyo-pathy (HCM) [83,85] and in congestive cardiac failure [86], two disorders in which sympathetic nervous system activation is chronically elevated.

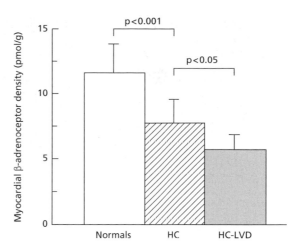

Fig. 9.10 Mean left ventricular β-adrenoceptor density in normal subjects and in patients with hypertrophic cardiomyopathy with preserved systolic function (HC) or with left ventricular dysfunction (HC-LVD).

It has been hypothesized that abnormal sympathetic activation may actually *precede* the development of systolic dysfunction in patients with HCM. To characterize the relationship between left ventricular function and changes in neural control of the heart in patients with HCM, we assessed left ventricular function by echocardiography and myocardial β-adrenoceptor density by PET in a group of patients with HCM, a subgroup with, and another without, heart failure [87]. Myocardial β-adrenoceptor density in the 17 patients was 7.00±1.90 pmol/g compared with 11.50±2.18 pmol/g in normal controls (*P*<0.01). β-Adrenoceptor density in the six patients with left ventricular failure was 5.61±0.88 pmol/g compared to 7.71±1.86 pmol/g in the 11 patients with normal ventricular function (*P*<0.05) (Fig. 9.10). Furthermore, there was a significant correlation (*r*=0.52; *P*<0.05) between left ventricular fractional shortening and myocardial β-adrenoceptor density. A positive correlation (*r*=0.51; *P*<0.05) was also found between myocardial β-adrenoceptor density and the E/A transmitral flow ratio, an index of left ventricular diastolic function. Thus, myocardial β-adrenoceptor downregulation was present in patients with HCM whether or not there were signs of heart failure.

Attempts have been made to study α_1 adrenoceptors *in vivo* with the use of carbon-11 labelled prazosin and PET [80], but to date studies in human subjects have not been performed. Investigations of the α-adrenergic system would be of interest because changes have been implicated in myocardial ischaemia, arrhythmogenesis [88] and the development of ventricular hypertrophy [89].

In addition to postsynaptic receptor studies, PET has been used to elucidate the integrity of presynaptic sympathetic innervation of the heart. Three tracers have been used for this purpose: fluorine-18 labelled fluorometaraminol [90], fluorine-18 labelled fluorodopamine [91] and carbon-11 labelled hydroxyephedrine (^{11}C-HED) [92]. These tracers compete with endogenous noradrenaline (norepinephrine) for the transport into the presynaptic nerve terminal via the neuronal uptake-1 transport system. Once within the neurone, these compounds are metabolized and trapped and hence serve as markers of sympathetic innervation. Recent studies have demonstrated decreased retention of carbon-11 labelled hydroxyephedrine in patients after cardiac transplant consistent with denervation of the heart [93]. However, with time, some sympathetic re-innervation occurred, particularly in anteroseptal regions. This change has been correlated with reappearance of angina pectoris [94]. Both pre- and postsynaptic myocardial autonomic function can be assessed non-invasively by combining different tracers, e.g. ^{11}C-HED and ^{11}C-(S)-CGP 12177 [95,96].

In addition to studies of the sympathetic nervous system, PET with carbon-11 labelled MQNB has been used to quantify the density of myocardial muscarinic cholinergic receptors in both experimental animals [97] and in human subjects. It would be desirable to extend such studies to patients given the possible pathophysiological role of muscarinic receptors in arrhythmogenesis and modulation of sympathetic function.

References

1 Jones T. The imaging science of positron emission tomography. *Eur J Nucl Med* 1996; 23: 807–13.

2 deKemp R, Nahmias C. Attenuation correction in PET using single photon transmission measurement. *Med Phys* 1994; 21: 771–8.

3 Ollinger J. Model-based scatter correction for fully 3D PET. *Phys Med Biol* 1996; 41: 153–76.

4 Klein GJ, Reutter BW, Ho MH, Reed JH, Huesman RH. *Real-time System for Respiratory-cardiac Gating in Positron Tomography*. IEEE Nuclear Science Symposium, Albuquerque NM, 1997.

5 Bailey DL, Miller MM, Spinks TJ *et al*. Experience with fully 3D PET and implications for future high-resolution 3D tomographs. *Phys Med Biol* 1998; 43: 777–86.

6 Spinks TJ, Jones T, Bloomfield PM *et al*. Physical characteristics of the ECAT EXACT 3D positron tomograph. *Phys Med Biol* 2000; 45: 2601–18.

7 Spinks TJ, Miller MM, Bailey DL, Bloomfield PM, Livieratos L, Jones T. The effect of activity outside the direct field of view in a 3D-only whole-body positron tomograph. *Phys Med Biol* 1998; 43: 895–904.

8 Smith T, Tong C, Lammertsma AA *et al*. Dosimetry of intravenously administered ^{15}O-labelled water in man: a model based on experimental human data from 21 subjects. *Eur J Nucl Med* 1994; 21: 1126–34.

9 Lammertsma AA, Brooks DJ, Frackowiak RSJ *et al*. Measurement of glucose utilisation with [^{18}F]2-fluoro-2-deoxy-D-glucose: a comparison of different analytical methods. *J Cereb Blood Flow Metab* 1987; 7: 161–72.

10 Karp JS, Muehllehner G, Mankoff DA *et al*. Continuous-slice PENN-PET: a positron tomograph with volume imaging capability. *J Nucl Med* 1990; 31: 617–27.

11 Lewellen TK, Miyaoka RS, Swan WL. PET imaging using dual-headed gamma cameras: an update. *Nucl Med Commun* 1999; 20: 5–12.

12 Bailey DL, Young H, Bloomfield PM *et al*. ECAT ART—a continuously rotating PET camera: performance characteristics, initial clinical studies, and installation considerations in a nuclear medicine department. *Eur J Nucl Med* 1997; 24: 6–15.

13 Bailey DL, Zito F, Gilardi M-C, Savi AR, Fazio F, Jones T. Performance comparison of a state-of-the-art neuro-SPECT scanner and dedicated neuro-PET scanner. *Eur J Nucl Med* 1994; 21: 381–7.

14 Bailey DL, Meikle S. A convolution-

subtraction scatter correction method for 3D PET. *Phys Med Biol* 1994; 39: 411–24.

15 Grootoonk S, Spinks TJ, Kennedy AM, Bloomfield PM, Sashin D, Jones T. The practical implementation and accuracy of dual window scatter correction in a neuro PET scanner with the septa retracted. *Phys Med Biol* 1996; 41: 2757–74.

16 Watson CC, Newport D, Casey ME, deKemp RA, Beanlands RS, Schmand M. Evaluation of simulation-based scatter correction for 3-D PET cardiac imaging. *IEEE Trans Nucl Sci* 1997; 44: 90–7.

17 Huang S-C, Hoffman EJ, Phelps ME, Kuhl DE. Quantitation in positron emission computed tomography: 2. Effects of inaccurate attenuation correction. *J Comput Assist Tomogr* 1979; 3: 804–14.

18 Hoffman EJ, Huang S-C, Phelps ME, Kuhl DE. Quantitation in positron emission computed tomography: 4. Effect of accidental coincidences. *J Comput Assist Tomogr* 1981; 5: 391–400.

19 Williams CW, Crabtree MC, Burgiss SG. Design and performance characteristics of a positron emission axial tomograph—ECAT II. *IEEE Trans Nucl Sci* 1979; NS-26: 619–27.

20 Spinks TJ, Jones T, Gilardi MC, Heather JD. Physical performance of the latest generation of commercial positron scanner. *IEEE Trans Nucl Sci* 1988; 35: 721–5.

21 Herman GT. *Image Reconstruction from Projections; The Fundamentals of Computerized Tomography*. New York: Academic Press, 1980.

22 Spinks TJ, Jones T, Bailey DL *et al*. Physical performance of a positron tomograph for brain imaging with retractable septa. *Phys Med Biol* 1992; 37: 1637–55.

23 Bailey DL, Jones T, Spinks TJ, Gilardi M-C, Townsend DW. Noise equivalent count measurements in a neuro-PET scanner with retractable septa. *IEEE Trans Med Imaging* 1991; 10: 256–60.

24 Casey ME, Hoffman EJ. Quantitation in positron emission computed tomography: 7. A technique to reduce noise in accidental coincidence measurements and coincidence efficiency calibration. *J Comput Assist Tomogr* 1986; 10: 845–50.

25 Badawi RD, Miller MP, Bailey DL, Marsden PK. Random variance reduction in 3D PET. *Phys Med Biol* 1999; 44: 941–54.

26 Casey ME, Nutt R. A multicrystal two dimensional BGO detector system for positron emission tomography. *IEEE Trans Nucl Sci* 1986; NS-33: 570–4.

27 Melcher CL, Schweitzer JS. A promising new scintillator: cerium-doped lutetium oxyorthosilicate. *Nucl Instr Meth Phys Res A* 1992; 314: 212–14.

28 Townsend DW, Geissbuhler A, Defrise M *et al*. Fully three-dimensional reconstruction for a PET camera with retractable septa. *IEEE Trans Med Imag* 1991; 10: 505–12.

29 Defrise M, Kinahan PE. Data acquisition and image reconstruction for 3D PET. In: Bendriem B, Townsend DW, eds. *The Theory and Practice of 3D PET*. Dordrecht: Kluwer Academic Publishers, 1998.

30 Shepp LA, Vardi Y. Maximum likelihood reconstruction for emission tomography IEEE. *Trans Med Imag* 1982; MI-1: 113–122.

31 Ganz W, Tamura K, Marcus HS, Donoso R, Yoshida S, Swan HJC. Measurement of coronary sinus blood flow by continuous thermodilution in man. *Circulation* 1971; 44: 181.

32 Hartley CJ, Cole JS. An ultrasonic pulsed Doppler system for measuring blood flow in small vessels. *J Appl Physiol* 1974; 37: 626.

33 Cole JS, Hartley CJ. The pulsed Doppler coronary artery catheter. Preliminary report of a new technique for measuring rapid changes in coronary artery flow velocity in man. *Circulation* 1977; 56: 1.

34 van der Waal EE. *Nuclear Cardiology and Cardiac Magnetic Resonance*. The Netherlands: Hans Soto Productions, 1992.

35 Hoffman EJ, Phelps ME. Positron emission tomography: principles and quantitation, In: Phelps ME, Mazziotta JC, Schelbert HR, eds, *Positron Emission Tomography and Autoradiography: Principles and Applications for the Brain and the Heart*. New York: Raven Press, 1986: 113–48.

36 Araujo LI, Lammertsma AA, Rhodes CG *et al*. Non-invasive quantification of regional myocardial blood flow in normal volunteers and patients with coronary artery disease using oxygen-15 labeled carbon dioxide inhalation and positron emission tomography. *Circulation* 1991; 83: 875–85.

37 Iida H, Kanno I, Takahashi A *et al*. Measurement of absolute myocardial blood flow with $H_2{}^{15}O$ and dynamic positron emission tomography: strategy for quantification in relation to the partial-volume effect. *Circulation* 1989; 78: 104–15.

38 Bergmann SR, Fox KAA, Rand AL *et al*. Quantification of regional myocardial blood flow *in vivo* with $H_2{}^{15}O$. *Circulation* 1984; 70: 724–33.

39 Bergmann SR, Herrero P, Markham J, Weinheimer CJ, Walsh MN. Noninvasive quantification of myocardial blood flow in human subjects with O-15 labelled water and positron emission tomography. *J Am Coll Cardiol* 1989; 14: 639–52.

40 Schelbert HR, Phelps ME, Hoffman EJ, Huang SC, Selin CE, Kuhl DE. Regional myocardial perfusion assessed by N-13 labelled ammonia and positron computerized axial tomography. *Am J Cardiol* 1979; 43: 209–18.

41 Krivokapich J, Smith GT, Huang SC *et al*. Nitrogen-13 ammonia myocardial imaging at rest and with exercise in normal volunteers: quantification of coronary flow with positron emission tomography. *Circulation* 1989; 80: 1328–37.

42 Bellina CR, Parodi O, Camici P *et al*. Simultaneous *in vitro* and *in vivo* validation of nitrogen-13 ammonia for the assessment of regional myocardial blood flow. *J Nucl Med* 1990; 31: 1335–43.

43 Hutchins GD, Schwaiger M, Rosenspire KC, Krivokapich J, Schelbert H, Kuhl DE. Noninvasive quantification of regional blood flow in the human heart using N-13 ammonia and dynamic positron emission tomographic imaging. *J Am Coll Cardiol* 1990; 15: 1032–42.

44 Herrero P, Markham J, Shelton ME, Weinheimer CJ, Bergmann SR. Noninvasive quantification of regional myocardial perfusion with rubidium-82 and positron emission tomography. Exploration of a mathematical model. *Circulation* 1990; 82: 1377–86.

45 Beller GA, Alten WJ, Cochavi S, Hnatowich D, Brownell GL. Assessment of regional myocardial pefusion by positron emission tomography after intracoronary administration of Ga-68 labeled albumin microspheres. *J Comput Assist Tomogr* 1979; 3: 447–52.

46 Wilson RA, De Shea MJ, Landsheere CH *et al*. Validation of quantification of regional myocardial blood flow *in vivo* with ${}^{11}C$-labeled human albumin microspheres and positron emission tomography. *Circulation* 1984; 70: 717–23.

47 Johnson JA, Cavert HM, Lifson N. Kinetics concerned with distribution of isotopic water in isolated dog heart and skeletal muscle. *Am J Physiol* 1952; 171: 687–93.

48 Yipintsoi T, Bassingthwaite JB. Circulatory transport of iodoantipyrine and water in the isolated dog heart. *Circ Res* 1970; 27: 461–7.

49 Bergmann SR, Hack S, Tewson T, Welch MJ, Sobel BE. The dependence of accumulation of ${}^{13}NH_3$ by myocardium on metabolic factors and its implications for the quantitative assessment of perfusion. *Circulation* 1980; 61: 34–43.

50 Hoffmann JIE. Maximal coronary flow and the concept of coronary vascular reserve. *Circulation* 1984; 70: 153–9.

51 Rossen JD, Simonetti I, Marcus ML, Winniford MD. Coronary dilatation with standard dose dipyridamole and dipyridamole combined with handgrip. *Circulation* 1989; 79: 556–72.

52 Czernin J, Müller P, Chan S *et al*. Influence of age and haemodynamics on myocardial blood flow and flow reserve. *Circulation* 1993; 88: 62–9.

53 Uren NG, Camici PG, Melin JA *et al*. The effect of ageing on the coronary vasodilator reserve in man. *J Nucl Med* 1995; 36: 2032–6.

54 Lorenzoni R, Rosen SD, Camici PG. Effect of selective α_1 blockade on resting and hyperemic myocardial blood flow in normal humans. *Am J Physiol* 1996; 271: H1302–6.

55 Uren NG, Melin JA, De Bruyne B, Wijns W, Baudhuin T, Camici PG. Relation between myocardial blood flow and the severity of coronary artery stenosis. *N Engl J Med*, 1994; 330: 1782–8.

56 Choudhury L, Rosen SD, Patel DP, Nihoyannopoulos P, Camici PG. Coronary flow reserve in primary and secondary left ventricular hypertrophy: a study with positron emission tomography. *Eur Heart J* 1997; 18: 108–16.

57 Choudhury L, Radvan J, Sheridan DJ, Oakley CM, Camici PG. Coronary flow reserve measurement allows differentiation of hypertrophic cardiomyopathy from the athlete's heart. *J Am Coll Cardiol* 1994; 160A: 885–67.

58 Rosen SD, Uren NG, Kaski J-C, Tousoulis D, Davies GJ, Camici PG. Coronary va-

sodilator reserve, pain perception and gender in patients with syndrome X. *Circulation* 1994; 90: 50–60.

59 Choudhury L, Elliott P, Rimoldi O, Ryan M, Lammertsma AA, Boyd H *et al.* Transmural myocardial blood flow distribution in hypertrophic cardiomyopathy during stress: effect of high-dose verapamil therapy. *Basic Res Cardiol* 1999; 94: 49–59.

60 Camici PG, Ferrannini E, Opie LH. Myocardial metabolism in ischemic heart disease: basic principles and applications to imaging by positron emission tomography. *Prog Cardiovasc Dis* 1989; 32: 217–38.

61 Camici PG, Marraccini P, Marzilli M *et al.* Coronary haemodynamics and myocardial metabolism during and after pacing stress in normal humans. *Am J Physiol* 1989; 257: E309–17.

62 Schelbert HR, Henze E, Schon HR *et al.* C-11 Palmitic acid for the noninvasive evaluation of regional myocardial fatty acid metabolism with positron computed tomography. IV. *In vivo* demonstration of impaired fatty acid oxidation in acute myocardial ischaemia. *Am Heart J* 1983; 106: 736–50.

63 Buxton DB, Schwaiger M, Nguyen A, Phelps ME, Schelbert HR. Radiolabeled acetate as a tracer of myocardial tricarboxylic acid cycle flux. *Circ Res* 1988; 63: 628–34.

64 Armbrecht JJ, Buxton DB, Schelbert HR. Validation of [1–^{11}C]acetate as a tracer for noninvasive assessment of oxidative metabolism with positron emission tomography in normal, ischemic, postischemic, and hyperemic canine myocardium. *Circulation* 1990; 81: 1594–605.

65 Brown MA, Myears DW, Bergmann SR. Noninvasive assessment of canine myocardial oxidative metabolism with carbon-11 acetate and positron emission tomography. *J Am Coll Cardiol* 1988; 12: 1054–63.

66 Buxton DB, Nienaber CA, Luxen A *et al.* Noninvasive quantitation of regional myocardial oxygen consumption *in vivo* with [1–^{11}C]acetate and dynamic positron emission tomography. *Circulation* 1989; 79: 134–42.

67 Armbrecht JJ, Buxton DB, Brunken RC, Phelps ME, Schelbert HR. Regional myocardial oxygen consumption determined noninvasively in humans with [^{11}C]

acetate and dynamic positron tomography. *Circulation* 1989; 80: 863–72.

68 Walsh MN, Geltman EM, Brown MA *et al.* Noninvasive estimation of regional myocardial oxygen consumption by positron emission tomography with carbon-11 acetate in patients with myocardial infarction. *J Nucl Med* 1989; 30: 1798–808.

69 Iida H, Rhodes CG, Araujo LI *et al.* Noninvasive quantification of regional myocardial metabolic rate for oxygen by use of $^{15}O_2$ inhalation and positron emission tomography. Theory, error analysis and application in humans. *Circulation* 1996; 94: 792–807.

70 Yamamoto Y, De Silva R, Rhodes CG *et al.* Noninvasive quantification of regional myocardial metabolic rate for oxygen by use of $^{15}O_2$ inhalation and positron emission tomography. Experimental validation. *Circulation* 1996; 94: 808–16.

71 Gallagher BM, Fowler JS, Gutterson NI, MacGregor RR, Wan C-N, Wolf AP. Metabolic trapping as a principle of radiopharmaceutical design: Some factors responsible for the biodistribution of [^{18}F] 2-deoxy-2-fluoro-D-glucose. *J Nucl Med* 1978; 19: 1154–61.

72 Huang SC, Phelps ME. Principles of tracer kinetic modeling in positron emission tomography and autoradiography, In: Phelps ME, Mazziotta JC, Schelbert HR, eds. *Positron Emission Tomography and Autoradiography Principles and Applications for the Brain and Heart.* New York: Raven Press, 1986: 287–346.

73 Ferrannini E, Santoro D, Bonadonna R, Natali O, Parodi O, Camici PG. Metabolic and haemodynamic effects of insulin on human hearts. *Am J Physiol* 1993; 264: E308–E315.

74 Camici PG, Wijns W, Borgers M *et al.* Pathophysiological mechanisms of chronic reversible left ventricular dysfunction due to coronary artery disease (hibernating myocardium). *Circulation* 1997; 96: 3205–14.

75 Wijns W, Vatner SF, Camici PG. Chronic reversible left ventricular dysfunction in patients with coronary artery disease a.k.a. hibernating myocardium. *N Engl J Med* 1998; 339: 173–81.

76 Fath-Ordoubadi F, Pagano D, Marinho NVS, Keogh BE, Bonser RS, Camici PG. Coronary revascularisation in the treatment of moderate and severe post-

ischaemic left ventricular dysfunction. *Am J Cardiol* 1998; 82: 26–31.

77 Tillisch J, Brunken R, Marshall R *et al*. Reversibility of cardiac wall-motion abnormalities predicted by positron tomography. *N Engl J Med* 1986; 314: 884–8.

78 Marinho NVS, Keogh BE, Costa DC, Lammertsma AA, Ell PJ, Camici PG. Pathophysiology of chronic left ventricular dysfunction: New insights from the measurement of absolute myocardial blood flow and glucose utilization. *Circulation* 1996; 93: 737–44.

79 Fath-Ordoubadi F, Beatt KJ, Spyrou N, Camici PG. Efficacy of coronary angioplasty for the treatment of hibernating myocardium. *Heart* 1999; 82: 210–16.

80 Syrota A. Positron emission tomography: Evaluation of cardiac receptors. In: Marcus ML, Schelbert HR, Skorton DJ, Wolf GL, eds. *Cardiac Imaging. A Companion to Braunwald's Heart Disease*. Philadelphia: WB Saunders Company, 1991; 1256–70.

81 Staehelin M, Hertel C. [^{3}H]CGP-12177: a β-adrenergic ligand suitable for measuring cell surface receptors. *J Recept Res* 1983; 3: 35–43.

82 Delforge J, Syrota A, Lançon J-L *et al*. Cardiac beta-adrenergic receceptor density measured *in vivo* using PET, CGP-12177, and a new graphical method. *J Nucl Med* 1991; 32: 739–48.

83 Choudhury L, Rosen SD, Lefroy D, Nihoyannopoulos P, Oakley CM, Camici PG. Myocardial beta adrenoceptor density in primary and secondary left ventricular hypertrophy. *Eur Heart J* 1996; 17: 1703–9.

84 Brodde O-E. β$_1$ and β$_2$-adrenoceptors in the human heart: Properties, function and alterations in chronic heart failure. *Pharmacol Rev* 1991; 43: 203–42.

85 Lefroy DC, de Silva R, Choudhury L *et al*. Diffuse reduction of myocardial beta adrenoceptors in hypertrophic cardiomyopathy: a study with positron emission tomography. *J Am Coll Cardiol* 1993; 22: 1653–60.

86 Merlet P, Delforge J, Syrota A *et al*. Positron emission tomography with ^{11}C-CGP 12177 to assess beta-adrenergic receptor concentration in idiopathic dilated cardiomyopathy. *Circulation* 1993; 87: 1169–78.

87 Choudhury L, Guzzetti S, Lefroy DC *et al*. Myocardial beta-adrenoceptors and left ventricular function in hypertrophic cardiomyopathy. *Heart* 1996; 75: 50–4.

88 Sheridan DJ, Penkoske PA, Sobel BE, Corr PB. Alpha-adrenergic contributions to dysrhythmias during myocardial ischaemia and reperfusion in cats. *J Clin Invest* 1980; 65: 161–71.

89 Morgan HE, Baker KM. Cardiac hypertrophy: mechanical, neural and endocrine dependence. *Circulation* 1991; 83: 13–25.

90 Wieland D, Rosenspire K, Hutchins G *et al*. Neuronal mapping of the heart with 6-[F-18]-Fluorometaraminol. *J Med Chem* 1990; 33: 956–64.

91 Goldstein DS, Chang PC, Eisenhofer G *et al*. Positron emission tomographic imaging of cardiac sympathetic innervation and function. *Circulation* 1990; 81: 1606–21.

92 Schwaiger M, Kaliff V, Rosenspire K *et al*. Noninvasive evaluation of the sympathetic nervous system in the human heart by PET. *Circulation* 1990; 82: 457–64.

93 Schwaiger M, Hutchins GD, Kalff V *et al*. Evidence for regional catecholamine uptake and storage sites in the transplanted human heart by positron emission tomography. *J Clin Invest* 1991; 87: 1681–90.

94 Stark RP, McGinn AL, Wilson RF. Chest pain in cardiac-transplant recipients. Evidence for sensory reinnervation after cardiac transplantation. *N Engl J Med* 1991; 324: 1791–4.

95 Schafers M, Dutka D, Rhodes CG *et al*. Myocardial pre- and postsynaptic autonomic dysfunction in hypertrophic cardiomyopathy. *Circ Res* 1998; 82: 57–62.

96 Schafers M, Wichter T, Lerch H *et al*. Cardiac sympathetic innervation in patients with idiopathic right ventricular outflow tract tachycardia. *J Am Coll Cardiol* 1998; 32: 181–6.

97 Delforge J, Janier M, Syrota A *et al*. Noninvasive quantification of muscarinic receptors *in vivo* with positron emission tomography in the dog heart. *Circulation* 1990; 82: 1494–504.

98 Camici PG, Gropler RJ, Jones T *et al*. The impact of myocardial blood flow quantitation with PET on the understanding of cardiac diseases. *Eur Heart J* 1996; 17: 25–34.

10: Does stress testing have a role?

Jan Kyst Madsen and Hans Mickley

Stress testing in patients recovering from acute coronary syndrome has been the subject of numerous studies over the past 20 or more years. The main purpose of these studies has been to give prognostic information regarding later cardiac events; but, more recently, some studies have evaluated stress testing as a tool for selecting patients for invasive or medical treatment. The results of these studies are of great importance for daily practice, and thus stress testing has gained renewed importance in recent years. The purpose of this chapter is to review the prognostic importance of exercise testing and to discuss the clinical implications in the light of recent randomized trials.

Stress testing

This chapter will only cover exercise ECG stress testing and perfusion scintigraphy. Measurements obtained from exercise stress testing can be divided into variables estimating the degree of residual ischaemia and those evaluating the extent of left-ventricular dysfunction. Markers reflecting the severity of myocardial ischaemia include chest pain, ST-segment depression, and scintigraphic evidence of defect reversibility. Exercise-test variables reflecting the quality of left-ventricular systolic function include systolic blood pressure response and exercise workload. Despite numerous studies on risk-stratification, there is only a limited consensus. The differences between study results may be attributable to patient selection, sample size, timing and type of exercise testing, treatment strategies, definition of end-point, and publication bias. Studies in patients with non-Q-wave-AMI (NQMI) or unstable angina pectoris are few, and the main body of literature focuses on mixed populations of Q-wave-AMI (QMI) and NQMI.

The prognostic importance of exercise ECG testing after AMI

The general conclusion in most studies is that, in patients capable of performing exercise testing, an abnormal systolic blood pressure response and a poor exercise capacity predict an increased risk. Exercise-induced ST-segment depression only appears to be predictive of a poor outcome in patients with inferior–posterior acute myocardial infarction (AMI). This was the results of a meta-analysis of 24 studies published from 1973 to 1985, which included 5331 patients [1]. This analysis also showed that mortality rates in patients with contraindications for exercise testing were up to fivefold higher than in patients able to perform stress testing. Thus, being excluded for clinical reasons from exercise testing *per se* identified a group of patients at increased risk. The general conclusions in most studies published during 1980 through 1995 are that, in patients capable of performing exercise testing, an abnormal systolic blood pressure response and a poor exercise capacity predict an increased risk. Exercise-induced ST-segment depression only appears to be predictive of a poor outcome in patients with inferior–posterior AMI.

In a recent meta-analysis of 15 613 patients from 28 studies, published during 1980 through 1995, only reports including 2×2 frequency rates of cardiac death or non-fatal AMI were considered [2]. In patients who had exercise electrocardiography (ECG) performed within 6 weeks after AMI, the pooled 1-year mortality was 3.3%, and the combined rate of cardiac death or AMI was 7.8%. The positive predictive values for future hard cardiac events were low for most test variables, whereas the negative values were definitely higher (Table 10.1). The sensitivity of exercise ECG variables ranged from 23% to 56% for cardiac death. The summary odds ratios (OR) for cardiac death were highest for impaired systolic blood pressure (OR 4.0) or limited exercise duration (OR 4.0). Definitely lower values for exertional ST-segment depression were observed (OR 1.7). A similar pattern was noted for the combined endpoints of cardiac death or non-fatal AMI.

The role of thrombolytic therapy for exercise ECG results

Originally the observations of increased rates of re-infarction and post-AMI angina in thrombolysed patients, compared with patients having traditional

Table 10.1 Predictive valued for cardiac events in exercise testing [2].

	$Pv_{pos}\%$		$Pv_{neg}\%$	
	Cardiac death (%)	Cardiac death or AMI (%)	Cardiac death (%)	Cardiac death or AMI (%)
Exercise-induced ST-depression	4	16	98	91
Reduced systolic pressure	11	21	96	88
Limited exercise duration	10	18	95	91
Exercise chest pain	8	19	94	89

therapy, raised the hypothesis that the widespread use of thrombolysis might result in higher rates of exercise-induced myocardial ischaemia. In a retrospective analysis of 791 patients over a 5-year period, a significant increasing trend over time was found in several clinical parameters, including the frequency of patients receiving thrombolytic therapy and patients demonstrating significant ST-segment depression on exercise testing [3]. In other studies, however, no difference—or even lower frequencies of exercise-induced ST-segment depression—have been observed in thrombolysed, as compared with non-thrombolysed, patients [4–6]. In a meta-analysis thrombolytic therapy was given in 9 of 28 reports [2]. The 1-year cardiac mortality rate was substantially lower in studies that included patients receiving thrombolytic therapy than in those which did not (4% vs. 7%). Consequently it was not surprising that the positive predictive value of exercise-induced ST-segment depression for hard cardiac events was decreased for thrombolytic-treated as compared with non-thrombolysed patients (cardiac death or AMI rate 8% vs. 18%).

The *GISSI-2 data-base report* published in 1995 [7] is absolutely the largest prognostic exercise ECG study from the thrombolytic era. A total of 10 219 patients were considered for investigation; but, in 3923 patients, exercise testing was contraindicated. The remaining 6296 patients performed a maximal symptom-limited exercise test a mean of 4 weeks after AMI. The 6-month mortality rate in patients who did not have the exercise test was > 5 times higher (7.1%) than the mortality rate in patients who actually performed pre-discharge stress testing (1.3%). These observations emphasize that, even in the thrombolytic era, the ability to undertake a pre-discharge stress test has important prognostic implications. Patients with a normal test had an exellent outcome, with a 6-month mortality of 0.9%. Only induced symptomatic ischaemia and low work-capacity indicated a higher 6-month mortality, and exercise-induced angina was the only test variable predictive of non-fatal AMI.

The importance of silent vs. symptomatic exercise-induced ischaemia

Despite controversy [8–10], it appears that silent exercise-induced ischaemia is associated with a better prognosis than painful ischaemia. In 537 patients with ST-segment depression and chest pain, also in the GISSI-2 database, the mortality at 6 months was 2.6%, compared with 1.3% in 1089 patients with asymptomatic ST-segment depression [7]. In other studies addressing different subgroups of AMI patients, painful ischaemia during exercise testing has also been associated with an increased risk of subsequent combined cardiac events—mainly severe angina—when compared with silent ischaemia. This applies to survivors of first AMI during medium- [11] and long-term

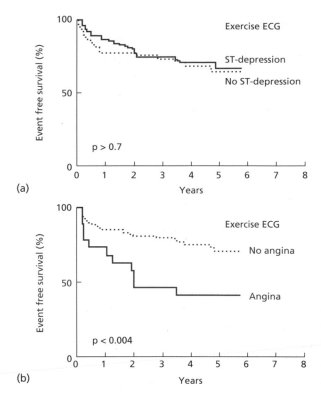

Fig. 10.1 Cumulative 5-year event-free (cardiac death, re-AMI, need for coronary revascularization) survival among 123 patients recovering from a first AMI. (a) Exercise-induced ST-segment depression. (b) Exercise-induced angina pectoris. (Reproduced with permission from the BMJ Publishing Group (*Br Heart J* 1995; 73: 320–26, Mickley *et al.* [12]).)

follow-up [12] (Fig.10.1), as well as to patients who had had a QMI years before [13].

Q-wave vs. non-Q-wave AMI

Information on the significance of stress testing in NQMI and QMI is scarce. In most previous studies, corresponding frequencies of exercise-induced ST-segment depression in QMI (27–55%) and NQMI (36–54%) have been reported [6,14–18]. Available data indicate that the frequences of exertional angina are comparable: 18–31% in QMI, and 16–33% in NQMI [14–18]. There is some evidence that the prognostic information from exercise-induced ST-segment depression in NQMI may be superior to the predictive accuracy of such changes after a recent QMI [19,20], but this issue needs to be tested in a large cohort.

The prognostic importance of exercise ECG in unstable angina

Studies addressing the clinical use of exercise testing in patients stabilized after an episode of unstable angina are limited. Many reports available contain both unstable angina and postinfarction patients [21–23]. The RISC study examined the use of pre-discharge exercise testing in 740 men admitted with unstable angina (51%) or NQMI (49%). The major independent predictors of 1-year infarction-free survival were the maximal workload achieved, and the number of leads with significant ST-segment depression [24]. The mere presence of exercise-induced ST-segment depression following unstable angina indicated an increased risk of AMI or death [25]. In a study of late exercise testing in 936 patients with an acute coronary event (30% with unstable angina, 26% with NQMI and 44% with QMI), the prognostic predictors for cardiac events did not differ in relation to the index event [21].

In conclusion: the prognostic importance of exercise ECG

- Patients who for clinical reasons are unable to perform exercise testing early after AMI comprise a high-risk group for future cardiac death.
- Patients with a normal pre-discharge exercise-test response have an excellent clinical outcome.
- Impaired systolic blood pressure response and low exercise-capacity are superior to ischaemic stress test variables in the prediction of subsequent cardiac death.
- Exercise-induced angina is associated with a worse clinical outcome than silent exertional ischaemia.
- Exercise-induced ST-segment depression may be a better prognostic marker in patients with NQMI than QMI. However, larger studies are needed.
- Thrombolytic therapy appears to result in lower positive predictive values for future hard cardiac events, when compared with the findings from non-thrombolysed patients.
- Studies addressing the prognostic use of exercise-testing in patients with a recent episode of unstable angina are limited.

The prognostic significance of perfusion scintigraphy

Perfusion scintigraphy is not as widely investigated as exercise ECG testing. Furthermore several techniques are used, which makes comparison more difficult. At one time thallium was the predominant tracer; but today, particularly in Europe, Tc-Sestamibi is taking over. Stress is applied either on a bicycle or treadmill or by pharmacological means using dipyridamole or adenosine. The interpretation of results is carried out by different types of computer analysis, and furthermore abnormal lung uptake is used in some studies but not in others, and is seldom used in Europe.

Despite these shortcomings, an analysis of the available studies is pertinent. Table 10.2 presents 8 studies of 1003 almost only post-AMI patients

Table 10.2 Prognostic information from post-AMI scintigraphy.

Study	Year	n	% with ischaemia	Event rate %	Pv_{pos} %	Pv_{neg}	Test	Predictive scintigraphic variable
Tilkemeier [26]	90	171	60	27*	33–36	n/a	ex-TI	Reversible defect/ Increased lung
Hendel [27]	91	71	51	14‡	17	11	DIPY-ti	None
de Cock [28]	92	100	54	20‡	28	89	ex-TI	Reversible defect
Mahmarian [29]	95	146	n/a	21†	n/a	n/a	adenosin-TI	Reversible defect
Miller [30]	95	210	66	17*	n/a	n/a	EX-ti	None
Travin [31]	95	134	70	10†	39	93	ex-MIBI	Reversible defect
Basu [32]	96	100	68	37†	49	88	EX-MIBI	Reversible defect
Dadik [33]	96	71	38	37†	n/a	n/a	ex-TI	Reversible defect/ increased lung

End-point for event rate:
* AMI, death, revascularization.
† AMI, death, unstable angina, heart failure.
‡ AMI, death.
n/a, not available.

from the thrombolytic era [26–33]. The differences are more striking than the similarities. In all studies the patient populations are small, from 71 to 210, and the events are defined differently. Besides re-infarction and death, they may include revascularization, unstable angina, and heart failure. The presence of transient defects is high, from 40 to 70% of all patients, and, in all but two studies, this is indicative of an increased risk of cardiac events. The predictive value of a positive or negative test is only available, or can be calculated, in a few studies, and the different use of end-points makes comparison of these values meaningless.

A recent meta-analysis of studies from 1980 to 1995 [2], disregarding the obvious differences quoted above, also indicated that transient defects have prognostic information, with different, though not significant, predictive values for exercise vs. pharmacological stress testing.

In general, however, it is clear that a transient defect on a perfusion scintigraphy post-AMI is indicative of a later cardiac event. The sensitivity, though not presented here, is high; but the frequent presence of transient defects in these populations limits their usefulness as a predictor for cardiac events. Increased lung uptake is used in some studies, and appears to have prognostic information too [26, 33]. Comparison of ST-segment depression in the exercise test and transient defects are performed in some studies [26,28,31–33]. They all show that, even though ST-segment depression also has prognostic information, the prognostic significance is stronger for a transient defect on perfusion scintigraphy, compatible with the data presented in Tables 10.1 and

10.2. In the VANQWISH trial it is noteworthy that in patients who have a NQMI, but who are without recurrent angina and do not have ischaemia on exercise thallium scintigraphy, the 1-month and 1-year risk of death or re-infarction was 1.3% and 11%—clearly lower than for patients with ischaemia who were treated invasively [34].

Only a few studies of the prognostic information obtained with perfusion scintigraphy in unstable angina have been published. In a study from 1991, which included 52 patients, a multivariate analysis of ECG stress testing and catheterization variables showed that a transient thallium defect was the only significant predictor of death or re-infarction [35]. The positive predictive value was 26% and the negative value was 97%. This result is in accordance with earlier observations [36], and altogether the findings point to a similar profile for perfusion scintigraphy in patients who have recovered from unstable angina, as for post-AMI patients.

The conclusions drawn below, therefore, seem to apply to all patients with unstable coronary syndrome.

In conclusion: the prognostic importance of scintigraphy

- A transient defect at perfusion scintigraphy is frequently found in patients with unstable coronary syndrome.
- There are no definitive indicators of differences between the tracer or the mode of stress used.
- Perfusion scintigraphy allows detection of the ischaemic location, but the clinical importance of this observation is not clarified.
- In comparison with exercise ECG testing, perfusion scintigraphy is more sensitive and has a higher predictive value of an abnormal test result.
- Pharmacological stress scintigraphy may be used in patients who are unable to exercise; however the clinical implications and prognostic information is not fully clarified.
- Stress perfusion scintigraphy is three times more expensive than exercise ECG stress testing.

Stress testing as a guide for treatment following unstable coronary syndrome

Medical treatment following Q- and non-Q-wave-AMI

Prospective, controlled studies linking exercise test stratified post-AMI patients with different strategies of medical therapy are extremely few. In one substudy from the DAVIT II trial [37], 298 AMI patients, who all performed pre-discharge exercise-testing, were double-blindly randomized to treatment with either verapamil or placebo. End-points were first major events (non-fatal re-infarction or death). During a mean follow-up of 17 months, 12.4% of patients had a cardiac end-point. The event rate in patients with exercise-induced ST-segment depression and placebo treatment was 15.4% as compared with 9.1% in patients with exercise-induced ST-segment depression, who received verapamil, altogether a non-significant reduction of 41%. The event rates in patients without exertional ST-segment depression were practically identical in both treatment strategies. The results available do not fully support the hypothesis that anti-ischaemic medical treatment can reduce the risk of future cardiac events in patients with ischaemic response during exercise testing.

Medical or invasive treatment following Q- and non-Q-AMI

Based on experience, it has become generally accepted that, in patients with angina refractory to medical therapy, those with a poor haemodynamic exercise test response or those with objective evidence of severe residual ischaemia should have coronary angiography performed with a view to revascularization.

Two recent randomized studies have used exercise testing to evaluate the prognostic impact of revascularization following AMI.

In the DANAMI study [38], 1008 patients with post-AMI angina and/or silent or symptomatic ST-segment change during a pre-discharge exercise test, were randomized to either deferred invasive treatment (in median percutaneous transluminal coronary angioplasty (PTCA) after 18 and coronary artery by-pass grafting (CABG) after 38 days respectively) or to conservative treatment. The majority (75%) had QMI. The protocol adherence was high: 80% in the invasive group were revascularized, whereas only 1.6% in the conservative group had PTCA or CABG during the first 2 months. The invasive strategy resulted in an almost 50% reduction in re-infarction from 10.5% to 5.6% (Fig. 10.2) and admission rate for unstable angina after 1 year, but no influence on mortality was demonstrated. Unpublished data, however, show a significant decrease in 5-year mortality in the patients with angina who were treated invasively (personal communication).

The DANAMI study shows that a deferred invasive strategy is beneficial in post-AMI patients with recurrent angina or stress-induced ischaemia, whereas the effect in those without ischaemia or a non-diagnostic test remains speculative.

In the VANQWISH trial [34], 920 patients with a NQMI were randomized to an early invasive, compared to an early ischaemia-guided, strategy in which those with spontaneous angina or ischaemia on stress thallium scintigraphy, were treated with PTCA or CABG if possible. Revascularization

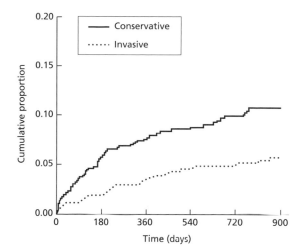

Fig. 10.2 Risk of re-infarction in the DANAMI study, a comparison of deferred invasive strategy and a conservative strategy in 1008 AMI patients with recurrent angina or exercise induced ischaemia, $P=0.0038$. (Reproduced with permission from *Circulation* 1997; 96: 748–55 [38].)

Table 10.3 Studies comparing invasive and conservative treatment strategies in patients recovering from acute coronary syndromes.

	n	QMI (%)	NQMI (%)	Unstable angina (%)	Thrombolytic (%)	Revascularization	
						Invasive (%)	Conservative (%)
TIMI IIIB [22]	1473	–	33	67	50	64	58
DANAMI [38]	1008	77	23	–	100	80	1.6
VANQUISH [34]	920	–	100	–	13	44	33
FRISC II [23]	2457	–	57	43	0	78	37

was performed in 44% in the early invasive group at a median of 8 days following AMI, compared with 33% at a median of 24.5 days in the ischaemia-guided group (Table 10.3). After 1 year there were significantly fewer primary end-points, death, or reinfarction, in the ischaemia-guided group, mainly due to a high perioperative mortality following CABG. During an average follow-up of 23 months, there was no difference in mortality of re-infarction-free survival between the two groups (Fig. 10.3). The VANQWISH trial indicates that an ischaemia-guided approached to revascularization in NQMI is at least or perhaps better than a routine invasive approach. It should be emphasized that the invasive strategy in the DANAMI study is largely similar to the conservative strategy in the VANQWISH trial.

As shown earlier in this chapter, the event rate is without doubt even lower in the patients *without* recurrent ischaemia than *with* ischaemia. The event rate in patients without ischaemia is probably only half of the event rate in the conservatively treated groups. In the DANAMI study of patients with

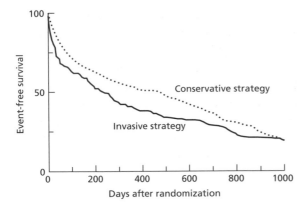

Fig. 10.3 Reinfarction-free survival in 920 non-Q-AMI patients randomized to early invasive strategy compared to a conservative strategy, i.e. ischaemia-guided invasive treatment. *P*-values after 1-year and mean follow-up, 23 months, were 0.25 and 0.35, respectively. (Reproduced with permission from *N Engl J Med*. 1998; 338: 1785–92. [34], copyright © 1998, Massachusetts Medical Society, all rights reserved.)

ischaemia, the 1-year mortality was 2.5% and reinfarction rate 7.5% in the conservative group. This means that the chance of a beneficial effect of revascularization in post-AMI patients without recurrent ischaemia is most unlikely, and revascularization is not generally recommended. In patients with non-diagnostic exercise tests, there is no information available about the effect of revascularization. A practical approach could be to do perfusion scintigraphy of any kind and perform revascularization in cases of ischaemia.

Medical treatment following unstable angina

At present there are no studies where exercise testing is used as a tool to address this issue. The ACIP study [39] included patients with stable ischaemic heart disease, and the results indicate that a maximally anti-ischaemic treatment has a prognostic benefit, and, as a parallel to this observation, it is tempting to suggest that ischaemia induced during stress testing warrants intensified medical treatment if invasive treatment is not indicated.

Medical or invasive treatment following unstable angina or non-Q-AMI

In the TIMI IIIB trial [22] a total of 1473 patients were included, 33% with NQMI and 67% with unstable angina (Table 10.3). Patients allocated to an early invasive strategy had cardiac catheterization performed 18–48h after randomization with immediate PTCA or CABG carried out as soon as possible. Patients assigned to an early conservative strategy did not have catheterization performed during the first 6 weeks, except where there was a failure of aggressive medical therapy or the presence of a positive exercise test, including thallium scintigraphy. One-year risk of death or AMI was 10.8% in the invasive arm, compared with 12.2% in the conservative arm. However, due to a high cross-over rate, the frequency of revascularization was almost identical in the two groups (Table 10.3). The outcome data were similar for patients with unstable angina and those with NQMI.

In the FRISC II study [23] a total of 2457 patients with unstable angina or NQMI, who received open dalteparin treatment, were randomized to an early invasive ($n = 1222$) or an early conservative ($n = 1235$) strategy. At study entry, 81% of the patients had chest pain at rest, 45% exhibited ST-segment depression in the resting ECG and 57% had significant troponin-T rise. Thus, from these numbers, a maximum of 57% of the patients had NQMI (Table 10.3). According to the protocol, patients in the invasive group should have coronary angiography and revascularization procedures performed <7 days, and this took place in 71%. In the non-invasive group, coronary angiography and revascularization were reserved for patients with: (1) severe residual ischaemia during exercise-testing; (2) low work-capacity; or (3) the development of refractory angina or AMI (90%). At 6-month follow-up, death or AMI had occurred in 12.1% of non-invasively-treated patients vs. 9.4% of patients in the invasive group: death alone 3.2% and 1.5%, respectively, both differences significant. In women, however, no difference in either death or AMI was observed. The FRISC II trial is the first report that has indicated an early, unselective invasive approach to be superior to a conservative, selective ischaemia-guided strategy in patients with acute coronary syndromes—at least when men are considered.

When the results of the FRISC II trial is put into context with previous studies, it should be noticed that the in-hospital mortality rate in patients undergoing CABG was very low (1.2%). Also of interest is the finding of a normal coronary angiography in 30% of women. The observations from this large-scale trial are very different from the results of the TIMI IIIB, but the two studies also vary considerably concerning the use of thrombolytics and revascularization procedures during follow-up (Table 10.3). A comparison with the findings from the VANQWISH or DANAMI reports does not seem appropriate either, because of the obvious differences in the proportions and types of acute coronary syndromes and in the use of thrombolysis (Table 10.3).

The OASIS registry [40] prospectively compared clinical outcomes for 7987 patients with unstable angina or suspected AMI without ST-elevation in countries with an aggressive use of invasive procedures and in those with a more conservative approach. Additionally, outcomes for patients initially admitted to hospitals with cardiac catheterization facilities and to hospitals without were studied. Data from 95 hospitals in 6 countries were collected, and patients were followed for 6 months. For the countries with the highest rates of invasive procedures (59%) vs. the rest (21%) there was no difference in the rate of cardiovascular death or AMI. Occurrences of strokes were higher in countries with high intervention rates, but the frequences of refractory angina at 7 days and re-admissions for unstable angina at 6 months were lower. Hospitals without cardiac catheterization facilities had lower rates of cardiovascular death, AMI or stroke at 1 month. In another database analysis of 8905 patients [41] who underwent elective catheterization during their initial hospitalization for acute coronary syndrome, the results were analysed using multivariate modelling to compare an invasive empirical to a conservative ischaemia-guided strategy. The incidence of death or AMI was greater in invasively treated patients at both 30 days (14.7% vs. 5.7%) and 6 months (17.2% vs. 8.5%). After adjusting for baseline differences, risk ratios confirmed that the invasive group had the worse prognosis.

The indications from these two recent registry studies are that early, routine cardiac catheterization in patients with unstable angina or NQMI may not be beneficial.

Conclusions regarding stress-testing-guided treatment

• From a prognostic point of view there is no solid evidence to support the routine use of cardiac catheterization and revascularization after QMI.

• An ischaemia-guided strategy with catheterization in cases of angina- or stress-induced ischaemia is associated with an improved survival and fewer re-infarctions.

• Stress testing with exercise-ECG or perfusion scintigraphy, the latter in particular in cases of non-diagnostic exercise-ECG, identifies patients with a possible beneficial effect of revascularization.

• QMI patients without angina and with a normal pre-discharge exercise test result are not likely to benefit from early catheterization and revascularization.

• Patients recovering from unstable angina and NQMI may benefit from an early non-selective invasive strategy, according to the FRISC II trial.

Conclusions

Exercise stress testing after acute coronary syndromes provides information for assessing the prognosis of the patient's functional capacity for activity after discharge from hospital. It can be used as a basis for advising patients about what levels of activity would be appropriate after leaving hospital and evaluating their capacity to return to work. It can also provide a guideline for cardiac rehabilitation, as well as being used in the evaluation of the efficacy of post-event treatment strategies.

Finally, and most importantly, the stress test can help to identify patients in whom revascularization is indicated for prognostic reasons:

- A normal stress test prior to discharge in QMI is associated with an excellent prognosis and gives no indication for catheterization and revascularization.
- An abnormal stress test with angina pectoris, ST-segment depression or reversible defects on perfusion scintigraphy indicates an increased risk in QMI and NQMI.
- Elective, ischaemia-guided catheterization and subsequent revascularization results in lower risk of death and reinfarction rates in QMI.
- Patients who are unable to perform an exercise test are at high risk, and pharmacological perfusion scintigraphy may be considered with a view to revascularization in the presence of ischaemia.
- The prognostic information from stress testing in unstable angina is limited, but ischaemia during exercise testing appears to be associated with a higher risk in this setting as well.
- In patients with acute coronary syndromes, revascularization is fully warranted in the presence of ongoing ischaemia.
- Data from the FRISC II trial indicate that revascularization leads to an improved prognosis in all patients with unstable angina and NQMI, regardless of the results of stress testing

References

1 Froelicher VF, Perdue S, Pewen W, Risch M. Application of meta-analysis using an electronic spread sheet to exercise testing in patients after myocardial infarction. *Am J Med* 1987; 83: 1045–54.

2 Shaw LJ, Peterson ED, Kesler K, Hasselblad V, Califf RM. A meta-analysis of predischarge risk stratification after acute myocardial infarction with stress electrocardiographic, myocardial perfusion, and ventricular function imaging. *Am J Cardiol* 1996; 78: 1327–37.

3 Lavie CJ, Gibbons RJ, Zinsmeister AR, Gersh BJ. Interpreting results of exercise studies after acute myocardial infarction altered by thrombolytic therapy, coronary angioplasty or bypass. *Am J Cardiol* 1991; 67: 116–20.

4 Svendsen JH, Madsen JK, Saunamäki KI, Grande P, Pedersen F, Clemmensen P, Hædersdal C, Granborg J. Effect of thrombolytic therapy on exercise response during early recovery from acute myocardial infarction: a placebo controlled study. *Eur Heart J* 1992; 13: 33–8.

5 Mickley H, Pless P, Nielsen JR, Berning J,

Møller M. Thrombolysis significantly reduces transient myocardial ischaemia following first acute myocardial infarction. *Eur Heart J* 1992; 13: 484–90.

6 Juneau M, Theroux P, Colles P, deGuise P, Lam J, Pelletier G, Waters D. Maximal versus low level exercise testing after Q and non-Q wave myocardial infarction. *J Am Coll Cardiol* 1991; 17: 214A (Abstract).

7 Villella A, Maggioni AP, Villella M *et al.* on behalf of the GISSI-2 investigators. Prognostic significance of maximal exercise testing after myocardial infarction treated with thrombolytic agents: the GISSI-2 data-base. *Lancet* 1995; 346: 523–9.

8 Pepine CJ. Prognostic implications of silent myocardial ischemia. *N Engl J Med* 1996; 334: 113–14.

9 Mickley H. Silent myocardial ischaemia in 1996. *Br J Cardiol* 1996; 3: 39–42.

10 Fox KM. Silent ischaemia: clinical implications. *Br Heart J* 1988; 60: 363–6.

11 Bigi R, Galati A, Curti G *et al.* Different clinical and prognostic significance of painful and silent myocardial ischemia

detected by exercise electrocardiography and dobutamine stress echocardiography after uncomplicated myocardial infarction. *Am J Cardiol* 1998; 81: 75–8.

12 Mickley H, Nielsen JR, Berning J, Junker A, Møller M. Prognostic significance of transient myocardial ischaemia after first acute myocardial infarction: five year follow-up study. *Br Heart J* 1995; 73: 320–6.

13 Casella G, Pavesi PC, Medda M, diNiro M *et al.* Long-term prognosis of painless exercise-induced ischemia in stable patients with previous myocardial infarction. *Am Heart J* 1998; 136: 894–904.

14 Mickley H, Pless P, Nielsen JR, Møller M. Residual myocardial ischaemia in first non-Q versus Q wave infarction: maximal exercise testing and ambulatory ST-segment monitoring. *Eur Heart J* 1993; 14: 18–25.

15 Jespersen CM, Kassis E, Edeling CJ, Madsen JK. The prognostic value of maximal exercise testing soon after first myocardial infarction. *Eur Heart J* 1985; 6: 769–72.

16 Schwartz KM, Turner JD, Sheffield LT *et al.* Limited exercise testing soon after myocardial infarction. Correlation with early coronary and left ventricular angiography. *Ann Intern Med* 1981; 94: 727–34.

17 Gibson RS, Beller GA, Gheorghiade M *et al.* The prevalence and clinical significance of residual myocardial ischaemia 2 weeks after uncomplicated non-Q wave infarction: a prospective natural history study. *Circulation* 1986; 73: 1186–98.

18 Fox JP, Beattie JM, Salih MS *et al.* Non Q wave infarction: exercise test characteristics, coronary anatomy, and prognosis. *Br Heart J* 1990; 63: 151–3.

19 Klein J, Froelicher VF, Detrano R, Dubach P, Yen R. Does the rest electrocardiogram after myocardial infarction determine the predictive value of exercise-induced ST depression? A 2 year follow-up study in a veteran population. *J Am Coll Cardiol* 1989; 14: 305–11.

20 Krone RJ, Gillespie JA, Weld FM, Miller JP, Moss AJ. Low-level exercise testing after myocardial infarction: usefulness in enhancing clinical risk stratification. *Circulation* 1985; 71: 80–90.

21 Moss AJ, Goldstein RE, Hall WJ *et al.* for the Multicenter Myocardial Ischemia Research Group. Detection and significance of myocardial ischemia in stable patients

after recovery from an acute coronary event. *JAMA* 1993; 269: 2379–85.

22 Anderson HV, Cannon CP, Stone PH *et al.* One-year results of the thrombolysis in myocardial infarction (TIMI) IIIB clinical trial. A randomised comparison of tissue-type plasminogen activator versus placebo and early invasive versus early conservative strategies in unstable angina and non-Q wave myocardial infarction. *J Am Coll Cardiol* 1995; 26: 1643–50.

23 Fragmin and fast revascularisation during instability in coronary artery disease (FRISC II) Investigators. Invasive compared with noninvasive treatment in unstable coronary-artery disease: FRISC II prospective randomised multicentre study. *Lancet* 1999; 354: 708–15.

24 Nyman I, Larsson H, Areskog M, Areskog NH, Wallentin L. The predictive value of silent ischemia at an exercise test before discharge after an episode of unstable coronary artery disease. RISC Study Group. *Am Heart J* 1992; 123: 324–31.

25 Fruergaard P, Lauenbjerg J, Jacobsen HL, Madsen JK. Seven-year prognostic value of the electrocardiogram at rest and an exercise test in patients admitted for, but without confirmed myocardial infarction. *Eur Heart J* 1993; 14: 499–504.

26 Tilkemeier PL, Guiney TE, LaRaia PJ, Boucher CA. Prognostic value of predischarge low-level exercise thallium testing after thrombolytic treatment of acute myocardial infarction. *Am J Cardiol* 1990; 66: 1203–7.

27 Hendel RC, Gore JM, Alpert JS, Leppo JA. Prognosis following interventional therapy for acute myocardial infarction: utility of dipyridamole thallium scintigraphy. *Cardiology* 1991; 79: 73–80.

28 De Cock CC, Visser FC, van Eenige MJ, Bezemer PD, Roos JC, Roos JP. Prognostic value of thallium-201 exercise scintigraphy in low-risk patients after Q-wave myocardial infarction: comparison with exercise testing and catheterization. *Cardiology* 1992; 81: 342–50.

29 Mahmarian JJ, Mahmarian AC, Marks GF, Pratt CM, Verani MS. Role of adenosine thallium-201 tomography for defining long-term risk in patients after acute myocardial infarction. *JACC* 1995; 25 (6): 1333–40.

30 Miller TD, Gersh BJ, Christian TF, Bailey KR, Gibbons RJ. Limited prognostic value

of thallium-201 exercise treadmill testing early after myocardial infarction in patients treated with thrombolysis. *Am Heart J* 1995; 130: 259–66.

31 Travin MI, Dessouki Amr Cameron T, Heller GV. Use of exercise technetium-99m sestamibi SPECT imaging to detect residual ischemia and for risk stratification after acute myocardial infarction. *Am J Cardiol* 1995; 75: 665–9.

32 Basu S, Senior R, Dore C, Lahiri A. Value of thallium-201 imaging in detecting adverse cardiac events after myocardial infarction and thrombolysis: a follow-up of 100 consecutive patients. *BMJ* 1996; 313: 844–8.

33 Dakik HA, Mahmarian JJ, Kimball KT, Koutelou MG, Medrano R, Verani MS. Prognostic value of exercise thallium-201 tomography in patients treated with thrombolytic therapy during acute myocardial infarction. *Circulation* 1996; 94: 2735–48.

34 Boden WE, O'Rourke RA, Crawford MH *et al.* for the Veterans Affairs Non-Q-Wave Infarction Strategies in Hospital (VANQWISH) Trial Investigators. Outcomes in patients with acute non-Q-wave myocardial infarction randomly assigned to an invasive as compared with a conservative management strategy. *N Engl J Med* 1998; 338: 1785–92.

35 Brown K. Prognostic value of thallium-201 myocardial perfusion imaging in patients with unstable angina who respond to medical treatment. *JACC* 1991; 17: 1053–7.

36 Launbjerg J, Fruergaard P, Jacobsen HL, Utne HE, Reiber J, Madsen JK. The long-term predictive value of an exercise thallium-201 scintigraphy for patients with acute chest pain but without myocardial infarction. *Coron Artery Dis* 1993; 4: 195–200.

37 Jespersen CM, Hagerup L, Holländer N *et al.* and the Danish Study Group on verapamil in myocardial infarction. Does exercise-induced ST-segment depression predict benefit of medical intervention in patients recovering from acute myocardial infarction? *J Int Med* 1993; 233: 33–7.

38 Madsen JK, Grande P, Saunamäki K *et al.* Danish multicenter randomized study of invasive versus conservative treatment in patients with inducible ischemia after thrombolysis in acute myocardial infarction (DANAMI). *Circulation* 1997; 96: 748–55.

39 Rogers WJ, Bourassa MG, Andrews TC, Bertolet BD, Blumenthal RS, Chaitman BR, Forman SA, Geller NL *et al.* for the ACIP Investigators. Asymptomatic cardiac ischemia pilot (ACIP) study: outcome at 1 year for patients with asymptomatic cardiac ischemia randomized to medical therapy or revascularization. *J Am Coll Cardiol* 1995; 26: 594–605.

40 Yusuf S, Flather M, Pogue J *et al.* for the OASIS (Organisation to Assess Strategies for Ischaemic Syndromes) Registry Investigators. Variations between countries in invasive cardiac procedures and outcomes in patients with suspected unstable angina or myocardial infarction without initial ST elevation. *Lancet* 1998; 352: 507–14.

41 Roe MT, Lauer MA, Houghtaling P *et al.* An ischemia-guided strategy of cardiac catheterisation in patients with non-ST-segment elevation acute coronary syndromes may be associated with improved outcomes. *J Am Coll Cardiol* 1999; 33: 391A (Abstract).

11: What is the role of echocardiography in acute coronary syndromes?

Petros Nihoyannopoulos

Introduction

There are five major types of phenomena that can affect patients with coronary artery disease and result in clinical syndromes: (1) the presence of reversible myocardial ischaemia, which is typically an imbalance between oxygen demand and supply, coupled with the accumulation of notorious metabolites; (2) myocardial infarction; (3) myocardial stunning, the consequence of an ischaemic episode with persistent myocardial dysfunction despite reperfusion; (4) hibernating myocardium, reflecting a chronically limited myocardial blood flow, but preserved cell membrane integrity and metabolic characteristics; and (5) the development of irreversible fibrosis replacing necrotic or apoptotic myocardium.

The term 'acute coronary syndrome' encompasses a wide spectrum of clinical presentations from unexpected sudden death, through unstable angina, to non-Q-wave and Q-wave myocardial infarction.

Unfortunately, diagnostic uncertainty, and delay in instituting appropriate treatment are common in patients with acute coronary syndromes. Echocardiography is the most widely available imaging technique that can be used to detect and differentiate the various phenomena described above. It is highly versatile, and because of its high spatial (2 mm) and temporal (400 frames/s) resolution, it can be used safely for: (1) monitoring global and regional left ventricular function at rest and with stress; (2) assessing valve morphology and the presence and severity of valvular leaks; and (3) recently, with the use of second- and third-generation intravenous contrast agents, it has even been used for assessing myocardial perfusion. Echocardiography is evolving as a 'one-stop strategy' for assessing cardiac anatomy, function, and perfusion in patients with suspected acute coronary syndromes.

Assessing left ventricular function

The assessment of left ventricular function, both global and regional, can be delivered with great accuracy using two-dimensional echocardiography [1]. Although ventricular volume calculations can be used to assess global left ventricular function, the high spatial resolution that echocardiography offers can provide additional detailed assessment of regional myocardial contraction, with mapping of the entire region served by coronary blood flow (Fig. 11.1). This is important for patients with coronary artery disease, particularly those in whom acute ischaemia is present, since in acute ischaemia one or more myocardial regions can be affected, while overall volumes may remain normal.

To assess regional left ventricular function, the left ventricle is typically divided into 16 regions, which correspond to the various coronary vascular beds [1]. If each of the 16 segments appears normal, there is usually no need to proceed with further volume calculations. A number of methods for the determination of overall ventricular volumes exist, but all rely on making geometric assumptions of the left ventricle, which may or may not be valid in every clinical condition [1,2]. In practice, the most common way to assess left ventricular function is visually (eye-balling). Most clinicians can clearly differentiate a good from a bad ventricle in this fashion. Therefore, making echocardiographic images readily available to clinicians for review at any time is crucial.

Detecting myocardial ischaemia

Several experimental studies have assessed regional wall-motion changes in response to ischaemia with the use of two-dimensional echocardiography [3–6]. They have demonstrated a linear reduction in regional wall thickness, that parallels the reduction of myocardial blood flow in the same territory. The extent and velocity of shortening associated with graded ischaemia roughly parallel an increase in local lactate production. Indexes of global left ventricular function are affected only with more severe ischaemia, and electrocardiographic changes are often absent with mild ischaemia.

Regional myocardial function is assessed by defining systolic wall thickening between sequentially recorded images in every myocardial segment. As the ventricle contracts, the endocardial surface moves inward towards the centre of the left ventricle (endocardial excursion) while the myocardium thickens. The cavity area decreases (area shrinkage), the cavity perimeter becomes smaller, and the distance between the endocardial and epicardial surfaces increases (wall thickening). With myocardial ischaemia, the amplitude of wall thickening increases, becoming apparent within seconds in the area supplied by the diseased vessel. In the previously normal ventricle, these changes are sufficiently distinct to be visualized easily in comparison with the behaviour of the adjacent normally contracting muscle. Once established, the severity of

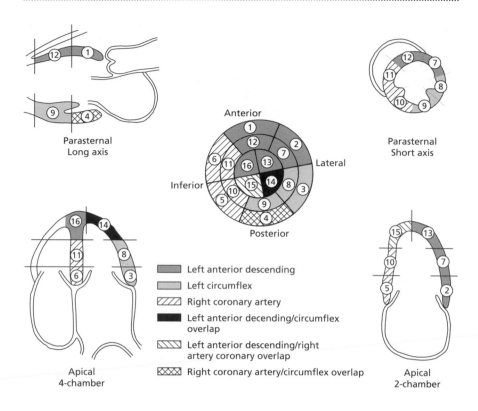

Parasternal
Long axis

Anterior

Lateral

Inferior

Posterior

Parasternal
Short axis

Apical
4-chamber

Left anterior descending

Left circumflex

Right coronary artery

Left anterior decending/circumflex
overlap

Left anterior descending/right
artery coronary overlap

Right coronary artery/circumflex overlap

Apical
2-chamber

Wall motion abnormalities detection						
Segment	Rest			Peak-stress		
	Basal	Middle	Apex	Basal	Middle	Apex
Anterior IVS	1	12	13	1	12	13
Ant. Free Wall	2	7	14	2	7	14
Lateral	3	8		3	8	
Posterior Wall	4	9	15	4	9	15
Inferior	5	10	16	5	10	16
Post IVS	6	11		6	11	
Score: Normokinetic = 1; Hypokinetic = 2; Akinetic = 3; Dyskinetic = 4						

Fig. 11.1 Regional wall-motion assessment in patients with coronary artery disease.
Parasternal and apical views with the corresponding coronary artery vascular beds are shown.
Below: the corresponding semiquantitative assessment of regional function. Each region is
assessed as normal (graded 1), hypokinetic (graded 2), akinetic (graded 3), and dyskinetic
(graded 4). The sum of all 16 segments gives the wall-motion score, which, when divided by the
number of evaluable regions, provides the wall-motion score index.

Table 11.1 Possible aetiologies of regional wall-motion abnormalities.

Coronary artery disease (myocardial infarction, reversible
    ischaemia, myocardial stunning, hibernation)
Acute myocarditis
Left bundle branch block
Wolff–Parkinson–White syndrome (WPW)
Permanent ventricular pacing
Post cardiac surgery
Cardiac sarcoidosis
Aortic regurgitation

contractile dysfunction can be defined semi-quantitatively as hypokinetic (normal direction but reduced magnitude), akinetic (absent), or dyskinetic (systolic expansion). The extent of abnormal wall-motion within a single tomographic section can be determined visually by defining the junctional points between the normally moving myocardium and the abnormal segment.

Once a regional wall-motion abnormality has been detected at rest, the diagnosis of coronary artery disease is highly likely. However, myocardial ischaemia is not the only cause for resting regional myocardial dysfunction. Abnormal septal motion can occur also in several other conditions such as abnormal intracardiac conduction (bundle branch block, Wolff–Parkinson–White syndrome (WPW)), right ventricular volume or pressure overload, focal myocarditis, and cardiac sarcoidosis (Table 11.1).

Acute coronary syndromes

Separating angina from other causes of chest pain

Patients presenting to the accident and emergency department complaining of acute chest pain often pose a diagnostic dilemma. When a typical history of angina is accompanied by characteristic ST-segment elevation on the electrocardiogram (ECG), a diagnosis of evolving myocardial infarction can be made rapidly. Often however, coronary artery occlusion can be clinically and electrocardiographically non-specific (Table 11.2). Subarachnoid haemorrhage, acute pericarditis, myocarditis, hypertrophic cardiomyopathy, and aortic dissection can all mimic acute coronary occlusion and vice versa, with potentially catastrophic results for the patient, because treatment for each of these conditions is fundamentally different. A potentially catastrophic scenario would be to give a thrombolytic drug for treatment of suspected evolving myocardial infarction in a patient with aortic dissection, subarachnoid haemorrhage, or acute pericarditis. Conversely, not giving such a drug

Table 11.2 Clinical questions that echocardiography can answer.

1 Is the pain due to myocardial ischaemia?
2 How much myocardium is in jeopardy?
3 Is an angiographic coronary artery lesion functionally significant?
4 Has there been a myocardial infarction?
5 Is there right ventricular infarction?

6 What is the cause of a given complication:
    Hypotension
    Cardiac failure
    Recurrent chest pain
    New systolic murmur

7 What are the post-myocardial-infarction risks?
    ?Remote areas of ischaemia
    ?Left ventricular aneurysm
    ?Ventricular thrombi

8 What has been achieved after revascularization?

quickly enough in a patient with evolving myocardial infarction because of a diagnostic uncertainty, may condemn the patient to sustain extensive myocardial damage.

Echocardiography can readily recognize each of the above clinical conditions and provide the diagnosis based on the presence or absence of regional wall-motion abnormalities, therefore guiding appropriate and speedy intervention. However, the detection of a regional wall-motion abnormality at rest alone does not differentiate between acute ischaemia and old myocardial infarction, or myocardial stunning or hibernation. Thus, echocardiographic information should always be evaluated with respect to the clinical context.

Unstable angina

As mentioned above, echocardiography can demonstrate the presence of regional wall-motion abnormalities, both permanent and transient. In the setting of an acute episode of unstable angina in a patient without previous ischaemic insult, myocardial thickness will be normal throughout the left ventricle. However, a lack of contraction (systolic thickening) will be evident. With the use of the segmental wall-motion score and score index (Fig. 11.1, p. 190), definition of the extent of the ischaemic zone can be ascertained. However, it is very difficult to differentiate between acute ischaemia, myocardial stunning, and acute infarction, since regional myocardial dysfunction appears similar in all these conditions.

The importance of immediate echocardiographic assessment of left ventricular systolic function and the extent of the ischaemic zone in emergency facilities has been emphasized by Sabia *et al.* [7]. Only 6% of their unselected patients had to be excluded because of poor quality imaging. Exclusion can be reduced further by regular training of a team whose role is to perform echocardiographic examinations in this setting. The presence of regional wall-motion abnormalities was the only echocardiographic finding that had a significant positive association with cardiac events occurring within the subsequent 48 hours, such as myocardial infarction (91%) and serious dysrhythmias (9%). The event rate was significantly higher in patients presenting with a high wall-motion score compared with those who had a low score. One third of all patients presenting to the emergency room with symptoms suggestive of a cardiac aetiology suffered a major cardiac event within the ensuing two years. Conversely, for those with no resting wall-motion abnormalities, less than 10% had a subsequent cardiac event [7].

Myocardial infarction and its complications

The development of acute myocardial infarction is the most dreaded consequence of acute myocardial ischaemia in patients who survive sudden death. Speedy diagnosis and the rapid institution of appropriate therapy can be life-saving. Echocardiography, because of its wide availability, should be used to reduce diagnostic uncertainty. Because of the absence of any ionizing radiation or radioactive materials, it can be used repetitively to assess the extent of myocardial damage and its potential resolution over time. Should myocardial infarction occur, echocardiography can assess its extent. Increased echodensity with regional thinning would imply myocardial scar. Its absence could imply salvageable myocardium.

Diverse complications of myocardial infarction are associated with increased morbidity and mortality (Table 11.3). Echocardiography is well suited for detection and detailed assessment of the vast majority of them.

Table 11.3 Complications after myocardial infarction.

Ventricular aneurysm
Pseudoaneurysm
LV thrombus
Ventricular septal rupture
Papillary muscle dysfunction
   Flail mitral valve
    Papillary muscle rupture
Post infarction pericarditis
   (Dresler's syndrome)
Right ventricular infarction
Ischaemic mitral regurgitation

Congestive heart failure can be caused by extensive left ventricular dysfunction involving a large myocardial segment or by the presence of ventricular aneurysm. An important differential diagnosis is between true and false aneurysm. The latter entails immediate risk of rupture and mortality. Transoesophageal imaging can help to define the presence of a ruptured free wall, as opposed to a true aneurysm in which the left ventricular wall remains intact.

Ventricular septal rupture or papillary muscle dysfunction can be identified rapidly with two-dimensional and colour-flow imaging in a patient who develops a heart murmur, heart failure, or shock. Such events occur usually within a few days to a week after myocardial infarction and should be considered to constitute a surgical emergency. Papillary muscle dysfunction and rupture can cause severe mitral regurgitation with pulmonary oedema and a fall in systemic arterial blood pressure. Echocardiography, particularly transoesophageal imaging with its high spatial resolution, can readily detect the cause and assess the severity of mitral regurgitation.

Right ventricular infarction can cause hypotension, necessitating fluid administration rather than the use of agents with positive inotropic effects or ventricular unloading agents, and can be very difficult to diagnose clinically or by ECG alone. Conversely, the right ventricle can readily be imaged using echocardiography, and, similar to the case with left ventricular dysfunction, right ventricular asynergy is a sensitive marker of myocardial infarction.

Detection of left ventricular thrombus can also readily be achieved. Its incidence has been diminished with the early use of anticoagulants and thrombolytic agents and other approaches designed to reduce infarct expansion (early use of angiotensin converting enzyme (ACE) inhibitors, β-blockers).

Myocardial stunning and hibernation

Myocardial ischaemia leads to a prompt cessation of contraction. If persistent, it leads to cell damage and irreversible myocardial necrosis or apoptosis [8]. The tight coupling of coronary flow, myocardial oxygen consumption, and contractile performance is a fundamental principle of cardiac physiology. A decrease in coronary blood flow rapidly translates into decreased contractile performance in the ipsilateral territory. Reperfusion after very short periods of low coronary flow (<10 min) usually results in rapid and complete restoration of cardiac performance with no necrosis. Myocardial ultrastructure remains normal. More prolonged periods of coronary flow reduction however (up to 20 minutes) though not usually causing necrosis, may be associated with prolonged but completely reversible dysfunction that has been called 'myocardial stunning' [9]. Further increases in the duration of ischaemia ultimately results in variable degrees of irreversible cell damage, including necrosis [10]. An elegant demonstration of myocardial stunning in humans was recently reported by Gerber *et al.* [11]. They have demonstrated a persisting left ventricular dysfunction by echocardiography at a time when positron emission tomography showed normal myocardial blood flow in the left anterior descending artery territory 4 days (median, range 1–23) after successful angioplasty in 14 patients with unstable coronary syndromes. Importantly, they showed that, following the successful revascularization, contractile function recovered progressively over a 36-week period, as could be seen from serial echocardiography.

With the advent of revascularization procedures, it has been demonstrated that prolonged regional myocardial dysfunction does not always reflect irreversible tissue damage, such as myocardial scarring, and that it can often be reversed after the restoration of blood flow, resulting in tissue that is recognized as being 'viable myocardium' [12–14]. The detection of myocardial viability in patients with resting ventricular dysfunction is important, because, when it is present, left ventricular function and survival can be improved by successful revascularization [15–17].

Diagnostic methods capable of delineating myocardial viability within the dysfunctioning regions have been based on the detection of either: (1) metabolic activity by Positron Emission Tomography (PET); (2) cell membrane integrity by rest/redistribution ^{201}Tl Single-Photon Emission Computed Tomography (Tl-SPECT); or (3) contractile reserve by dobutamine stress echocardiography. Echocardiography, with its wide availability and high spatial resolution, can serve well, when it is used in combination with low-dose dobutamine infusion.

The detection of viable myocardium with dobutamine echocardiography is based on the principle that, whereas regional contractile function may be abnormal at rest, improved contractility following stimulation of the heart and reduction of peripheral vascular resistance may differentiate viable (presence of contractile reserve), from non-viable (absence of contractile reserve), scarred myocardium [18].

The potential value of dobutamine echocardiography was first tested in patients with recent myocardial infarction. Pierard *et al.* [19] were the first to use low-dose dobutamine echocardiography to identify reversible myocardial dysfunction after reperfusion.

In contrast to the early postinfarction myocardium, in which stunning is probably predominant, chronic myocardial hibernation is associated with both the loss of contractile material and a severe limitation of residual coronary flow reserve—two factors that may profoundly affect its ability to respond to an agent with positive inotropic effects.

Chronic stable angina

Often patients with known coronary artery disease have angina or transient episodes of breathlessness, an angina equivalent. Echocardiography can be used in combination with stress (exercise or pharmacological) to detect reversible ischaemia. Pharmacological stress is used for patients who are unable to exercise sufficiently or who have resting ECG abnormalities that prohibit the accurate interpretation of ECG-exercise testing (left bundle branch block (LBBB), ventricular hypertrophy).

Stress echocardiography

The occurrence of abnormal regional systolic wall thickening with stress is perhaps the most specific marker of myocardial ischaemia [20]. Stress echocardiography combines cardiovascular stress with two-dimensional echocardiographic imaging of the heart in order to detect the consequences of ischaemia. The use of transient regional asynergy as a marker for ischaemia evolved after it was demonstrated that progressive coronary artery ligation in animals produced progressive regional hypokinesia of the respective myocardial segment when myocardial oxygen consumption was increasing. When demand exceeds supply in one or more myocardial regions, the wall ceases to contract [21,22].

There are several types of stress that can be combined with echocardiography. The fundamental advantage of exercise echocardiography over pharmacological stress is that it uses physiological cardiovascular stress and the physician's familiarity with ECG changes and symptoms with cross-sectional echocardiography to detect ischaemia-induced wall-motion abnormalities. Its diagnostic accuracy has been documented in patients with atherosclerotic coronary artery disease, in contrast to the case of patients with cardiac syndrome X in whom no regional wall-motion abnormalities are induced [22–24].

Dobutamine stress has emerged as the best pharmacological stressor, and a good alternative to exercise, with very similar diagnostic accuracy [25–27]. It is possible, however, that in patients with single-vessel disease or with mild stenosis, tests using exercise may be more sensitive [28]. Dobutamine stress is used for the detection of myocardial viability, particularly in patients unable to exercise, but in others also. During the course of stress echocardiography, dobutamine is given intravenously starting from 5 mgr/kg/min in increments of 5 or 10 mgr/kg/min up to 40 µg/kg/min for 3 min each. At these doses myocardial oxygen demand increases through an increase in heart rate, systolic blood pressure and contractility. Often, if the heart rate fails to increase, atropine, up to 1.8 mg, is given to increase the heart rate and thus the overall workload.

The detection of myocardial ischaemia with dobutamine stress has been shown to be associated with an adverse prognosis in patients with known or suspected coronary artery disease [29]. Patients having an entirely normal dobutamine stress echocardiogram and who do not exhibit any wall-motion abnormalities at rest have a low risk for future (5 years) cardiac events. Their annual event rate of cardiac death or myocardial infarction is 1.2%, with a total cumulative risk of 8% over a 5-year period. Conversely, patients with no resting wall-motion abnormalities but with a positive dobutamine stress test, exhibit a moderate risk with an annual events rate of 5.4% and a total cumulative risk over the 5 years of 12%. The group with the poorest prognosis is the one with resting wall-motion abnormalities and a positive dobutamine stress test with the development of new wall-motion abnormalities, for these patients the annual event rate mounts to 6.8%, with a total 5-year cumulative risk of >30% [28].

Contrast echocardiography

Contrast enhancement is used extensively in diagnostic and clinical radiology. Modalities such as X-rays, computed tomography, magnetic resonance imaging, and nuclear scintigraphy regularly rely on the introduction of foreign material into tissue in order to improve the contrast resolution in the image. The development of contrast media in echocardiography has been slow and sporadic. It is only recently that transpulmonary contrast agents have become readily available for clinical use [30]. The primary indication for the use of contrast echocardiography is at present for the improvement of endocardial border delineation in patients in whom adequate imaging is difficult. In patients with coronary artery disease where particular attention should be focused on regional myocardial contraction, clear endocardial definition is crucial. Intravenous contrast agents can improve endocardial delineation at rest [31] and with stress [32].

Detection of myocardial perfusion. The major use of transpulmonary contrast agents is in the detection of myocardial perfusion, or lack of it. We recently proposed that this is indeed possible in patients following myocardial infarction [33]. Intravenous injection of Sonazoid™ (Nycomed-Amersham, Oslo, Norway) consistently produced myocardial opacification in patients with previous myocardial infarction, and allowed the delineation of myocardial perfusion abnormalities. The anatomical location of each myocardial perfusion abnormality detected by contrast echo correlated well with that of SPECT perfusion imaging and wall-motion abnormalities. However, the results indicated also that assessment of myocardial perfusion by either SPECT or myocardial contrast is subject to attenuation artefacts, that predominate in the inferior wall for SPECT and the anterior and lateral walls for echocardiography.

Conclusions

Echocardiography is an important tool for patients with acute coronary syndromes. It can be used to differentiate regional myocardial ischaemia from other aetiologies of chest pain; to evaluate the extent of myocardial dysfunction, at rest and with stress; and to ascertain the presence of complications in patients with acute myocardial infarction. With the prospect of identifying myocardial perfusion defects, echocardiography is clearly an approach that can provide a 'one-stop' strategy for assessing cardiac anatomy, function and perfusion.

References

1 Schiller NB, Shah PM, Crawford M, De-Maria A, Devereux R, Feigenbaum H *et al.* American Society of Echocardiography Committee on Standarts, Subcommittee on Quantitation of Two-dimensional Echocardiograms. Recommendations for quantitation of the left ventricle by two-dimensional echocardiography. *J Am Soc Echocardiogr* 1989; 2: 358–67.

2 Schiller NB, Foster E. Analysis of left ventricular systolic function. *Heart (Suppl)* 1996; 75: 17–26.

3 Goldstein S, de Jong JW. Changes in LV wall dimensions during regional myocardial iscaemia. *Am J Cardiol* 1974; 34: 56.

4 Theroux P, Franklin D, Ross J Jr. *et al.* Regional myocardial function during acute coronary artery occlusion and its modification by pharmacologic agents in the dog. *Circ Res* 1974; 35: 896.

5 Kerber RE, Marcus ML, Ehrhardt J *et al.* Correlation between echocardiographically demonstrated segmental dyskinesis and regional myocardial perfusion. *Circulation* 1975; 52: 1097.

6 Battler A, Froelicher VF, Gallagher KP *et al.* Dissociation between regional myocardial dysfunction and ECG changes during ischaemia in the conscious dog. *Circulation* 1980; 62: 735.

7 Sabia P, Abbott RD, Afrookteh A, Keller MW, Touchtstone DA, Kaul S. Importance of two-dimensional echocardiographic assessment of left ventricular systolic function in patients presenting to the emergency room with cardiac-related symptoms. *Circulation* 1991; 84: 1615–24.

8 Tennant R, Wiggers CJ. The effects of coronary occlusion on myocardial contraction. *Am J Physiol* 1935; 112: 351–61.

9 Nesto RW, Kowalchunck GJ. The ischaemic cascade: temporal response of haemodynamic, electrocardiographic and symptomatic expression of iscaemia. *Am J Cardiol* 1987; 57: 23C–30C.

10 Vanoverschelde JLJ, Pasquet A, Gerber B, Melin JA. Pathophysiology of myocardial hibernation. Implications for the use of dobutamine echocardiography to identify myocardial viability. *Heart* 1999; 82 (Suppl. 3): 13–17.

11 Gerber BL, Wijns W, Vanoverschelde J-LJ, Heyndrickx GR, De Bruyne B, Bartunek J, Melin JA. Myocardial perfusion and oxygen consumption in reperfused noninfarcted dysfunctional myocardium after unstable angina. *J Am Coll Cardiol* 1999; 34: 1939–46.

12 Heyndrickx GR, Millard RW, McRitchie RJ, Maroko PR, Vatner SF. Regional myocardial functional and electrophysiological alterations after brief coronary occlusions in conscious dogs. *J Clin Invest* 1975; 56: 978–85.

13 Braunwald E, Rutherford J. Reversible ischaemic left ventricular dysfunction: evidence for 'hibernating myocardium'. *J Am Coll Cardiol* 1986; 8: 1467–70.

14 Rahimtoola S. A perspective on the three large multicentre randomised clinical trial of coronary bypass surgery for stable angina. *Circulation* 1985; 72: V123–35.

15 Di Carli MF, Asgrzadie F, Schelbert H *et al.* Quantitative relation between myocardial viability and improvement in heart failure symptoms after revascularisation in patients with ischaemic cardiomyopathy. *Circulation* 1995; 92: 3436–44.

16 Senior R, Kaul S, Lahiri A. Myocardial viability on echocardiography predicts long-term survival after revascularisation in patients with ischaemic congestive heart failure. *J Am Coll Cardiol* 1999; 33: 1848–54.

17 Pasquet A, Robert A, D'Hondt A-M, Dion R, Melin JA, Vanoverschelde J-LJ. Prognostic value of myocardial ischaemia and viability in patients with chronic left ventricular ischaemic dysfunction. *Circulation* 1999; 100: 141–8.

18 Mertes H, Segar DS, Johnson M, Ryan T, Sawada SG, Feigenbaum H. Assessment of hibernating myocardium by dobutamine stimulation in a canine model. *J Am Coll Cardiol* 1995; 26: 1348 55.

19 Pierard LA, Landsheere CM, Berthe C, Rigo P, Kulbertus HE. Identification of viable myocardium by echocardiography during dobutamine infusion in patients with myocardial infarction after thrombolytic therapy: comparison with positron emission tomography. *J Am Coll Cardiol* 1990; 15: 1021–31.

20 Ross J Jr. Assessment of ishaemic regional myocardial dysfunction and its reversibility. *Circulation* 1986; 74: 1186–90.

21 Gallagher KP, Matsuzaki M, Koziol JA, Kemper WS, Ross J Jr. Regional myocardial perfusion and wall thickening during ischaemia in conscious dogs. *Am J Physiol* 1984; 16: H727.

22 Marwick TH, Nemec JJ, Pashkow FJ, Stewart WJ, Salcedo EE. Accuracy and limitations of exercise echocardiography in a routine clinical setting. *J Am Coll Cardiol* 1992; 19: 74–81.

23 Nihoyannopoulos P, Kaski JC, Crake T, Maseri A. Absence of myocardial dysfunction during stress in patients with syndrome X. *J Am Coll Cardiol* 1991; 18: 1463–70.

24 Armstrong WF. Exercise echocardiography. Ready, willing able. *J Am Coll Cardiol* 1988; 11: 1359–61.

25 Sawada SG, Segar DS, Ryan T *et al.* Echocardiographic detection of coronary artery disease during dobutamine infusion. *Circulation* 1991; 83: 1605–14.

26 Sear DS, Brown SE, Sawada SG, Ryan T, Feigenbaum H. Dobutamine stress echocardiography: correlation with coronary lesion severity as determined by quantitative angiography. *J Am Coll Cardiol* 1992; 19: 1197–202.

27 Marwick T, Willemart B, D'Hondt A *et al.* Selection of the optimal myocardial dysfunction and malperfusion. Comparison of dobutamine and adenosine using echocardiography and ^{99m}Tc-MIBI single photon emission computed tomography. *Circulation* 1993; 87: 345–54.

28 Rallidis L, Cokkinos P, Tousoulis D, Nihoyannopoulos P. Comparison of dobutamine and treadmill exercise echocardiography in inducing ischaemia in patients with coronary artery disease. *J Am Coll Cardiol* 1997; 30: 1660–8.

29 Poldermans D, Fioretti PM, Boersma E, Bax JJ, Thomson IR, Roelandt JRTC, Simoons ML. Long-term prognostic value of dobutamine-atropine stress echocardiography in 1737 patients with known or suspected coronary artery disease. *Circulation* 1999; 99: 757–62.

30 Feinstein SB, Cheirif J, Ten Cate FJ, Silverman PR, Heidenreich PA, Dick C *et al.* Safety and efficacy of a new transpulmonary ultrasound contrast agent: initial multicenter clinical results. *J Am Coll Cardiol* 1990; 16: 316–24.

31 Crouse LJ, Cheirif J, Hanly DE, Kisslo JA, Labovitz AJ, Raichlen JS *et al.* Opacification and border delineation improvement in patients with suboptimal endocardial border definition in routine echocardiography: results of phase III Albunex multicenter trial. *J Am Coll Cardiol* 1993; 22: 1494–500.

32 Ikonomidis I, Holmes E, Narbuvold H, Bolstad B, Muan B, Nihoyannopoulos P. Left ventricular wall motion assessment and endocardial border delineation after intravenous injection of Infoson™ during dobutamine stress echocardiography. *Coronary Artery Disease*, 1998; 9: 567–76.

33 Jucquois I, Nihoyannopoulos P, D'Hontdt A-M, Roelants V, Robert A, Melin JA, Glass D, Vanoverschelde J-LJ. Comparison of myocardial contrast echocardiography with NC100100 and Tc-99 m sestamibi single photon emission computed tomography for detection of resting myocardial perfusion abnormalities in patients with previous myocardial infarction. *Heart* 2000; 83: 518–24.

Part 3: Treatment

12: Treatment of acute coronary syndromes: which heparin and for how long?

Sonia S. Anand and Jack Hirsh

Introduction

Acute coronary syndromes (ACS) are clinical disorders that include acute myocardial infarction (MI) with or without ST elevation and unstable angina. All the conditions in the spectrum have in common lesions of the coronary arteries often with atherosclerotic narrowing with superimposed acute thrombosis. The key pathophysiological components of this syndrome are atherosclerosis, plaque disruption, and intraluminal thrombi [1]. The most dire clinical consequences of ACS are irreversible myocardial damage from MI and death. Given the critical role of thrombosis in its pathogenesis, the acute medical management of ACS involves antiplatelet therapy, fibrinolytic therapy, and anticoagulant therapy [1].

Anticoagulants modulate thrombin generation and/or inhibit thrombin activity. Inhibition of thrombin generation or activity can be achieved with the use of direct or indirect inhibitors. Unfractionated and low-molecular-weight heparin are indirect inhibitors [2]. In this chapter we review the roles of unfractionated heparin (UFH) and low-molecular-weight heparin (LMWH) in the treatment of patients with ACS.

Pharmacokinetic properties of unfractionated heparin and low-molecular-weight heparin

Unfractionated heparin is a glycosaminoglycan with a mean molecular weight (MW) of 15 000 (approximately 50 monosaccharide units) and a MW range of 5000–30 000. LMWHs are derived from UFH by chemical or enzymatic depolymerization. These glycosaminoglycans have mean MWs of 4000–5500 (about 13 and 18 saccharide units) and have a range of molecular weights of 1000–10 000. Both agents produce their major anticoagulant effect by binding to and activating antithrombin, thereby inactivating thrombin and factor Xa. UFH inhibits factor Xa and IIa in a ratio of 1 : 1, whereas LMWHs inhibit factor Xa and IIa in ratios between 4 : 1 and 2 : 1, depending on their MW

203

distribution [2]. There are a number of important differences between UFH and LMWH that make LMWH compounds more attractive than their parent compound for the treatment of venous and arterial thromboembolic disease. LMWHs exhibit: (i) reduced non-specific binding to plasma proteins that results in a more predictable anticoagulant response and usually makes their monitoring unnecessary; (ii) an increased plasma half-life that allows once or twice daily subcutaneous (SC) administration; (iii) reduced binding to platelets and platelet factor IV, which may explain the lower incidence of heparin-induced thrombocytopenia (HIT); and (iv) reduced bone loss when used over the long term [2]. UFH has been evaluated extensively and is used routinely in the treatment of patients with ACS. Based on their superior properties and their safety and effectiveness in the prevention and treatment of venous thrombosis, LMWHs have also been evaluated recently in the setting of ACS.

Acute coronary syndromes with ST elevation

Acute coronary syndromes that are associated with persistent elevation of the ST segments on a 12-lead electrocardiogram (ECG) are frequently acute myocardial infarctions (AMI). AMI with ST elevation accounts for approximately 10% of all patients who present to hospital with chest pain [3]. In this setting, fibrinolytic therapy and aspirin are clearly indicated [4]. Before the role of fibrinolytic therapy and aspirin had been established, intravenous (IV) UFH had been evaluated in the treatment of patients with AMI and found to reduce mortality significantly. However, the role of IV UFH as adjunctive therapy to fibrinolytic therapy and aspirin remains controversial [5].

Unfractionated heparin without aspirin

Trials of UFH therapy in patients with AMI have been too small to detect moderate reductions of important outcomes such as death, recurrent MI and stroke. However, a pooled analysis of 5459 patients who did not routinely receive aspirin (of whom only 14% received fibrinolytic agents) showed that treatment with UFH resulted in a 23% reduction in death (11.4% vs 14.9%, $P = 0.002$), 18% reduction in MI (6.7% vs 8.2%, $P = 0.08$), 47% reduction in stroke (1.1% vs 2.1%, $P = 0.01$), and 86% reduction in pulmonary embolism (2.0% vs 3.8%, $P < 0.001$) [5]. The benefit from UFH occurred at the 'cost' of a significant, two-fold increase in major bleeding (1.9% vs 0.9%, $P = 0.01$).

Unfractionated heparin with fibrinolytic therapy and aspirin

There is clear evidence that fibrinolytic therapy and aspirin are effective in the treatment of AMI with ST elevation. In contrast, there is uncertainty whether UFH adds to the benefit achieved by these therapies. Although angiographic studies which evaluated IV UFH and aspirin given together with fibrinolytic therapy reported improved coronary artery patency for up to 81 h after fibrinolysis [6], the additional benefit of UFH (either IV or SC) in patients with AMI who routinely receive aspirin and fibrinolytic therapy is not as clear. Studies comparing UFH and aspirin to aspirin alone, where over 90% of patients received fibrolynic therapy (streptokinase, tissue plasminogen activator (t-PA), or anistreplase), indicate that the combination is associated with small and marginally significant reductions in death (8.6% vs 9.1%, $P = 0.03$), and reinfarction (3.0% vs 3.3%, $P = 0.04$), yet the combination is associated with a significant increase in major bleeding (1.0% vs 0.7%, $P < 0.001$). The majority of patients in this overview came from two large trials, GISSI-2 in which UFH was given subcutaneously (12 500 U twice a day) beginning 12 h after fibrinolytic therapy [7], and ISIS-3 in which 12 500 U twice a day of SC UFH was given but started 4 h after fibrinolytic therapy [8].

In the GUSTO-1 trial ($n = 20 173$), IV UFH was compared to SC UFH with fibrinolytic therapy and aspirin [9]. Four strategies were compared: (i) accelerated t-PA plus IV UFH for 48 h; (ii) streptokinase plus IV heparin for 48 h; (iii) streptokinase and 12 500 U SC UFH for 7 days starting 4 h after streptokinase had finished; and (iv) reduced-dose t-PA plus streptokinase plus IV heparin for 48 h. No advantage of IV UFH over SC UFH in patients who received streptokinase was observed for death (7.4% vs 7.3%), MI (4.2% vs 3.5%), or stroke (1.4% vs 1.2%). Of the four treatment regimens, patients who received t-PA and IV UFH had the lowest mortality rate at 30 days (6.3%), and showed a significant 14% relative risk reduction over the streptokinase regimens. In addition, in an angiographic sub-study ($n = 1210$) of GUSTO-1, improved patency (TIMI grade 3 flow) at 90 min with t-PA and IV UFH over the other regimens was observed [10]. On the basis of GUSTO-1, the accelerated-dose t-PA protocol has been widely adopted for use in patients with AMI.

In summary, overall, only small and marginally significant reductions in death, MI, and stroke are observed with UFH compared with no UFH, in patients who receive fibrinolytic therapy (e.g. streptokinase, t-PA, and anistreplase) and aspirin for AMI, and these benefits may be offset by an increase in major bleeding. The data evaluating the role of adjunctive IV UFH vs control are sparse, and in the absence of further direct comparisons, its role remains inconclusive [11]. Despite the limited data supporting the routine use of IV UFH as adjunctive therapy to fibrinolytic therapy, trials conducted after GUSTO-1 [12] have used IV UFH routinely for approximately 48 h after administration of fibrinolytic therapy [3], and IV UFH is widely used with fibrin-specific fibrinolytic agents (e.g. t-PA) in usual practice, at least in the United States.

Low-molecular-weight heparin

Research evaluating the role of LMWH as adjunctive therapy to fibrinolytic therapy and aspirin in the setting of ACS with ST elevation is on-going. BIO-MACS-II is a Phase III clinical trial being conducted in Scandinavia to evaluate this question [13].

Acute coronary syndrome without electrocardiographic ST segment elevation

Acute coronary syndromes occur in a large spectrum of patients who have chest pain which is not associated with ST elevation on the ECG. They may (non-Q wave MI) or may not (unstable angina) sustain myocardial necrosis manifested by biochemical criteria [14]. In the United States, in 1996, approximately 700 000 men and women were discharged from hospital with a diagnosis of unstable angina, and the incidence of ACS without ST elevation is increasing as the population ages [15]. Before the routine use of antithrombotic therapy, the in-hospital rate of MI and death in patients with ACS without ST elevation was about 10% [16,17]. With the routine use of UFH and aspirin this rate was reduced by about 50%. Such reductions in important clinical outcomes have a large impact in reducing the burden of cardiovascular disease in a population, given the high prevalence of this condition.

Aspirin

For patients with unstable angina or non-Q wave MI, meta-analyses of randomized trials confirm that aspirin significantly reduces the rate of cardiovascular (CV) death and recurrent MI [5], therefore aspirin should be used in all patients with ACS. Conversely, randomized trials of fibrinolytic therapy in patients with ACS without ST elevation have not demonstrated any significant benefit of fibrinolytic therapy in this setting, and its use is not generally recommended [18].

Unfractionated heparin

Most patients with unstable angina are treated with IV UFH and aspirin initially [14]. Whether UFH produces additional improvement in clinical outcomes in patients with ACS without ST elevation cannot be answered from the results of single randomized trials because individually they lack sufficient power to detect important clinical differences. A meta-analysis of published data from six small randomized trials (n = 1353) reported a risk reduction of 33% (95% CI: –2–56%) in cardiovascular death and MI with the combination of IV UFH and aspirin. However, this was of borderline significance [19]. Given the potential limitations of meta-analysis and the relatively small numbers of patients included, this finding may represent an overestimation of the true relative benefit of the combination of UFH and aspirin over aspirin (Fig. 12.1). More recently however, trials that evaluated the combination of LMWH and aspirin compared to aspirin alone in the setting of ACS without ST elevation [20,21] have reported large reductions in clinical events with the combined antithrombotic therapy. Addition of these data to the original meta-analysis evaluating heparin ($n = 2919$) leads to an estimated 47% reduction (95% CI: 27–62%) in CV death and MI in patients treated with combination antithrombotic therapy (UFH or LMWH and aspirin) compared with aspirin alone [22].

Low-molecular-weight heparin

LMWHs have been evaluated in patients with ACS without ST elevation as short-term (< 7 days) and longer-term (14–60 days) therapy, and have been compared directly with both placebo and to IV UFH against a background of aspirin therapy (Table 12.1).

Short-term trials of LMWH vs placebo

Two trials have evaluated LMWH compared with placebo in the presence of aspirin [20,21]. A small three-arm randomized trial conducted by Gurfinkel *et al.* compared nadroparin calcium with placebo and with UFH in 219 patients. A 63% relative risk reduction (RRR) was observed (compared with placebo) for the composite of MI, recurrent angina, and urgent revascularization (15/68 (22%) vs 43/73 (59.0%), $P < 0.001$). These differences were attributed primarily to differences in the incidence of recurrent episodes of angina that

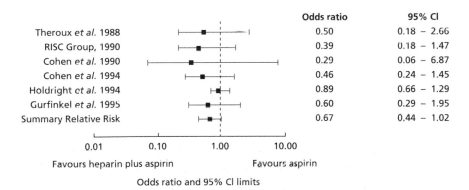

Fig. 12.1 Relative risk of myocardial infarction or death during hospitalization [10].

Table 12.1 Trials of LMWH in ACS without ST elevation.

Trial	n	Short-term comparison	Long-term comparison
Gurfinkel 1995 [20]	279	Nadroparin 214 IU SC b.i.d. vs placebo	N/A
FRISC 1996 [26]	1506	Dalteparin 120 IU/kg SC b.i.d. vs placebo	Dalteparin 7500 IU SC o.d. vs placebo
FRIC 1997 [23]	1482	Dalteparin 120 IU/kg SC b.i.d. vs UFH 5000 IU B, 1000 IU i.v./h then 12500 iu SC b.i.d.	Dalteparin 7500 IU SC o.d. vs placebo
ESSENCE 1997 [24]	3171	Enoxaparin 1 mg/kg SC b.i.d. 2–8 d vs UFH 5000 IU APTT 55–85 s	N/A
TIMI 11B 1998 [29]	3912	Enoxaparin 3000 IU B, 100 IU/kg b.i.d. vs UFH 70 IU B, 15 U/kg APTT 1.5–2 ×	Enoxaparin 4500 IU–6000 IU SC b.i.d. vs placebo
FRAXIS 1998 [30]	3468	Nadroparin 87 IU SC b.i.d. vs UFH 5000 B 1250/h target local APTT	Nadroparin 87 IU SC vs placebo
FRISC II 1999 [28]	2457	Dalteparin 120 IU/kg b.i.d. vs placebo	Dalteparin 5000 IU or 7500 IU SC b.i.d. vs placebo

SC, subcutaneous; IU, international units; o.d., once daily; b.i.d, twice daily; UFH, unfractionated heparin; B, bolus.

were defined as chest pain at rest lasting greater than 10 min in patients being treated with anti-ischaemic medications [20]. In the second trial, FRISC ($n =$ 1506), dalteparin was compared with placebo for 6 days in the presence of aspirin, and an 81% RRR was demonstrated with dalteparin over placebo for death and MI (1.8% vs 9.7%, $P < 0.001$) [20].

Short-term trials of LMWH vs UFH

Once it was established that LMWH added to the benefits of antiplatelet agents, attention focused upon whether LMWHs were superior to UFH. In the trial by Gurfinkel *et al.*, nadroparin was compared directly with UFH, and a 63% RRR in favour of LMWH was observed (15/68 (22%) vs 42/70 (60%), $P < 0.001$) at 7 days [20]. Subsequently, two large trials, FRIC [23] and ESSENCE, [24] were conducted. The FRIC trial compared dalteparin (120 U/kg b.i.d. vs IV UFH) in an open comparison in the short term (1–6 days), and dalteparin (7500 IU o.d.) or placebo in a double-blind comparison in the long-term phase (6–45 days) (Table 12.1). No differences in the short-term (9.3% vs 7.6%) or long-term rates (12.3% vs 12.3%) of death, MI or recurrent angina were observed between the groups. The study was powered to detect large reductions (e.g. 50%) in death, MI, and recurrent angina over the long term. Therefore, the results cannot exclude the possibility that modest, (e.g. 15–20%) but clinically important, differences exist between these agents.

In ESSENCE [24], enoxaparin (1 mg/kg (100 U/kg) q 12 h) was directly compared with IV UFH for approximately 72 h in a randomized double-blind comparison. A significant 17% reduction in death, MI, and recurrent angina with enoxaparin was observed at 14 days (16.6% vs 19.8%, $P < 0.02$), and this benefit persisted up to 30 days (19.8% vs 23.3%, $P < 0.02$). Furthermore, a significant 16% reduction in revascularization rates with enoxaparin was observed (27% vs 32.2%, $P = 0.001$). There was no difference in the incidence of major bleeds, but a significant increase in minor bleeds was seen in the enoxaparin group (11.9% vs 7.2%, $P = 0.001$); most being attributed to puncture wounds at the injection sites. The promising results in the ESSENCE study contrast with those of the FRIC trial. The differences could reflect important methodological differences. Unlike FRIC, ESSENCE was a double-blind placebo-controlled trial adequately powered to detect a difference in CV death, MI and recurrent angina in the acute phase. Whether the observed benefits of enoxaparin in ESSENCE are indicative of a superior class effect of LMWHs over IV UFH, a unique benefit of enoxaparin over dalteparin, or to chance, is not yet clear.

Long-term trials of LMWH compared to placebo

Biochemical and clinical data indicate that ACS are an acute manifestation of a chronic disease that results in persistent activation of coagulation [25,26], and sustained clinical event rates over the long term [27]. Because the clinical events are precipitated by the development of thrombosis, LMWHs have been evaluated for long-term use in patients with ACS. Three recent trials FRISC-2 [28], TIMI [29], and FRAXIS [30] have evaluated prolonged LMWH therapy in this condition.

TIMI-11B

This randomized double-blind placebo-controlled trial in 3912 patients with ACS without ST elevation compared the LMWH enoxaparin with IV UFH [29]. The primary end-point was the composite of CV death, MI and recurrent ischaemia requiring revascularization at 43 days. Initially, patients who were randomized to enoxaparin received 3000 IU bolus IV, followed by 100 IU/kg b.i.d. for 3–8 days or IV UFH 5000 IU bolus followed by 15 IU/kg IV infusion to target an activated partial thromboplastin time (APTT) of 1.5–2.0 times control. Patients who did not require immediate revascularization or did not experience bleeding in the acute phase were continued on enoxaparin 4500–6000 IU SC b.i.d. for an additional 35 days, and the IV UFH patients continued to receive placebo injections. At 14 days, the rate of CV death, MI, and recurrent ischaemia requiring revascularization was 277/1953 (14.2%) in the enoxaparin group compared with 325/1957 (16.6%) with IV UFH, resulting in a RRR of 18%, $P < 0.03$. Although an early benefit of enoxaparin was observed, by 43 days the initial absolute difference of 2.3% persisted without additional benefit from long-term LMWH (17.3% vs 19.6%, RRR = 12%, $P < 0.049$), and at a cost of a significant excess of major bleeding with LMWH (2.9% vs 1.5%. $P < 0.02$).

FRAXIS

The FRAXIS trial was a three-arm double-blind randomized comparison in which 3468 patients with ACS without ST elevation received 6 days of IV UFH in systemic doses (5000 IU bolus, followed by 1250 U/hr IV infusions to a target APTT) or nadroparin (87 IU/kg SC b.i.d.) for 6 days or nadroparin (87 IU/kg SC b.i.d.) for 14 days. The primary end-point was a composite of death, MI, and refractory or recurrent angina at 6 days. No differences between short-term IV UFH heparin or LMWH were observed at 6 days, and no difference between long-term LMWH (14 days) and short-term (6 days) antithrombotic therapy was observed by 14 days [30] (Table 12.2).

FRISC II

This was a randomized placebo-controlled trial of dalteparin in 2267 patients with ACS without ST elevation [28]. All patients received dalteparin 120 IU/kg q 12 h for the acute phase (5–7 days), and after the acute treatment patients were randomized to dalteparin 5000–7500 IU q 12 h or placebo for

Table 12.2 FRAXIS results.

Efficacy	IV UFH ($n = 1151$)	LMWH × 6 days ($n = 1166$)	LMWH × 14 days ($n = 1151$)
6 days	172 (14.9%)	161 (13.8%)	182 (15.8%)
14 days	208 (18.1%)	207 (17.8%)	230 (20%)
Major bleed			
6 days	13 (1.1%)	8 (0.7%)	15 (1.3%)
14 days	28 (2.4%)	22 (1.9%)	46 (4%)

UFH, unfractionated heparin; LMWH, low molecular weight heparin.

90 days in a double-blind manner. The primary end-point was a composite of death and MI at 3 months, and the rates did not differ significantly between dalteparin and placebo (6.7% vs 8.0%, $P = 0.17$). The rates of major and minor bleeding were significantly higher in the dalteparin compared with the placebo group (3.3% vs 1.5%, $P < 0.01$ and 23.0% vs 8.4%, $P < 0.001$), respectively.

Summary results

By pooling results of all trials that compared short-term LMWH with UFH ($n = 12\,171$), an odds ratio = 0.88 (95% CI: 0.69–1.12) is observed that indicates that a modest, 12% reduction with LMWH over UFH may exist (Fig. 12.2). However, the upper border of the 95% CI crosses 1, indicating that more data are needed to provide a conclusive answer. In a pooled analysis of results in all long-term trials, data from approximately 12 099 patients do not indicate a benefit of LMWH over placebo in reducing MI or death OR = 0.98 (95% CI: 0.81–1.7) (Fig. 12.3). Possible reasons for the lack of benefit of long-term LMWH treatment are outlined in Table 12.3.

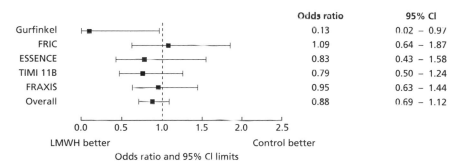

Fig. 12.2 Heparin meta-analysis. Short-term trials: death/recurrent MI.

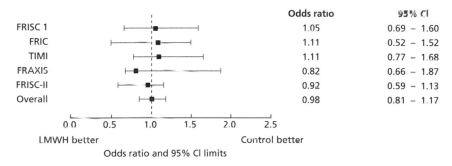

Fig. 12.3 Heparin meta-analysis. Long-term trials: death/recurrent MI.

Table 12.3 Possible reasons for lack of effect thus far observed with prolonged anticoagulant therapy in ACS without ST elevation.

Selection of low-risk patients
ACS is a heterogeneous condition — some benefit, others do not
Anticoagulant therapy was inadequate — unlikely as the rates of bleeding are increased as expected in AC treated patients.
Anti-platelet action is more important to turn off to prevent chronic events than antithrombotics
Study design/Play of chance

Differences between LMWHs

Although there are differences in the pharmacokinetic and anticoagulant profiles of various LMWHs, there is no evidence that they are clinically important [31]. Proponents of enoxaparin suggest that this LMWH is more effective than other preparations because it was shown in the short term, in both the ESSENCE [24] and TIMI-11B [29] trials, to be more effective than IV UFH. This contrasts with the neutral results observed with dalteparin, and nadroparin. Although it is possible that one LMWH preparation might be better than another, the superiority of one LMWH preparation over another can be reliably assessed only by direct comparisons of different LMWH agents in randomized trials [8]. However such trials would require very large sample sizes (e.g. $n = 20\,000$), and to our knowledge none are currently planned.

Which heparin and for how long?

In patients with AMI with ST elevation there is no clear role for the regular use of IV UFH after initial treatment with fibrinolytic agents plus aspirin. Low-molecular-weight heparin is in the early stages of evaluation in this setting. For patients with ACS without ST elevation, either short-term use of LMWH or IV UFH appears to be effective against a background of aspirin therapy, and LMWH may be easier to administer, with consequently shorter hospitalizations. Despite the biochemical and clinical evidence that the risk of MI and death in ACS persists for weeks after the acute event, there is no firm evidence to date that extending heparin (LMWH) treatment beyond the short-term results in additional clinical benefit.

References

1 Theroux P, Fuster V. Acute Coronary Syndromes. *Circulation* 1998; 97: 1195–206.
2 Hirsh J. Low-molecular-weight heparin: a review of the results of recent studies of the treatment of venous thrombo-embolism and unstable angina. *Circulation* 1998; 98: 1575–82.
3 Cairns JA, Theroux P, Lewis HD Jr, Ezekowitz M, Meade TW, Sutton GC. Antithrombotic agents in coronary artery

disease. *Chest* 1998; 114 (5 Suppl.): 611S–633S.

4 Collins R, Peto R, Baigent C, Sleight P. Aspirin, heparin, and fibrinolytic therapy in suspected acute myocardial infarction. *N Engl J Med* 1997; 336: 847–53.

5 Collins R. Clinical effects of anticoagulant therapy in suspected acute myocardial infarction: Systematic overview of randomized trials. *BMJ* 1996; 313 (7058): 652–9.

6 Hsia J, Kleinman N, Aguirre F, Chaitman BR, Roberts R, Ross AM. Heparin-induced prolongation of partial thromboplastin time after thrombolysis: relation to coronary artery patency. HART Investigators. *JACC* 1992; 20 (1): 31–5.

7 GISSI-2. a factorial randomized trial of alteplase versus streptokinase and heparin versus no heparin among 12 490 patients with acute myocardial infarction. Gruppo Italiano per lo Studio della Sopravvivenza nell'Infarto Miocardico. *Lancet* 1990; 336 (8707): 65–71.

8 ISIS-3. A randomised comparison of streptokinase vs tissue plasminogen activator vs anistreplase and of aspirin plus heparin vs aspirin alone among 41 299 cases of suspected acute myocardial infarction. ISIS-3 (Third International Study of Infarct Survival) Collaborative Group. *Lancet* 1992; 339 (8796): 753–70.

9 Anonymous. An international randomized trial comparing four thrombolytic strategies for acute myocardial infarction. The GUSTO Investigators. *N Engl J Med* 1993; 329: 673–82.

10 Simes RJ, Topol EJ, Holmes DR Jr. *et al.* Link between the angiographic substudy and mortality outcomes in a large randomized trial of myocardial reperfusion. Importance of early and complete infarct artery reperfusion. GUSTO-I Investigators. *Circulation* 1995; 91: 1923–8.

11 Ridker PM, Hebert PR, Fuster V, Hennekens CH. Are both aspirin and heparin justified as adjuncts to thrombolytic therapy for acute myocardial infarction? [Review] *Lancet* 1993; 341 (8860): 1574–7.

12 International Joint Efficacy Comparison of Thrombolytics. Randomised double-blind comparison of reteplase double-bolus administration with streptokinase in acute myocardial infarction (INJECT). trial to investigate equivalence. *Lancet* 1995; 346 (8971): 329–36.

13 Frostfeldt G. Low molecular weight heparin (dalteparin) as adjuvant treatment of thrombolysis in acute myocardial infarction – a pilot study: Biochemical markers in acute coronary syndromes (BIOMACS II). *J Am Coll Cardiol* 1999; 33 (3): 627–33.

14 Theroux P, Fuster V. Acute Coronary Syndrome: unstable angina and non-Q-wave myocardial infarction [Review]. *Circulation* 1998; 97: 1195–206.

15 American Heart Association. *American Heart Association Heart and Stroke Statistical Update 1998.* Dallas, Texas, 1999.

16 Anonymous. Risk of myocardial infarction and death during treatment with low dose aspirin and intravenous heparin in men with unstable coronary artery disease. The RISC Group. *Lancet* 1990; 336 (8719): 827–30.

17 Theroux P, Waters D, Qiu S, McCans J, de Guise P, Juneau M. Aspirin versus heparin to prevent myocardial infarction during the acute phase of unstable angina. *Circulation* 1993; 88 (5: Part 1): 2045–8.

18 The TIMI IIIB Investigators. Unstable angina/myocardial infarction: effects of tissue plasminogen activator and a comparison of early invasive and conservative stategies in unstable angina and non-Q wave myocardial infarction: results of the TIMI IIIB trial. *Circulation* 1994; 89: 1545–56.

19 Oler A, Whooley MA, Oler J, Grady D. Adding heparin to aspirin reduces the incidence of myocardial infarction and death in patients with unstable angina: a meta-analysis. *JAMA* 1996; 276: 811–15.

20 Gurfinkel EP. Low molecular weight heparin versus regular heparin or aspirin in the treatment of unstable angina and silent ischemia. *J Am Coll Cardiol* 1995; 26: 313–18.

21 Wallentin L, Ohlsson J, Swahn E. and the FRISC study group. Low-molecular-weight heparin during instability in coronary artery disease. *Lancet* 1996; 347: 561–8.

22 Eikelboom JW, Anand SS, Malmberg K, Weitz J, Ginsberg JS, Yusuf S. Unfractionated heparin and low-molecular weight heparin in acute coronary syndromes without ST elevation: A systematic overview of the randomized trials. *Lancet* 2000; 355 (9219): 1936–42.

23 Klein W. Fragmin in unstable angina pectoris or in non-Q-wave acute myocardial infarction (the FRIC study). Fragmin in unstable coronary artery disease. *Am J Cardiol* 1997; 80 (5A): 30E–4E.

24 Cohen M. A comparison of low-molecular-weight heparin with unfractionated heparin for unstable coronary artery disease. Efficacy and Safety of Subcutaneous Enoxaparin in Non-Q-Wave Coronary Events Study Group. *N Engl J Med* 1997; 337 (7): 447–52.

25 Merlini PA, Bauer KA, Oltrona L *et al.* Persistent activation of coagulation mechanism in unstable angina and myocardial infarction. *Circulation* 1994; 90: 61–8.

26 Toss H. Prognostic influence of increased fibrinogen and C-reactive protein levels in unstable coronary artery disease. FRISC Study Group. Fragmin during Instability in Coronary Artery Disease. *Circulation* 1997; 96: 4204–10.

27 Yusuf S, Flather M, Pogue J *et al.* Variations between countries in invasive cardiac procedures and outcomes in patients with suspected unstable angina or myocardial infarction without initial ST elevation.

OASIS (Organization to Assess Strategies for Ischaemic Syndromes) Registry Investigators. *Lancet* 1998; 352 (9127): 507–14.

28 FRISC II Investigators. Long-term low molecular mass heparin in unstable coronary artery disease: FRISC II prospective randomized multicentre study. *Lancet* 1999; 354: 701–7.

29 Elliott M, Antman, Carolyn H. *et al.* Enoxaparin prevents death and cardiac ischemic events in unstable angina/non–q-wave myocardial infarction: results of the thrombolysis in myocardial infarction (TIMI) 11B trial. *Circulation* 1999; 100: 1593–601.

30 The FRAXIS Study Group. Comparison of two treatment durations (6 days and 14 days) of a low-molecular-weight heparin with a 6-day treatment of unfractionated heparin in the initial management of unstable angina or non-Q-wave myocardial infarction. *Eur Heart J* 1999; 20: 1553–62.

31 Weitz JI, Califf RM, Ginsberg JS, Hirsh J, Theroux P. New antithrombotics [Review]. *Chest* 1995; 108 (Suppl. 4): 471S–485S.

13: What about the novel antiplatelet agents?

Freek W. A. Verheugt

Introduction

Thrombosis plays a major role in the pathogenesis of cardiovascular diseases. Thrombosis in both coronary and cerebral arteries are complications of atherosclerosis, the most important single cause of mortality in the Western world. Both myocardial and cerebral infarction cause significant mortality and morbidity in millions of patients each year.

Acute coronary syndrome is usually caused by thrombosis on a pre-existing coronary atherosclerotic plaque. Rapidly progressive narrowing, or even acute total occlusion, is the common consequence of this thrombotic process. Both platelets and activation of the coagulation cascade play a pivotal role in the initiation and propagation of this process [1]. The presence of platelet thrombi in the coronary vessel distal to the site of active coronary disease and the presence of layers of platelet thrombi at the site of coronary occlusion indicate that platelets play a major role in the pathogenesis of unstable angina [2,3]. It is well recognized that unstable angina pectoris is associated with a high risk of myocardial infarction and sudden death. In addition, it was shown that about 80% of episodes of chest pain in patients with angina are associated with increased platelet activity resulting in an increased thromboxane and prostacyclin synthesis [4]. Platelets are known to release vasoactive substances such as thromboxane A_2, serotonin and platelet-derived growth factors which induce vasoconstriction thereby further reducing the coronary flow [5].

Since the 1960s, antiplatelet therapy has been used with great success to prevent these frequently fatal thrombotic complications. This chapter will deal with the use of antiplatelet therapy in acute coronary syndrome in general and with the new therapeutic agents in particular.

Pharmacology of antiplatelet agents

First generation antiplatelet drugs

The most regularly used antiplatelet agents in cardiovascular disease are aspirin (acetylsalicylic acid) and dipyridamole [6]. Aspirin irreversibly blocks cyclo-oxygenase in the blood platelet, and thereby prevents the formation of the proaggregatory and vasoconstrictive thromboxane A_2. Because endothelial cells are nucleated, the blockage of cyclo-oxygenase in these cells is almost immediately reversible. The anti-aggregatory and vasodilating endothelial prostaglandin (PGI_2 or prostacyclin) is not blocked by low-dose aspirin, and a favourable imbalance in the interaction between platelet and vessel wall is achieved. The most widely used and effective dosage of aspirin in cardiovascular disease is between 75 and 325 mg daily. Lifelong administration of aspirin is usually recommended in cardiac patients. Since the 1980s, low-dose aspirin has been introduced and found to be as effective as high-dose aspirin [6]. High-dose aspirin is related to gastrointestinal ulceration and subsequent bleeding.

Dipyridamole inhibits phosphodiesterase in the platelet and therefore diminishes platelet adhesion and possibly subsequent aggregation. Its clinical efficacy as a single agent is questionable [6]. It is almost uniformly used in combination with aspirin; however, the benefit of its addition to aspirin therapy is also debatable [6]. The usual dosage of dipyridamole is 75–100 mg three times daily.

Second generation antiplatelet drugs

Ticlopidine (a thienopyridine) inhibits platelet aggregation independently from the cyclo-oxygenase and thromboxane pathway, the phosphodiesterase metabolism or intracellular cyclic AMP. It inhibits mainly ADP-induced platelet aggregation, probably by interfering with the platelet membrane ADP receptor. It takes 4–7 days after the initiation of treatment before the maximum effect on ADP platelet aggregation is achieved. It also takes several days after withdrawal of the drug to achieve normal platelet aggregation. The usual dose is 250 mg twice daily. Neutropenia is seen in 2% of patients, with most during the first weeks of treatment. Recently, clopidogrel has been introduced; this is also a thienopyridine, but lacks the side-effects of ticlopidine (see below). The usual dose is 75 mg daily and clopidogrel has, like ticlopidine, a slow onset of action. This may be overcome by a single loading dose of 300 mg.

Side-effects of the second generation antiplatelet drugs

Ticlopidine use may lead to early neutropenia, thrombocytopenia and rash.

The mechanisms involved are not fully understood. Neutropenia is seen in up to 2% of patients within 2 weeks after treatment initiation. Fatal agranulocytosis has been described, but is rare. Severe infection, however, may occur, but drug withdrawal restores white blood cell count within days. Thrombocytopenia under 100 000 platelets per ml may occur in up to 2% of patients. A rare, but potentially fatal, side-effect is thrombotic thrombocytopenic purpura [7]. Finally, severe rashes are sometimes seen following ticlopidine treatment, which slowly resolve after drug withdrawal. These infrequent, but sometimes potentially fatal side-effects of ticlopidine have forced regulatory bodies to withdraw the agent from registration in several Western countries. The beneficial effects of ticlopidine after stent implantation [8] have led only partially to a rebirth of the agent.

Clopidogrel lacks the side-effects of ticlopidine and seems even safer than aspirin [9]. It has been registered in most Western countries and is used by hundreds of thousands of patients, most of whom use it for a short period of time after stent implantation. It appears to be the 'ideal' second generation antiplatelet drug. Its efficacy in ischaemic heart disease, however, remains to be established.

Third generation antiplatelet drugs

The platelet glycoprotein IIb/IIIa receptor binds fibrinogen during the aggregation process. Inhibition of this binding prevents platelet aggregation independently of the stimulus (ADP, thrombin, arachidonic acid, adrenalin (epinephrine)). Glycoprotein IIb/IIIa receptor-blocking agents therefore inhibit the final pathway of platelet aggregation and prolong bleeding time profoundly. Chimaeric mouse–human monoclonal antibodies (c7E3) to this receptor are available for clinical use under the name abciximab (Reopro[R]). Non-antibody blockers have also been developed, they mimic the fibrinogen molecule by its RGD or KGD sequences and therefore bind to the receptor. They are meant for intravenous use and some are available (tirofiban or Aggrastat[R] and eptifibatide or Integrilin[R]). Finally, oral glycoprotein IIb/IIIa receptor antagonists are currently being tested in patients. They have a longer plasma half-life than the intravenous non-antibody agents, but their clinical pharmacology is quite similar: competitive receptor binding and renal clearance. The latter may be of interest when severe bleeding occurs. Usually in that case renal drug clearance is diminished, while plasma drug levels remain constant, making platelet transfusions useless [10,11].

Side-effects of glycoprotein IIb/IIIa receptor antagonists

Due to unknown mechanisms, glycoprotein IIb/IIIa receptor antagonists may produce thrombocytopenia, which may lead to excess bleeding complications. Bleeding is the most common complication of glycoprotein IIb/IIIa receptor antagonists. Since most trials have been performed in angio-plasty patients, access site bleeding is the most commonly described bleeding complication. Fatal bleeding due to this class of drugs is extremely rare. Excess cerebral bleeding, a fairly common complication of thombolytic agents and oral anticoagulants, has not been described [11]. On the other hand minor ('nuisance') bleeding is common, especially during longer-term treatment with the oral glycoprotein blockers. Gingival bleeding occurs frequently with these agents, leading to early withdrawal of the drug.

Trials with antiplatelet therapy in acute coronary syndrome

Antiplatelet agents have been proved to be effective in the primary and sec-ondary prevention of myocardial infarction, as well as in unstable angina, coronary artery bypass grafting, percutaneous transluminal coronary angio-plasty, atrial fibrillation and in patients with prosthetic heart valves. These data are summarized in the overview published by the Antiplatelet Trialists' Collaboration [6]. This overview consists of a meta-analysis of nearly 300 randomized controlled trials in over 100 000 patients with vascular disease. One should realize that meta-analytic documentation necessarily includes publication bias and might overestimate drug efficacy and safety. Antiplatelet agents may reduce the risk of myocardial infarction and sudden death in patients with unstable angina. The effectiveness of the first generation antiplatelet agent aspirin in unstable angina has been investigated in four large-scale randomized double-blind placebo-controlled trials [12–15]. As-pirin in doses of between 75 and 1300 mg daily prevents myocardial infarction and death in 30–50% of patients admitted with unstable coronary artery disease.

Second generation antiplatelet agents in the treatment of acute coronary syndrome

To date, the only trial of second generation antiplatelet agents in the treatment of acute coronary syndrome has been done by Balsano and colleagues [16]. Over 600 patients with unstable angina were randomized to ticlopidine 250 mg twice daily or to control treatment, the nature of which is not completely clear. Ticlopidine reduced death and myocardial infarction with the same magnitude as aspirin in the above placebo-controlled trials. The effect of ticlo-pidine became clear only after the first week. This finding is in line with its pharmaco-dynamic profile and is a drawback of the second-generation an-tiplatelet agents in the treatment of acute coronary syndrome. The efficacy of ticlopidine relative to aspirin in acute coronary syndrome has not been established. The outcome of the postmyocardial infarction patient cohort in the CAPRIE-trial [9] is not in favour of the second generation platelet inhibitors, i.e. clopidogrel, when compared to aspirin.

Since the first and second generation platelet aggregation inhibitors have completely different modes of action, they should not be compared to each other, but on top of each other vs aspirin alone. This hypothesis is currently tested in the CURE study, in which clopidogrel (with a loading dose) plus aspirin is compared to aspirin alone in patients admitted with acute coronary syndrome.

Third generation antiplatelet agents in the treatment of acute coronary syndrome

The third generation antiplatelet agents have been clinically tested initially in patients undergoing percutaneous coronary interventions indicated for various forms of ischaemic heart disease. The landmark trial was the EPIC investigation [17], in which patients with high-risk angioplasty were treated with abciximab bolus (250 µg per kg), bolus plus infusion (10 µg per min for 12 h), or placebo. Major cardiac events were reduced by over 30% by bolus and infusion, which has become the standard abciximab regimen. The benefit is extended for at least 6 months [18]. Bolus therapy alone was inferior to this regimen. The beneficial effects of abciximab in general and high-risk angioplasty has been confirmed in several large trials, one of which addressed the issue of 24h pre-treatment with abciximab prior to angioplasty for unstable angina [19]. In that study, the CAPTURE trial, pre-treatment with abciximab tended to reduce early major coronary events before the actual angioplasty was performed. Trials with abciximab in primary angioplasty for acute transmural myocardial infarction also tend to be positive [20,21]. Abciximab for acute coronary syndrome without the intention of coronary angioplasty has hardly been studied to date, but this issue is currently being addressed in the GUSTO-4 Acute Coronary Syndrome megatrial.

The other intravenous glycoprotein IIb/IIIa receptor antagonists have been shown to be efficacious in patients admitted with acute coronary syndrome in three mega-trials: PRISM [22] and PRISM-PLUS [23] with tirofiban, and PURSUIT [24] with eptifibatide. The subset of patients in need of coronary angioplasty had the most benefit in these studies. A smaller trial (PARAGON, with over 2200 patients) tested lamifiban in acute coronary syndrome and did not find any benefit in the short term, however, paradoxically, showed reduction of major coronary events on the longer term [25].

The mechanism by which the intravenous glycoprotein IIb/IIIa receptor antagonists reduce coronary events is probably the reduction of thrombus load in the culprit coronary artery. The high cost of these agents, however, prevents them being used on a large scale, especially in low-risk patients and in those admitted to hospitals without angioplasty facilities. Furthermore, the drugs are short acting and the benefit of more permanent glycoprotein IIb/IIIa receptor blockade is not achieved by these agents. Therefore, oral glycoprotein IIb/IIIa receptor blockade has recently been tested in coronary patients. The most long-term experience so far has been collected with xemilofiban and orbofiban. Neither in patients undergoing coronary angioplasty in the large EXCITE study [26] using xemilofiban, nor in those admitted with acute coronary syndrome (the OPUS TIMI-16 megatrial with orbofiban [27]) was any clinical benefit observed. On the contrary, in some sub-groups mortality was increased, although not significantly, as well as non-fatal major and minor bleeding. The manufacturer of these agents halted their further development. In a smaller dose-finding trial (FROST [28] in over 600 patients) with another oral glycoprotein blocker, lefradafiban, bleeding was increased as a dose response, but clinical benefit was not. Also, neutropenia was seen for the first time with this class of agents; this occurred in 5% of patients. Sibrafiban is the only agent currently tested on a large scale, in the SYMPHONY studies in patients with acute coronary syndrome.

It is too early to determine the place of the oral glycoprotein IIb/IIIa receptor antagonists in ischaemic heart disease, since the mechanism of possible harm has not been elucidated. The receptor occupancy during trough periods may be too low to provide protection and may even cause rebound by paradoxical stimulation of the receptor.

Conclusions

Antiplatelet therapy is probably the most efficacious treatment of acute coronary syndrome. New agents have been developed beyond aspirin. The second generation platelet inhibitors (the thienopyridines), ticlopidine and clopidogrel, are promising when used on top of aspirin, but the role of the safer clopidogrel in acute coronary syndrome has to be established. The glycoprotein IIb/IIIa receptor antagonists form the third generation antiplatelet drugs and the short-acting intravenous agents have been shown to be superior to aspirin alone in acute coronary syndrome both in the short and long term, especially in patients undergoing early percutaneous coronary interventions. However, this form of antiplatelet therapy is expensive and its cost-effectiveness is not yet clear. The oral glycoprotein IIb/IIIa receptor antagonists have so far not shown beneficial results in patients with ischaemic heart disease with or without coronary interventions.

The current indications for the new and newer antiplatelet agents in acute coronary syndrome are listed in the Table 13.1.

Table 13.1 Indications for the new and newer antiplatelet agents in acute coronary syndrome.

Generation	Agent(s)	Indication
Second	Ticlopidine	Coronary stent implantation*
	Clopidogrel	Post-myocardial infarction in case of aspirin intolerance
Third	Abciximab	High-risk coronary angioplasty*
	Eptifibatide	Any acute coronary syndrome*
	Tirofiban	Any acute coronary syndrome

* Together with aspirin.

References

1 Davies MJ, Path FRC, Thomas AC *et al.* Intramyocardial platelet aggregation in patients with unstable angina suffering sudden ischemic cardiac death. *Circulation* 1986; 73: 418–27.

2 Sherman CT, Litvack F, Grundfest W *et al.* Coronary angioscopy in patients with unstable angina pectoris. *N Engl J Med* 1986; 315: 913–19.

3 Falk E. Unstable angina with fatal outcome: dynamic coronary thrombosis leading to infarction and/or sudden death. *Circulation* 1985; 71: 699–708.

4 Fitzgerald DJ, Roy L, Catella F, FitzGerald GA. Evidence of marked platelet activation following thrombolytic therapy in acute myocardial infarction in man. *Circulation* 1986; 74 (Suppl. II:): 234–9.

5 Lam JYT, Chesebro JH, Badimon L, Fuster V. Serotonin and thromboxane A$_2$ receptor blockade decrease vasoconstriction but not platelet deposition after deep arterial injury. *Circulation* 1987; 76 (Suppl. II:): 97–104.

6 Antiplatelet Trialists' Collaboration. Collaborative overview of randomised trials of antiplatelet therapy I. Prevention of death, myocardial infarction, and stroke by prolonged antiplatelet therapy in various categories of patients. *BMJ* 1994; 308: 81–106.

7 Bennett CL, Weinberg PD, Rozenberg BDK, Yarnold PR, Kwaan HC, Geen D. Thrombotic thrombocytopenic purpura associated with ticlopidine. A review 60 cases. *Ann Intern Med* 1998; 128: 51–44.

8 Schömig A, Neumann FJ, Kastrati A *et al.* A randomized comparison of antiplatelet and anticoagulant therapy after the placement of coronary-artery stents. *N Engl J Med* 1996; 334: 1084–9.

9 CAPRIE Steering Committee. A randomised, blinded, trial of clopidogrel versus aspirin in patients at risk of ischaemic events (CAPRIE). *Lancet* 1996; 349: 1329–39.

10 Simpfendorfer C, Kottke-Marchant K, Lowrie M *et al.* First chronic platelet glycoprotein IIb/IIIa integrin blockade. A randomized placebo-controlled pilot study of xemilofiban in unstable angina with percutaneous coronary interventions. *Circulation* 1997; 96: 76–81.

11 Verheugt FWA. In search of the super aspirin for the heart. *Lancet* 1997; 349: 1409–10.

12 Lewis HD, Davis JW, Archibald DG *et al.* Protective effects of aspirin against acute myocardial infarction and death in men with unstable angina. *N Engl J Med* 1983; 309: 396–403.

13 Cairns JA, Gent M, Singer J *et al.* Aspirin, sulfinpyrazone, or both in unstable angina. *N Engl J Med* 1985; 313: 1369–75.

14 Théroux P, Ouimet H, McCans J *et al.* Aspirin, heparin, or both to treat acute unstable angina. *N Engl J Med* 1988; 319: 1105–11.

15 The RISC Group. Risk of myocardial infarction and death during treatment with low dose aspirin and intravenous heparin in men with unstable coronary artery disease. *Lancet* 1990; 336: 827–30.

16 Balsano F, Rizzon P, Violi F *et al.* Antiplatelet treatment with ticlopidine in unstable angina. A controlled multicenter clinical trial. *Circulation* 1990; 82: 17–26.

17 The EPIC Investigation. Use of a monoclonal antibody directed against the platelet glycoprotein IIb/IIIa receptor in high-risk coronary angioplasty. *N Engl J Med* 1994; 330: 956–61.

18 Topol EJ, Califf RM, Weisman HF *et al.*
Randomised trial of coronary intervention
with antibody against platelet IIb/IIIa integrin for reduction of clinical restenosis:
results at six months. *Lancet* 1994; 343:
881–6.

19 The CAPTURE investigators. Randomised placebo-controlled trial of abciximab before, during and after coronary
intervention in refractory unstable angina:
the CAPTURE study. *Lancet* 1997; 349:
1429–35.

20 Brener SJ, Barr LA, Burchenal JEB *et al.*
Randomized, placebo-controlled trial of
platelet glycoprotein IIb/IIIa blockade
with primary angioplasty for acute
myocardial infarction. *Circulation* 1998;
98: 734–41.

21 Van den Merkhof LFM, Zijlstra F, Grip L
et al. Abciximab in the treatment of acute
myocardial infarction eligible for primary
PTCA. results of the GRAPE pilot study.
J Am Coll Cardiol 1999; 33: 1528–32.

22 PRISM Study Investigators. A comparison
of aspirin plus tirofiban with aspirin plus
heparin for unstable angina. *N Engl J Med*
1998; 338: 1498–505.

23 PRISM-PLUS. Study Investigators. Inhibition of platelet glycoprotein IIb/IIIa receptor with tirofiban in unstable angina and
non-Q wave myocardial infarction. *N
Engl J Med* 1998; 338: 1488–97.

24 PURSUIT Investigators. Inhibition of
platelet glycoprotein IIb/IIIa with eptifibatide in patients with acute coronary
syndromes. *N Engl J Med* 1998; 339:
436–43.

25 Moliterno DJ, Van de Werf F, Diaz R *et al.*
International, randomized, controlled
trial of lamifiban (a glycoprotein IIb/IIIa
inhibitor), heparin, or both in unstable
angina. *Circulation* 1998; 97: 2386–95.

26 O'Neill, Serruys P, Knudtson M *et al.*
Long-term treatment with platelet
glycoprotein-receptor antagonist after
percutaneous coronary revascalarization.
N Engl J Med 2000; 342: 1316–24.

27 Cannon CP, McCabe CH, Wilcox RG,
Langer A *et al. Circulation* 2000; 102:
149–56.

28 Wilcox RG. FROST trial. Presented 48th
Annual Scientific Session American College of Cardiology, New Orleans, March
1999.

14: What is the value of novel thrombolytic drugs and combination therapies in acute coronary syndromes?

Alan J. Tiefenbrunn

Background

Although activation of the fibrinolytic system for the treatment of acute myocardial infarction was reported as early as 1958 [1], preliminary studies were hampered by relatively late treatment, lack of angiographic data, sample sizes too small to assess an impact on mortality, and lack of understanding of the relationship between thrombosis and myocardial infarction. The modern thrombolytic era began in approximately 1980 with the angiographic demonstration of thrombotic occlusion in the majority of patients presenting early after onset of acute myocardial infarction, as well as the angiographic demonstration of thrombolytic-drug-induced recanalization [2,3]. During the early 1980s, significant amounts of human tissue-type plasminogen activator (t-PA) were first isolated from cells and tissues [4]. Subsequent cloning of the gene expressing this protein ultimately led to the production of pharmacological quantities of the naturally occurring plasminogen activator (recombinant tissue-type plasminogen activator [rt-PA]) [5].

Somewhat surprisingly, thrombolysis does not benefit patients who present with refractory angina or with myocardial infarction which is without diagnostic electrocardiographic changes and documented only by changes in concentration or activity of macromolecular markers in blood [6]. These syndromes are associated often with non-occlusive epicardial thrombus and/or distal microemboli. However, in patients presenting with symptoms of myocardial infarction with concomitant ST segment elevation or left bundle branch block, usually associated with acute thrombosis superimposed on a pre-existing atherosclerotic plaque resulting in total obstruction of an epicardial vessel, marked improvement in clinical outcome is readily demonstrable. Several large controlled trials performed during the 1980s documented lower mortality rates in patients treated with a thrombolytic drug, with early benefit sustained over medium-term follow-up [7–9]. The importance of achieving early recanalization to maximize the amount of myocardium salvaged is intuitively obvious, and supported by studies in animals [10,11]. Clinical trials confirmed the essentiality of prompt implementation of therapy. Earlier treatment was found to be associated consistently with more favourable clinical outcome [7,8,12–14].

It is the prompt restoration of normal antegrade blood flow (Thrombolysis in Myocardial Infarction (TIMI) grade 3) that is the most powerful descriptor of reduction in mortality. Patients with retarded antegrade blood flow (TIMI grade 2) may have incomplete thrombolysis. Conversely, they may have excellent recanalization of the epicardial vessel, but limited nutritive reperfusion because of distal microembolization and/or downstream tissue damage manifested as the 'no reflow' phenomenon. In the Global Use of Strategies to Open Occluded Coronary Arteries (GUSTO I) clinical trial of more than 41 000 patients with evolving myocardial infarction, patients treated with a 90-minute regimen of alteplase (rt-PA, ACTIVASE-Genentech, Inc., ACTILYSE-Boehringer Ingelheim) experienced a 1% absolute lower 30-day mortality compared with that in those treated with streptokinase [12]. In the angiographic sub-study of this trial, 54% of patients given rt-PA were found to have 90-minute angiographic TIMI 3 flow, compared with a 29% incidence in patients treated with streptokinase [15]. There was no significant difference in TIMI 3 flow rate in patients treated with rt-PA compared with those treated with streptokinase at the 180-minute time point. Thus, the difference in *early* TIMI 3 flow appears to be the determinant of the 1% absolute mortality reduction. A correlation between early TIMI 3 flow and reduced early mortality has been confirmed in numerous trials in which early angiographic and subsequent clinical follow-up data have been available, including TIMI 1, 4, 5, 10B and the Thrombolysis and Angioplasty in Myocardial Infarction (TAMI) trials 1–7 [16].

Unfortunately, calculations based on the GUSTO I results indicate that to achieve an additional 1% improvement in mortality (assuming a linear relationship), the incidence of early TIMI 3 flow would have to be approximately 80%. Increasing the dose of streptokinase has not been shown to improve efficacy [17]. Increasing the dose of rt-PA has been associated with an unacceptably high rate of intracranial bleeding [18]. Thus, recent efforts to improve therapy for patients with acute myocardial infarction have been directed at maximizing the frequency of early TIMI 3 flow by minimizing treatment delays, improving thrombolytic agents, and utilizing combination therapy.

Novel thrombolytic agents

Efforts to improve thrombolytic drug efficacy have led to development of multiple agents including saruplase (pro-urokinase, a single-chain plasminogen activator that is converted *in vivo* to urokinase) [19,20], staphylokinase, initially isolated from staphylococcus and subsequently synthesized in a recombinant form [21], and an agent isolated from the saliva of the vampire bat, ds-PA [22]. Promising work has entailed modifying the naturally occurring t-PA molecule to improve the rapidity and frequency of thrombolysis and/or ease of administration while maintaining a satisfactory safety profile. Three such agents developed in this context have been studied extensively in recently completed phase 3 trials.

Reteplase (r-PA, RETAVASE-Centocor)

Reteplase (r-PA, RETAVASE-Centocor), developed by Boehringer Mannheim and currently marketed by Centocor, has been clinically available in the United States since 1997. It is a deletion mutant of the naturally occurring t-PA molecule that has less fibrin specificity and a longer circulating half-life than naturally occurring t-PA that is administered as two boluses separated by a 30-minute time interval. In the International Joint Efficacy Comparison of Thrombolytics (INJECT) trial, 5936 patients were randomized to receive double bolus reteplase or a 1-hour infusion of 1.5 million units of streptokinase. The 30-day mortality after administration of double bolus r-PA was 8.9%, comparable to the 9.4% mortality observed in patients randomized to receive streptokinase (P = ns) [23]. Mortality at 6 months was not significantly different either, 11.0% for reteplase, 12.0% for streptokinase.

The Recombinant plasminogen activator Angiographic Phase II International Dose-finding (RAPID)-2 trial was an angiographic study randomizing 303 patients to double bolus Retevase (r-PA) or bolus and 90-minute infusion of alteplase (rt-PA). The incidence of TIMI 3 flow at 90 min was higher for r-PA (60%) than for rt-PA (45%, $P < 0.01$) [24]. Based largely on results from this study, the GUSTO III trial was undertaken to determine whether a mortality benefit would be observed in a large clinical study comparing r-PA with rt-PA. In this trial, 15 060 patients were enrolled and randomized in a 2:1 fashion to receive r-PA or rt-PA [25]. The results of the study were negative, with a 30-day mortality of 7.43% for patients treated with r-PA vs. 7.22% for those receiving rt-PA (P = ns). The confidence limits for the trial overlapped a 1% superiority value for rt-PA, indicating that these two agents cannot necessarily be considered equivalent.

Lanoteplase

Another product, developed by Bristol Meyers Squibb, is lanoteplase (n-PA, for novel plasminogen activator). It too is a deletion mutant of t-PA. This agent has a long enough half-life to allow for single bolus administration. In a dose ranging angiographic trial, the incidence of 90-minute TIMI 3 flow was 57% in the 124 patients who received the maximum dose used of

120 kU/kg. This frequency was significantly higher than that of 46% observed in the 124 patients treated with a 90-minute regimen of rt-PA in the same study [26].

The Intravenous n-PA for Treatment of Infarcting Myocardium Early (InTime) 2 trial randomized 15 078 patients 1 : 1 to receive single bolus lanoteplase (n-PA) or bolus and 90-minute infusion alteplase (rt-PA). This trial demonstrated comparable 30-day mortality for patients receiving n-PA compared with those receiving rt-PA (6.8% vs 6.6%, respectively, P = ns) [27]. However, the intracranial bleed rate was significantly higher in those patients treated with n-PA (1.1% vs 0.6% with rt-PA, P = 0.003). Lanoteplase development has been halted, in part because of the unacceptably high incidence of intracranial bleeding.

Tenecteplase (TNK t-PA, TNKase)

A third agent, developed by Genentech, Inc., is tenecteplase (TNK t-PA, TNKase). This is not a deletion mutant, but rather a molecule with six amino acids substituted at three different sites (T, N, and K refer to the names of the three amino acids at loci that were altered). This molecule has very high fibrin specificity, high plasminogen activator inhibitor resistance, and a prolonged half-life allowing single bolus administration [28]. In the TIMI 10B dose ranging angiographic study of TNK t-PA, patients treated with a single 40 mg bolus dose (approximately 0.5 mg/kg) experienced a 90-minute TIMI 3 flow rate of 63%, not significantly different from that in patients treated with a bolus and 90-minute infusion of rt-PA [29].

TNK t-PA was compared with rt-PA in a large clinical study, the Assessment of the Safety of a New Thrombolytic (ASSENT)-2 trial with results recently published [30]. In this study, 16 505 patients were randomized in a 1 : 1 ratio to receive single bolus TNK t-PA or bolus plus 90-minute infusion rt-PA. Thirty-day endpoints were identical for the two patient groups, 6.2% mortality, 0.9% intracranial bleed rate (P = ns). Univariate analysis showed a significantly lower 30-day mortality in those patients treated with TNK t-PA in whom treatment began more than 4 h after symptom onset, 7.0%, compared with 9.2% in comparable patients treated with rt-PA beginning after 4 h ($P <$ 0.02). The difference may reflect greater efficacy of TNK t-PA on older thrombi as a result of higher fibrin specificity. The incidence of non-intracranial major bleeding (requiring blood transfusions or other intervention) was lower in patients receiving TNK t-PA (4.68% vs 5.94%, $P <$ 0.01), also consistent with higher fibrin specificity. This agent became commercially available in the United States in June of 2000.

The novel thrombolytic agents make treatment easier and more convenient because of bolus administration. This may lead to earlier treatment, possibly before hospital arrival in selected patients. However, as indicated by the results of the above studies, overall mortality has not yet been decreased compared with that seen with bolus plus 90-minute infusion of rt-PA.

Combined pharmacological therapy

Another approach to improving the clinical efficacy of reperfusion is combined pharmacological therapy. In addition to attacking both the platelet and fibrin components of thrombus, combining an antiplatelet agent with a thrombolytic may help overcome the platelet aggregation that can be promoted by the thrombolytic drug. Antiplatelet therapy also may help prevent re-occlusion and limit tissue damage related to distal microemboli. This concept is not new: in the International Study of Infarct Survival (ISIS) 2 trial, which was published in 1988, patients were randomized to receive placebo, aspirin, streptokinase, or aspirin plus streptokinase [8]. In this trial, aspirin alone produced an improvement in survival similar to that observed following streptokinase alone, with a further improvement among patients receiving both agents. However, interpretation of this study is not easy because patients comprised those with unstable angina (in whom aspirin may well have been helpful independent of clot lysis) as well as acute myocardial infarction, since a qualifying electrocardiogram was not a requirement for entry into this study. Present enthusiasm for a combined approach is based, in part, on the availability of novel antiplatelet drugs, particularly the platelet glycoprotein IIb/IIIa inhibitors.

The combination of the IIb/IIIa inhibitor abciximab (REOPRO-Lilly) and full-dose rt-PA was explored in the TAMI 8 study, published in 1993 [31]. In 60 patients treated with a 3-h regimen of rt-PA for acute myocardial infarction, escalating doses of abciximab were added after completion of treatment with rt-PA. Late angiography (approximately 5 days after treatment) demonstrated TIMI 3 flow in 92% of patients who had received combination therapy compared with 56% in a small control group receiving a 3-h infusion of rt-PA alone. More recent trials have explored the concept of combining IIb/IIIa inhibition with a *reduced* dose of a thrombolytic drug in the hope of improving safety, while achieving TIMI 3 flow more frequently and more rapidly, and reducing the incidence of re-occlusion.

The TIMI 14 trial was an angiographic study of patients with acute ST segment elevation myocardial infarction treated with aspirin plus full-dose abciximab and reduced doses of either streptokinase or rt-PA [32]. Fourteen different dose regimens were studied. There were two reference groups, full-dose (weight adjusted) rt-PA bolus plus 90-minute infusion, and abciximab alone with no thrombolytic agent. All patients were treated with conjunctive intravenous heparin, although the dose of heparin was reduced for those patients receiving abciximab. Patients receiving rt-PA alone had a 90-minute

TIMI 3 flow rate of 58%, comparable to other angiographic trials. Those receiving abciximab alone had a 90-minute TIMI 3 flow rate of 32%. Patients receiving a reduced dose of rt-PA or streptokinase in combination with abciximab consistently had higher TIMI 3 flow rates at 90 min than conventionally observed with a full dose of either of these agents administered alone. The most promising regimen was a 15-mg bolus plus 60-minute infusion of a total of 50 mg of rt-PA (half the usual dose) plus abciximab, which resulted in a 90-minute TIMI 3 flow rate of 77% ($n = 87$, combining patients from the dose-finding and dose-confirming arms of the study) (Fig. 14.1). This TIMI 3 flow rate is 'competitive' with the 73% value observed in the core angiographic laboratory evaluation of patients undergoing primary angioplasty in the GUSTO IIB trial [33], but the pharmacological regimen allows more widespread availability and the potential for more prompt initiation of therapy. Although the number of patients in each group was relatively small, the angiographic patency rates were promising and were not associated with an unacceptably high rate of complications in patients treated with abciximab plus rt-PA.

In the Strategies to Promote Early reperfusion in the Emergency Department (SPEED) trial (the GUSTO IV pilot study) of patients with acute myocardial infarction, abciximab alone was shown to result in a relatively low rate of TIMI 3 flow (27% at 60–90 min, $n = 48$), but the combination of abciximab plus half dose r-PA (5 units plus 5 units) was found to be effective with a 63% TIMI 3 flow rate at 60–90 min ($n = 60$) in Phase A (dose-ranging) and a 54% TIMI 3 flow rate at 60–90 min in Phase B ($n = 100$) [34].

Larger trials to fully assess the safety and clinical benefits, if any, of combination pharmacological regimens are clearly needed: several are planned or under way. The ongoing GUSTO IV trial is comparing clinical outcome in a large number of patients with acute myocardial infarction randomized to

TIMI 3 flow @ 90 min.

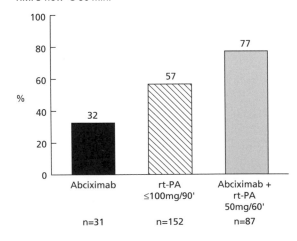

Fig. 14.1 Proportion of patients in whom TIMI 3 flow was observed angiographically at 90 min after treatment with abciximab alone, full dose weight adjusted rt-PA over 90 min (15 mg initial bolus), or abciximab plus 50 mg rt-PA over 60 min (15 mg initial bolus). (Data from TIMI 14 [32].)

receive reteplase (r-PA) alone or a combination of reduced-dose r-PA and abciximab. Phase 2 angiographic trials of reduced-dose Tenecteplase (TNK t-PA) in combination with each of the three currently available intravenous IIb/IIIa inhibitors (abciximab [REOPRO–Lilly], tirofiban [AGGRASTAT–Merck], eptifibatide [INTEGRILIN–Cor Therapeutics]) in comparison with full-dose TNK t-PA alone are also planned. A large, phase 3 study, ASSENT 3, will compare full-dose TNK t-PA plus unfractionated heparin, full-dose TNK t-PA plus low-molecular-weight heparin (enoxaparin [LOVENOX–Aventis Pharmaceuticals]) and reduced-dose TNK t-PA plus abciximab plus enoxaparin.

Combined pharmacological and mechanical therapy

Another approach to maximizing early recanalization is a combination of pharmacological and mechanical interventions. Although primary percutaneous coronary intervention (PCI) during evolving myocardial infarction is highly effective in achieving TIMI 3 flow, this therapeutic modality is hampered by limited availability, the requirement for highly skilled personnel, and unsatisfactory delays in implementation [33]. Pharmacological treatment of eligible patients on the way to the catheterization laboratory with IIb/IIIa-inhibiting agents, high-dose intravenous heparin, or thrombolytic drugs has been proposed as a potential way to achieve earlier reperfusion in responsive patients.

Several randomized trials in the 1980s demonstrated that PCI immediately after *successful* thrombolysis (performed in an attempt to minimize the rate of early re-occlusion) was associated with increased complications and no apparent benefit [35–37]. A pilot study published in 1992 randomizing 92 patients with evolving myocardial infarction to receive intravenous streptokinase or placebo on the way to the catheterization laboratory also showed only increased complications, high blood transfusion requirements, and longer length of stay for those patients treated with streptokinase [38]. These reports contributed to a belief that PCI immediately after administration of a thrombolytic is hazardous.

However, a more recent study indicates that thrombolysis may be a particularly promising adjunct to angioplasty in patients with evolving myocardial infarction. The Plasminogen Activator Angioplasty Compatibility Trial (PACT) was designed to assess the value of thrombolytic pretreatment of patients undergoing primary angioplasty and to determine the impact of such pretreatment on results achievable with angioplasty [39]. Patients under the age of 75 without prior bypass surgery with acute ST segment elevation myocardial infarction were randomized to receive a 50-mg bolus of alteplase (rt-PA) or placebo before angiography. All patients received oral aspirin and intravenous heparin. If subsequent angiography demonstrated TIMI grade 3 flow, a second dose of study drug was administered. Patients with less than TIMI grade 3 flow underwent angioplasty. For patients treated with placebo, this was 'primary PCI'. However, it should be noted that patients undergoing PCI after receiving rt-PA in this trial are not identical to those undergoing conventional 'rescue' angioplasty: they routinely went to the catheterization laboratory as part of the protocol; they were not selected because of evidence of thrombolytic drug failure; they were brought to the catheterization laboratory very early; and they had received only half of the usual dose of rt-PA.

Of those patients receiving rt-PA, 33% had TIMI 3 flow at the time of initial angiography and 61% had TIMI 2 or 3 flow. These rates were approximately twice as high as those observed in patients receiving placebo ($P <$ 0.001). There was no difference in success rates for angioplasty in patients who had received rt-PA compared with those who had received placebo. Of the patients with TIMI flow grade 0 or 1 after receiving rt-PA, 77% had TIMI 3 flow and 93% had TIMI 2 or 3 flow following angioplasty. These figures are not significantly different from 79% and 95%, respectively, for those receiving placebo. The median time until TIMI 3 flow was observed was 51 min for patients not requiring angioplasty vs 93 min for those undergoing PCI ($P <$ 0.0001). This study was not powered ($n = 606$) to assess mortality, but indexes of global and regional left ventricular function were better in patients who had a patent infarct-related artery at the time of the first angiogram. For example, global ejection fraction at 5–7 days after treatment was 0.62 in patients with TIMI 3 flow on their first angiogram, 0.58 in patients with TIMI 3 flow following PCI, and 0.55 in patients in whom TIMI 3 flow was never observed ($P < 0.01$). There was no excess of complications in the patients given the thrombolytic drug.

Results of angioplasty shortly after combined therapy with reduced-dose (5 units plus 5 units) reteplase (r-PA) plus abciximab are consistent with those in the PACT trial [40]. The SPEED investigators report an 88% core lab angiographic success rate in 161 non-randomized patients undergoing PCI 60–90 min after initiation of thrombolytic therapy. (Of these 161 patients, 47% had TIMI 3 flow before angioplasty.)

These reports suggest that pharmacological reperfusion therapy before angiography may be of value in selected patients, given that a significant proportion will respond early to pharmacological therapy, even at a reduced dose, and have an open vessel before mechanical intervention can be implemented. Outside of a clinical trial setting, angiography could be deferred in patients who respond clinically before reaching the catheterization laboratory. Those not responding quickly to a pharmacological regimen are likely to still benefit from relatively early mechanical reperfusion. Results in these studies emphasize the fact that thrombolytic therapy and early angioplasty are not mutually exclusive options for treating patients with myocardial infarction. Additional studies are required to evaluate this approach with the use of either full-dose thrombolytic drugs or reduced-dose thrombolytic drugs plus a IIb/IIIa inhibitor and to assess outcomes when initial angiography is delayed for clinically realistic time intervals, i.e. between 90 min and several hours.

Conclusions

It is clear that in the next few years novel approaches will improve the incidence of induction of TIMI 3 flow in infarct-related vessels and shorten the time interval within which it is achieved. Such therapeutic options, combined with efforts to maximize the number of eligible patients treated with appropriate therapy [41], should further enhance benefits conferred by therapies designed to induce reperfusion in patients with evolving myocardial infarction.

References

1 Fletcher AP, Alkjaersig N, Smyrniotis FE, Sherry S. The treatment of patients suffering from early myocardial infarction with massive and prolonged streptokinase therapy. *Trans Assoc Am Physicians* 1958; 71: 287–95.

2 DeWood MA, Spores J, Notske R et al. Prevalence of total coronary occlusion during the early hours of transmural myocardial infarction. *N Engl J Med* 1980; 303: 897–902.

3 Rentrop KP, Blanke H, Karsch KR et al. Acute myocardial infarction: intracoronary application of nitroglycerin and streptokinase. *Clin Cardiol* 1979; 2: 354–63.

4 Collen D, Rijken DC, Van Damme J, Billiau A. Purification of human tissue-type plasminogen activator in centigram quantities from human melanoma cell culture fluid and its conditioning for use *in vivo*. *Thromb Haemost* 1982; 48: 294–6.

5 Pennica D, Holmes WE, Kohr WJ et al. Cloning and expression of human tissue-type plasminogen activator cDNA in *E. coli*. *Nature* 1983; 301: 214–21.

6 The TIMI IIIB Investigators. Effects of tissue plasminogen activator and a comparison of early invasive and conservative strategies in unstable angina and non-Q-wave myocardial infarction. Results TIMI IIIB Trial. *Circulation* 1994; 89: 1545–36.

7 GISSI. (Gruppo Italiano per lo Studio della Streptochinasi nel'Infarto Miocardico). Effectiveness of intravenous thrombolytic treatment in acute myocardial infarction. *Lancet* 1986; 1: 397–401.

8 ISIS-2 Collaborative Group. Randomised trial of intravenous streptokinase, oral aspirin, both, or neither among 17187 cases of suspected acute myocardial infarction: ISIS-2. *Lancet* 1988; 2: 349–60.

9 Wilcox RG, Von der Lippe G, Olsson CG et al. Trial of tissue plasminogen activator for mortality reduction in acute myocardial infarction. Anglo-Scandinavian Study of Early Thrombolysis (ASSET). *Lancet* 1988; 2: 525–30.

10 Reimer KA, Lowe JE, Rasmussen MM et al. The wave front phenomenon of ischemic cell death, I. Myocardial infarct size versus duration of coronary occlusion in dogs. *Circulation* 1977; 56: 786–94.

11 Bergmann SR, Lerch RA, Fox KAA et al. Temporal dependence of beneficial effects of coronary thrombolysis characterized by positron tomography. *Am J Med* 1982; 73: 573–81.

12 GUSTO Investigators. An international randomised trial comparing four throm-

bolytic strategies for acute myocardial infarction. *N Engl J Med* 1993; 329: 673–82.

13 Weaver WD, Cerqueira M, Hallstrom AP *et al.* for the MITI Project Investigators. Prehospital initiated vs hospital initiated thrombolytic therapy. *JAMA* 1993; 270: 1211–16.

14 Fibrinolytic Therapy Trialists' Collaborative Group. Indications for fibrinolytic therapy in suspected acute myocardial infarction: collaborative overview of early mortality and major morbidity results from all randomised trials of more than 1000 patients. *Lancet* 1994; 343: 311–22.

15 GUSTO Angiographic Investigators. The effects of tissue plasminogen activator, streptokinase, or both on coronary-artery patency, ventricular function, and survival after acute myocardial infarction. *N Engl J Med* 1993; 329: 1615–22.

16 Timmis GC (ed). *Thrombolytic Therapy.* New York: Futura Publishing Company Inc., 2000: 167–204.

17 Six AJ, Louwerenburg HW, Braams R *et al.* A double-blind randomized multicenter dose-ranging trial of intravenous streptokinase in acute myocardial infarction. *Am J Cardiol* 1990; 65: 119–23.

18 Gore JM, Sloan M, Price T *et al.* Intracerebral hemorrhage, cerebral infarction, and subdural hematoma after acute myocardial infarction and thrombolytic therapy in the Thrombolysis in Myocardial Infarction Study. Thrombolysis in Myocardial Infarction, Phase II, pilot and clinical trial. *Circulation* 1991; 83: 448–59.

19 PRIMI Trial Study Group. Randomised double-blind trial of recombinant pro-urokinase against streptokinase in acute myocardial infarction. *Lancet* 1998; 1: 863–8.

20 Tebbe U, Michels R, Adgey J *et al.* Randomized double-blind study comparing saruplase with streptokinase therapy in acute myocardial infarction: the COMPASS equivalence trial. *J Am Coll Cardiol* 1998; 31: 487–93.

21 Vanderschueren S, Dens J, Kerdsinchai P *et al.* Randomized coronary patency trial of double-bolus recombinant staphylokinase versus front-loaded alteplase in acute myocardial infarction. *Am Heart J* 1997; 134: 213–19.

22 Witt W, Maass B, Baldus B *et al.* Coronary thrombolysis with *Desmodus* salivary

plasminogen activators in dogs. *Circulation* 1994; 90: 421–6.

23 International Joint Efficacy Comparison of Thrombolytics. Randomised, double-blind comparison of reteplase double-bolus administration with streptokinase in acute myocardial infarction (INJECT): trial to investigate equivalence. *Lancet* 1995; 346: 329–36.

24 Bode C, Smalling RW, Berg G *et al.* Randomized comparison of coronary thrombolysis achieved with double-bolus reteplase (recombinant plasminogen activator) and front-loaded, accelerated alteplase (recombinant tissue plasminogen activator) in patients with acute myocardial infarction. *Circulation* 1996; 72: 518–24.

25 The Global Use of Strategies to Open Occluded Coronary Arteries (GUSTO)-III Investigators. A comparison of reteplase with alteplase for acute myocardial infarction. *N Engl J Med* 1997; 337: 1118–23.

26 Heijer P, Vermeer F, Ambrosioni E *et al.* Evaluation of weight-adjusted single-bolus plasminogen activator in patients with myocardial infarction: a double-blind, randomized angiographic trial of lanoteplase versus alteplase. *Circulation* 1998; 98: 2117–25.

27 Neuhaus K-L. A phase three trial of novel bolus thrombolytic lanoteplase (nPA): intravenous nPA for treatment of infarcting myocardium early (Intime-II). Presented at the 48th Annual Scientific Sessions of the American College of Cardiology, New Orleans, March 1999.

28 Keyt BA, Paoni NF, Refino CJ *et al.* A faster-acting and more potent form of tissue plasminogen activator. *Proc Natl Acad Sci USA* 1994; 91: 3670–4.

29 Cannon CP, Gibson MC, McCabe CH *et al.* TNK-tissue plasminogen activator compared with front-loaded alteplase in acute myocardial infarction: results of the TIMI-10B trial. *Circulation* 1998; 98: 2805–14.

30 ASSENT-2 Trial. Single-bolus tenecteplase compared with front-loaded alteplase in acute myocardial infarction: the ASSENT-2 double-blind randomized trial. Assessment of the Safety and Efficacy of a New Thrombolytic investigators. *Lancet* 1999; 354: 716–22.

31 Kleiman NS, Ohman EM, Califf RM *et al.* Profound inhibition of platelet aggrega-

tion with monoclonal antibody 7E3 Fab after thrombolytic therapy: results of the Thrombolysis and Angioplasty in Myocardial Infarction (TAMI) 8 Pilot Study. *J Am Coll Cardiol* 1993; 22: 381–9.

32 Antman EM, Giugliano RP, Gibson CM *et al.* Abciximab facilitates the rate and extent of thrombolysis: results of the Thrombolysis in Myocardial Infarction (TIMI) 14 trial. *Circulation* 1999; 99: 2720–32.

33 GUSTO Investigators. A clinical trial comparing primary coronary angioplasty with tissue plasminogen activator for acute myocardial infarction: the Global Use of Strategies to Open Occluded Coronary Arteries in Acute Coronary Syndromes (GUSTO IIb) Angioplasty Substudy Investigators. *N Engl J Med* 1997; 336: 1621–8.

34 SPEED Group. Trial of Abciximab with and without low-dose Reteplase for acute myocardial infarction. *Circulation* 2000; 101: 2788–94.

35 Topol EJ, Califf RM, George BS *et al.* A randomized trial of immediate versus delayed elective angioplasty after intravenous tissue plasminogen activator in acute myocardial infarction. *N Engl J Med* 1987; 317: 581–8.

36 Rogers WJ, Baim DS, Gore JM *et al.* Comparison of immediate invasive, delayed invasive, and conservative strategies after tissue-type plasminogen activator. Results

of the Thrombolysis in Myocardial Infarction (TIMI) Phase II-A Trial. *Circulation* 1990; 81: 1457–76.

37 Simoons ML, Arnold AE, Betriu A *et al.* Thrombolysis with tissue plasminogen activator in acute myocardial infarction: no additional benefit from immediate percutaneous coronary angioplasty. *Lancet* 1988; 1: 197–203.

38 O'Neill WW, Weintraub R, Grines CL *et al.* A prospective, placebo-controlled, randomized trial of intravenous streptokinase and angioplasty versus lone angioplasty therapy of acute myocardial infarction. *Circulation* 1992; 86: 1710–7.

39 Ross AM, Coyne KS, Reiner JS *et al.* A randomized trial comparing primary angioplasty with a strategy of short-acting thrombolysis and immediate planned rescue angioplasty in acute myocardial infarction. The PACT Trial. *J Am Coll Cardiol* 1999; 34: 1954–62.

40 Hermann HC, Moliferno DJ, Bode C *et al.* Combination abciximab and reduced-dose reteplase facilitates early PCI in acute MI. Results from the SPEED trial 1999. *Circulation* 100 (Suppl. I): I-188 (Abstract).

41 Barron HV, Bowlby LJ, Breen T *et al.* Use of reperfusion therapy for acute myocardial infarction in the United States: data from the National Registry of Myocardial Infarction 2. *Circulation* 1998; 97: 1150–642.

15: Preconditioning: what is its potential?

Robert M. Bell and Derek M. Yellon

Introduction

Coronary artery disease, a huge problem in the Western world, accounts for a third of all deaths in the UK, and over 6 million deaths world wide per annum [1]. The introduction of therapeutic modalities designed to avoid the onset of irreversible myocyte damage in the context of myocardial ischaemia has brought genuine advances over the past 20 years. Rapid recanalization of an occluded coronary artery was demonstrated in the landmark GISSI-1 trial [2]. The rapid achievement of coronary patency is critical to avoid the progression of reversible ischaemic injury to infarction. The possibility of delaying the onset of myocyte death, thus allowing more time for successful recannalization, is of interest to all clinicians involved in the management of patients with acute coronary syndromes (ACS) and those undergoing cardiac surgery. The phenomenon of myocardial preconditioning has emerged as a potential candidate with which to achieve this goal.

Acute coronary syndromes

Acute coronary syndrome encompasses a range of clinical manifestations of coronary vascular disease. In essence, ACS describes any condition in which critical compromise of blood flow to the myocardium occurs. The two most common manifestations are acute myocardial infarction and unstable angina. The purpose of this chapter is to discuss novel methods for delaying the onset of irreversible myocardial injury and preserving myocardial function in the context of otherwise lethal ischaemia.

Preconditioning

Preconditioning was first described in 1986 by Murry, Jennings and Reimer [3], in a series of experiments in open chest dogs. The then current doctrine held that serial brief ischaemic insults, with intervening reperfusion to wash out catabolites, would result in depletion of high-energy phosphates. Conversely, it was found that ATP was preserved. It was noted that six of the seven dogs studied had no evidence of infarction [4]. The investigators hypothesized that a mechanism of rapid cellular adaptation might exist, which may result in myocyte protection against lethal ischaemia. Subsequent investigation demonstrated that following four 5-min coronary occlusions, a 75% reduction in infarct size after a subsequent 40-min ischaemic insult could be observed in comparison with the results in control animals [3]. They labelled this phenomenon 'preconditioning with ischaemia'. Thus, ischaemic preconditioning can be defined as increased myocardial resistance to ischaemia induced by preceding, intermittent sublethal ischaemia. As interest has grown in this field, it has been found that stimuli other than ischaemia can be used to elicit similar effects. Examples include endogenous agents, the 'autocoids' (adenosine, bradykinin, prostinoids, catecholamines), and exogenous stimuli such as heat stress and bacterial endotoxins (monophosphoryl lipid A).

The form of ischaemic preconditioning identified by Reimer *et al.* [3] develops within minutes, and has a finite duration of protection lasting approximately 2–3 h. This later became known as 'classical preconditioning' with the discovery of a second distinct temporal phase of protection in 1993 [5]. The latter phase, which we termed the 'second window of protection', or delayed preconditioning, occurs between 12 and 72 h after an initial preconditioning stimulus [6].

Over the 12 years since preconditioning's initial description, researchers have demonstrated classical preconditioning in a number of mammalian species (mouse [7], rat [8], rabbit [9], and dog [3]), including human beings (human trabeculae [10]). The second window has been found to be as equally widespread (rat [11,12], rabbit [13–15], dog [16]). This suggests that there are genotypically conserved protective mechanisms against cellular stress, present across a spectrum of species.

Preconditioning protects the heart from lethal ischaemic injury. The protection is described classically with respect to a reduction of infarct size, but preconditioning protects also against other sequelae of injurious ischaemic injury (summarized in Fig. 15.1). The preconditioned myocardium is resistant to arrhythmias [17], contractile dysfunction (stunning) [18], and apoptotic death [19]. The coronary vasculature is protected. In contrast to the case in non-preconditioned animals, the coronary arteries of preconditioned animals exhibit a normal vasodilatory response to acetylcholine [20]. Thus, the preconditioned animals demonstrate preserved endothelial function. If each of these protective features of preconditioning can be demonstrated in humans and particularly in patients with ACS, preconditioning will have the potential of becoming a useful clinical therapeutic modality.

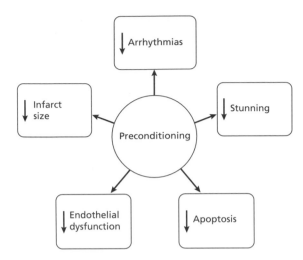

Fig. 15.1 Protective features of preconditioning.

Mechanisms of preconditioning

In investigating the mechanisms of preconditioning, it is important to distinguish between the two phases: classical preconditioning and the second window of protection. This is critical, in part because of the potentially different signalling pathways implicated in each phase. For example, classical preconditioning is demonstrable with or without inhibition of protein synthesis [21], whilst the second window of protection requires new protein synthesis and/or post-translational modification, as is evident from the attenuation of the second window by the protein synthesis inhibitor, cycloheximide [22].

The triggers of preconditioning

In classical preconditioning, an array of neuroendocrine and paracrine triggers have been identified that are released and/or operative during ischaemia. They exert their biological affect via specific receptors, and include: adenosine via A_1/A_3 receptors [23,24]; acetyl choline via muscarinic M-2 receptors [25]; catecholamines via α-1 receptors [26]; angiotensin II via AT-1 receptors [27]; bradykinin via B-2 receptors [28], and the opioids via δ opioid receptors [29]. Whilst these agents have been found to be active across a variety of different mammalian species, their concentration in the cellular microenvironment during periods of ischaemia may vary greatly. An example is adenosine. In the rat, adenosine is present at three times the concentrations in the myocardial microcirculation during ischaemia compared to the case in the rabbit under the same conditions [30]. It may be simply that different concentrations that explain why previous studies have failed to reproduce preconditioning with adenosine receptor agonists in the rat [31–36] whereas this agent had been un-equivocally demonstrated to do so in other species (such as the rabbit [23,26]). The involvement of adenosine preconditioning in the rat is alluded to by work demonstrating that the A_1 receptor agonist 2-chloro N6 cyclopentyl adeno-sine (CCPA), injected directly into the coronaries, produces preconditioning in the isolated rat heart [37].

When one preconditioning trigger is insufficient to generate protection, two or more triggers may summate signals to generate preconditioning. Downey's group has undertaken studies that suggest that a preconditioning 'threshold' needs to be reached [38]. This concept is supported by research from Yellon's group demonstrating that sub-threshold ischaemia can be made to precondition human trabeculae by the addition of an angiotensin-converting-enzyme inhibitor [10]. The protection is subsequently lost by following the addition of Hoc 140, an inhibitor of the bradykinin B2 receptor.

Whilst the triggers for the second window of protection have been less ex-tensively defined, adenosine appear to be a potent trigger in the rabbit [14–15]. Adenosine blockade concomitantly with a preconditioning stimulus inhibits the protection seen during the second window [14]. Conversely, administration of CCPA results in marked protection against infarction 24–72 h later [6,14,39]. In pigs subjected to myocardial stunning there is an exception to the adenosine-triggered second window phenomenon. In this case, free radicals and nitric oxide appear to be important triggers [40]. At present, it is not clear what the difference reflects, i.e. whether it is a species-dependent variant with the pig not demonstrating infarct size reduction with adenosine.

Other triggers of classical preconditioning may also induce a second win-dow of protection. In recent work, Gross' group [41,42] has found that δ opi-oid receptor agonists invoke both phases of preconditioning. Schultz et al. demonstrated that classical preconditioning in the rat can be triggered by δ opioid agonists via $G_{i/o}$ (inhibitory) linked receptors, and the protection mediated by K_{ATP} channel opening [41]. δ opioid agonist administered 24–48 h prior to the lethal ischaemic insult appears to mediate the second window of protection, also through K_{ATP} channel opening [42]. The significance of the K_{ATP} channel is addressed in more detail below.

The bacterially derived endotoxin, monophosphoryl lipid A (MLA), is a pharmacological alternative that can trigger the second window of protec-tion, as characterized by work in dogs [16]. MLA has been successfully ap-plied in other species, including rat (with cultured myocytes [43]) and rabbit [44]. MLA, unlike adenosine, is not endogenous in ischaemic myocardium. Nonetheless, MLA effects are mediated by similar end effectors, particularly K_{ATP} channels [16]. However, MLA does not increase the expression of the major heat shock protein, HSP72 [45]. This suggests that there are differences in the signalling cascade for 'endogenously' triggered preconditioning (with adenosine, bradykinin, etc.) and that induced by MLA.

The postreceptor signalling pathway

Many of the triggers of preconditioning signal via G-protein coupled receptors. This is evident from the ablation of their effect by pre-treatment with pertussis toxin [46]. G-proteins may be either inhibitory ($G_{i/o}$) or stimulatory (G_s) depending upon their regulatory properties affecting adenylate cyclase and hence influence on intracellular concentrations of cyclic adenosine monophosphate (cAMP). Adenosine A_1/A_3 and δ opioid receptors are mediated by $G_{i/o}$-linked receptors; bradykinin and noradrenaline (norepinephrine) via G_s-linked receptors (for review see [47]). It has been proposed that these G-proteins are coupled to phospholipase C and that the product, diacyl glycerol, activates protein kinase C (PKC) [48]. The role of this pathway is supported by evidence that phorbol myristate or diacyl glycerol analogues can independently activate PKC and precondition the heart [49,50]. (PKC's role in preconditioning is summarized in Fig. 15.2.)

The pivotal role of PKC in preconditioning appears to be confirmed by the attenuation of preconditioning by the PKC inhibitors staurosporine [49], polymyxin B [49,51], and chelerythrine [50,52]. Interestingly, whilst total

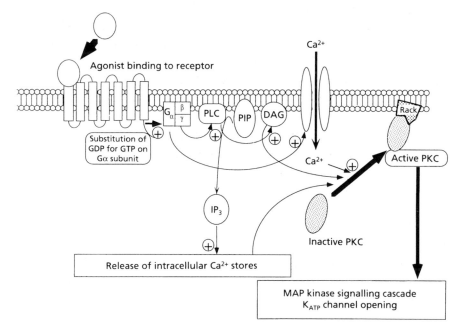

Fig. 15.2 Receptor mediated induction of preconditioning via PKC activation. DAG, diacylglycerol; PIP, phosphatidylinositol phosphate kinase; PLC, phospholipase C; MAP, mitogen-activated protein.

PKC activity may not be markedly increased in response to stress, two iso-forms of PKC, PKCε [53–55] and PKCη [54], translocate from the cytosolic to the particulate fraction in response to preconditioning and exhibit specific increases in enzymatic activity (PKCε). Furthermore, the particulate fraction of PKCε increases in a dose-dependent fashion in proportion to the intensity of the ischaemic stimuli administered. In contrast, maximal translocation of PKCη occurs at the preconditioning threshold [54]. Pharmacological stimulation of the novel ε isoforms with ingenol 3,20-dibenzoate (an δ, ε/δ-PKC isoform selective activator) protects incubated isolated rabbit myocytes against ischaemia, whereas stimulation of calcium dependent α/β/γ-PCK isoforms with thymeleatoxin exerts no protective effect [56]. Furthermore, with the use of a PKCε-selective antagonist, εV1–2 peptide, preconditioning can be ablated [57] suggesting that whilst PKCη may be involved in preconditioning in an as yet undetermined way, PKCε activation and translocation are essential to the induction of preconditioning.

Recent work has implicated protein kinases other than PKC in preconditioning; that may be either in parallel and/or downstream to this enzyme group. Experiments with the tyrosine kinase inhibitor, genistein, have demonstrated that tyrosine kinase (TK) activation is a crucial step in the preconditioning cascade [58]; the preconditioning effect of stimulation via the adenosine A_1 receptor can be attenuated both by chelerythine (PKC inhibitor) and lavendustin-A (TK inhibitor) [59]. Recent data suggest that TK's position in the signalling cascade is downstream of PKC [58].

Whilst mitogen-activated protein kinases (MAPK) are activated during classical preconditioning [60,61], these enzymes are thought also to be linked to the second window of protection. The characterization of the three major MAPK families and their pathways (p42/p44 extracellular receptor-linked kinase (ERK), p38-MAP kinase, and the stress activated c-jun N-terminal kinase, SAPK/JNK) remains incomplete. (The JNK, p38-MAPK families are reviewed in depth in [62], the ERK in [63].) PKC is known to phosphorylate raf-1 kinase [64] which provides a direct link to the p42/p44 MAPK family. Furthermore, the activation by ischaemia or reactive oxygen species of p38 kinase and JNK SAPK [65,66] phosphorylate factors that co-ordinate gene transcription and therefore protein synthesis. Post-translational modification of proteins by the MAPK pathways has been demonstrated; a good example of this is the induction of the p38 MAPK leading to MAPKAPK2 activation [60] with the subsequent phosphorylation of HSP27 [67]. These kinases are a focus for many working to elucidate the mechanisms of delayed preconditioning.

Metabolic modification in classical preconditioning

Whilst preconditioning with ischaemia was described initially in terms of preservation of high-energy phosphates, the relatively small reduction in the rate of energy consumption is unlikely to be sufficient to explain the anti-infarct effect that is observed. During brief periods of ischaemia, glycogen stores are depleted rapidly with a concomitant accumulation of lactate and protons. With reperfusion, these acidic catabolites are washed out. Glycogen storage recommences but at a reduced rate compared with that in tissue that has not been subjected to ischaemia. The glycogen stores remain depleted for a long time which mirrors the time over which the first window of protection occurs [68]. If glycogen depleted myocardium is exposed to further episodes of ischaemia, lactate accumulation is notably reduced [69]. This is the major explanation for the markedly reduced progression to ischaemic acidosis in preconditioned myocardium. In the preconditioned myocardium, the onset of pH decline is delayed compared with ATP depletion [70]. The process of glycogen depletion is not essential for induction of myocardial protection; it is still possible to precondition glycogen-depleted myocardium and further-more, catabolite washout is not required for protection either [71].

The accumulation of intracellular protons could have significant conse-quences for the ischaemic myocardium. An excess of protons in ischaemic or hypoxic myocardium can stimulate trans-sarcolemmal Na^+/H^+ exchange even in the absence of a proton gradient. In order to maintain sodium homeostasis, ATP would be required to drive the Na^+/K^+ ATPase. With early reperfusion, activation of the Na^+/Ca^{2+} exchanger could contribute to serious Ca^{2+} over-load. Blockade of the Na^+/H^+ exchanger is only partially additive to classical preconditioning [72] suggesting that the Na^+/H^+ is not the only or the major effector of preconditioning. None the less, it may be additive to other mechanisms.

Our understanding of cellular metabolism during ischaemia remains in-complete. More research is needed to elucidate the full ramifications of pre-conditioning on cellular energy content and storage, ionic concentrations and ion transport. Such research may identify effective pharmacological means to induce myocardial protection.

The effectors of the preconditioning response

Interestingly, mechanisms that generate myocardial resistance to injury are remarkably similar in the two phases of preconditioning, particularly with respect to the apparent shared dependence upon the activation/opening of the K_{ATP} channel.

In classical preconditioning, PKC is thought to translocate from the cytosol to the cellular membrane and activate the K_{ATP} channel; PKC can directly stimulate K_{ATP} as shown after application of purified constitutively active PKC to the intracellular surface of patch clamped isolated rabbit myocytes which produces an approximately threefold increase in the channel open probability [73]. The protection derived from the stimulation of PKC by dioctanoylglycerol in human muscle is lost with blockade of K_{ATP} by glibenclamide [74]. Numerous studies have been performed with both K_{ATP} channel openers [75] and K_{ATP} channel blockers (rats [76,77], rabbits [78,79], dogs [80], pigs [81,82] and man [74]) that demonstrate either preconditioning-mimetic behaviour or preconditioning attenuation, respectively.

K_{ATP} channels, when open, shorten the duration of the action potential [82]; this is thought to be linked to accelerated ion flux through the sarcolemmal K_{ATP} channel with consequent reduction of calcium overload and thus preservation of myocardial viability. However, the assumption that myocardial protection is mediated by sarcolemmal K_{ATP} channels has been challenged by the observation that low-dose bimakalim (a K_{ATP} channel opener) may induce cardioprotection without influencing the duration of the action potential [83]. Thus the involvement of other K_{ATP} channels in other membranes has been suggested, particularly those in the mitochondrial inner membrane (see review [84]). The most direct evidence derives from research utilizing the relatively selective mitochondrial K_{ATP} channel opener, diazoxide. This agent induces myocardial protection associated with a change of mitochondrial REDOX potential in the absence of activation of the sarcolemmal K_{ATP} channel [85]. Without the apparent opening of the sarcolemmal channel, myocardial protection can none the less be observed.

In delayed preconditioning, K_{ATP} channels have been linked with protection in rabbit 24 h after heat stress [86] and in dog 24 h after MLA administration [16]. The relationship with the product of the inducible isoform of nitric oxide synthase, nitric oxide with K_{ATP} [87], is discussed below.

The current hypothesis regarding divergence between the two windows of myocardial protection focuses on the time when new protein synthesis takes place or when post-transcriptional changes affect existing proteins. The identities of the protective proteins and pathways remain to be fully elucidated, but several candidates merit consideration.

Manganese-superoxide dismutase (Mn-SOD) [88], a mitochondrial free radical scavenger, and HSP72 [5], a major inducible heat shock protein, are two examples. Both are inducible and both have been implicated in delayed preconditioning. The temporal activity of Mn-SOD is biphasic after a preconditioning stimulus with a time course similar in onset and duration to first and second windows of protection [89]. Furthermore, in a study of cultured rat myocytes, oligonucleotide antisense to Mn-SOD abrogated the preconditioning response resulting in greater cardiac enzyme release following injurious ischaemia [88].

Similar circumstantial evidence exists for HSP72 in rabbits; HSP72 levels are elevated at 24 h [5] at the same time as the commencement of the second window [5]. Further, gene transfection studies (HSP72) [90] and transgenic mouse studies with constituitively over-expressed rat HSP72 [91], support heat stress protein's involvement in the second window of protection.

Heat stress proteins that are expressed constitutively may be modified in response to preconditioning stimuli. HSP27 is an example. HSP27 is phosphorylated by MAPKAPK2, part of the p38 MAPK signalling cascade that is induced as a result of preconditioning [60]. When activated, HSP27 binds to actin, altering actin microfilament dynamics [92,93] thus possibly explaining the increased osmotic strength that preconditioned isolated rabbit myocytes exhibit with a concomitant increase in p38 MAPK activation [61].

Preconditioning can therefore increase gene expression by elevation of levels of mRNA [94], increase protein synthesis [5], and modify proteins post-transcriptionally [60].

The inducible isoform of nitric oxide synthase (iNOS) is an enzyme that becomes expressed as a result of a preconditioning stimulus. iNOS (or NOSII) is a member of the nitric oxide synthase family that also includes two constituitively expressed isoforms, endothelial NOS (eNOS/NOSIII) and neuronal NOS (nNOS/NOSI). Pharmacological manipulation with agents such as dexamethasone can significantly attenuate iNOS expression [95] and in doing so abrogate the protective effects seen with the second window of protection [96]. Specific inhibition of nitric oxide synthase activity produces a similar result [44, 97–99]. The biologically active messenger synthesized by this enzyme is nitric oxide (NO) that can potentiate the opening of K_{ATP} channels [87] probably through intracellular accumulation of cGMP [100]. With the availability of transgenic mice genetically rendered deficient in iNOS, a more specific tool for examining the role of these inducible proteins has become available. In initial investigations with such mice, iNOS appears to be essential in the evolution of the second window of protection initiated by the prior administration of the bacterial endotoxin, monophosphoryl lipid A (MLA) [101].

The role of programmed cell death, apoptosis, is coming under scrutiny. Increasing evidence indicates that this form of cell death occurs during both the early stages of ischaemia, and during reperfusion (see review [102]). Whilst there are problems in quantifying the effect of apoptosis and distinguishing myocytes from other cell types (see review [103]), preconditioning may have an anti-apoptotic effect [19, 104–106]. Mechanisms by which the cell can become resistant to this form of cell death remain unknown, but by taking advantage of these by preconditioning, greater myocardial salvage from otherwise lethal ischaemia and reperfusion injury may be achievable.

Clinical applications of preconditioning

The potential for value of classical preconditioning in patients undergoing invasive coronary procedures [107–111] has been recognized. Whilst there is little evidence at present regarding the presence of a second window of protection in humans, recently, we and others have demonstrated that this delayed form of preconditioning occurs in human cultured myocyte cell lines [112,113] (see below).

The methods employed in inducing preconditioning have been aimed primarily at the triggers of preconditioning discussed above. As mechanisms of preconditioning are clarified, it may become possible to manipulate the signal transduction pathway or the end effectors of those pathways with the use of drugs that could be regarded as 'preconditioning-mimetics'.

The time at which preconditioning is applied in relation to an ischaemic event will mandate different therapeutic approaches: pre-empting a period of ischaemia of predictable onset; prior to thrombolysis; and salvage at the time of pharmacological or mechanical recanalization.

Preconditioning before invasive coronary procedures

Angioplasty, coronary artery bypass grafting, and invasive coronary imaging techniques employed in the diagnosis and treatment of ACS are not without risk of mortality or morbidity resulting from myocardial ischaemia. According to the USA Medicare figures published in 1992, mortality at 30 days and 1 year respectively were: for angioplasty 3.8% and 8.2%, and for coronary bypass grafting 6.4% and 11.8% [114]. During an invasive coronary procedure, patients are subjected to episodic attenuated coronary blood flow (ischaemia). As the time of myocardial ischaemia is predictable and short, myocardial resistance to potential injury can be induced preoperatively by classical preconditioning. By invoking myocardial protection in this manner it may be possible to reduce the risks associated with invasive procedures in combination with other effective strategies. In trials of preconditioning strategies to date, the chosen method of preconditioning induction has been via the modulation of the trigger mechanisms either through brief preprocedure ischaemia [107,111] or by the administration of adenosine [108,109]. Results have shown reduced Troponin-T release (an indirect measure of myocyte injury) in patients subjected to ischaemic preconditioning before bypass grafting [110,111] and better preservation of ATP [107,110] as judged from assays of sequential ventricular biopsies. A similar reduction of cardiac enzyme release has been seen with adenosine pretreatment with a concomitant improvement in postoperative haemodynamics [108]. When adenosine was administered to patients before percutaneous transluminal angioplasty, ST-segment shift decreased and post-surgical pain declined [109].

However, no study has yet demonstrated decreased morbidity or mortality. Further studies with preconditioning-mimetic drugs will be needed before preconditioning can be recommended routinely before coronary interventions.

The future for preconditioning: prolonging the window of protection

The first window of protection (classical preconditioning) diminishes after 2–3 hours. Until the onset of the second window of protection, the myocardium appears 'refractory' to further ischaemic preconditioning. Results of a recent study have suggested that this phenomenon is related to depletion of endogenous adenosine, at least in pigs [115]. With an infusion of an adenosine A_1 agonist during the refractory period, 'classical' preconditioning could be restored and protection against a subsequent, otherwise lethal duration of ischaemia could be re-established [115]. What has not been demonstrated is whether protection can be seamlessly prolonged over time in this manner. Problematically, we know from earlier research that a constant infusion of an adenosine A_1 agonist, CCPA, leads to a rapid fatigue and loss of the preconditioning response in rabbits [116]. Thus, design of a 'convenient' and acceptable drug may be extremely difficult; the short duration of classical preconditioning may necessitate a frequent and carefully timed dosing regime.

The 48-h duration of delayed preconditioning may be a more convenient therapeutic starting point.

In a recent investigation carried out in our laboratory, a regimen of adenosine A_1 agonist (CCPA) administered once every 48 h was used successfully in rabbits to prolong the second window of protection over a 10-day period. Its use yielded a 42% reduction in infarct size compared with those animals after vehicle alone [117]. Questions still remain, however. Over what duration can protection be prolonged? What will be an optimal dosing regimen? Can other triggers of preconditioning yield similar results? And most important, can the approach be effective in patients?

Drugs with potential 'preconditioning-mimetic' actions

Among the elements of the preconditioning pathway downstream of the cellular receptors, the end effector, K_{ATP} channel opening, has been studied most thoroughly with respect to the potential target for preconditioning-mimetric drugs. Nicorandil, a K_{ATP} channel opener, reduces infarct size in rabbits [118,119] and dogs [120].

Two pilot studies with nicorandil have been performed with patients admitted with acute myocardial infarction. The first, a small study by Sakata *et al.* [121], evaluated 20 patients presenting with anterior myocardial infarction treated with thrombolytic drugs or by primary angioplasty to whom nicorandil was administered. Contrast echocardiography demonstrated improved regional wall movement 1 month later. The other study by Sen *et al.* [122] demonstrated in 45 patients treated conventionally after infarction that nicorandil was apparently safe and well tolerated. The incidence of arrhythmia decreased, and a trend toward the reduction of development of Q-waves on the ECG was seen in those who had non-Q wave infarcts.

These results are encouraging, though preliminary. However, both studies have recruited only small numbers of patients and have somewhat soft endpoints. Large, carefully designed clinical trials will be needed to determine whether clinical outcomes, i.e. morbidity and mortality, can be reduced.

Preconditioning and acute coronary syndromes

The potential for preconditioning as a clinically useful therapy has not yet been defined, even though human myocardium can be preconditioned. One of the difficulties in the application of preconditioning lies in the identification of the patient who can benefit from a preconditioning intervention. By definition, preconditioning requires that the preconditioning stimulus be applied before the onset of otherwise lethal ischaemia. Among the acute coronary syndromes, an initial acute myocardial infarction is perhaps the most difficult to predict. Thus, preconditioning is unlikely to be applicable to an unheralded acute myocardial infarct. However, preconditioning could be applied to the patient with unstable angina who is hospitalized in a coronary care unit. Such patients are at significant risk of acute myocardial infarction (the PURSUIT investigators reported a 15.7% rate of infarction or death by 30 days after hospital admission [123]), and therefore comprise a population that could potentially benefit from preconditioning to diminish the sequelae of possible coronary occlusion. If the prolongation of the second window of protection, as described by Dana *et al.* [117], can be applied in man, preconditioning could be a useful myoprotective adjunct to conventional therapies in the days after hospital admission.

Conclusions

Since the original description of ischaemic preconditioning in 1986 our understanding of the mechanisms involved has grown. Several neuroendocrine and paracine agents have been identified as triggers of preconditioning. Their receptors are obvious pharmacological targets. The effectors that mediate myocyte resistance to injury may also be susceptible to therapeutic manipulation; the mitochondrial K_{ATP} channel is a prime example. That preconditioning may be applicable to patients has been explored in the context of invasive coronary procedures, in the TIMI4 and TIMI9B trials and other studies (references [124,125] and [126], respectively). However, the full potential of preconditioning as a therapeutic modality has yet to be defined. This is particularly true for delayed preconditioning, which as we have shown, can be prolonged over a period of days in the rabbit. Studies with human myocytes in culture indicate the likelihood of a second window of protection in human myocardium. Prolonged protection could have a role in the management of patients with unstable angina, however, the ramifications of prolonged 'stress' protein induction remain unknown. With the elucidation of the signalling pathways and effector mechanisms involved, such as the anti-apoptotic role of preconditioning in ischaemia and reperfusion, further progress can be made in exploring the utility of cellular protection against lethal injury. And thus, useful clinically applicable therapeutic modalities may evolve.

Ultimately, the effect upon morbidity and mortality will define the clinical usefulness of preconditioning. Outcome measures need to be interpreted in the context of other effective therapeutic strategies. However, preconditioning as an approach for improved management of patients with acute coronary syndromes deserves thorough exploration.

References

1 Murray C, Lopez A. Mortality by cause for eight regions of the world: Global Burden of Disease Study. *Lancet* 1997; 349: 1269–76.

2 Anonymous. Effectiveness of intravenous thrombolytic treatment in acute myocardial infarction. Gruppo Italiano per lo Studio della Streptochinasi nell' Infarto Miocardico (GISSI). *Lancet* 1986; 1 (8478): 397–402.

3 Murry CE, Jennings RB, Reimer KA. Preconditioning with ischemia: a delay of lethal cell injury in ischemic myocardium. *Circulation* 1986; 74: 1124–36.

4 Reimer KA, Murry CE, Yamasawa I, Hill ML, Jennings RB. Four brief periods of ischaemia cause no cumulative ATP loss or necrosis. *Am J Physiol* 1986; 251: H1306–15.

5 Marber MS, Latchman DS, Walker JM, Yellon DM. Cardiac stress protein elevation 24 hours after brief ischemia or heat stress is associated with resistance to

myocardial infarction. *Circulation* 1993; 88: 1264–72.

6 Baxter GF, Yellon DM. Time course of delayed myocardial protection after tansient adenosine A1 receptor activation in the rabbit. *J Cardiovasc Pharmacol* 1997; 29: 631–8.

7 Sumeray MS, Cohen MV, Downey J, Gelpi RJ, Slezak J, Yellon D. Characterisation of a new murine model of global ischaemia-reperfusion injury. *Mol Cell Biochem* 1998; in press.

8 Yellon DM, Alkhulaifi AM, Browne EE, Pugsley WB. Ischaemic preconditioning limits infarct size in the rat heart. *Cardiovasc Res* 1992; 26: 983–7.

9 Tsuchida A, Miura T, Miki T, Shimamoto K, Iimura O. Role of adenosine receptor activation in myocardial infarct size limitation by ischaemic preconditioning. *Cardiovasc Res* 1992; 26: 456–61.

10 Morris SD, Yellon DM. Angiotensin-converting enzyme inhibitors potentiate preconditioning through bradykinin B_2

receptor activation in human heart. *J Am Coll Cardiol* 1997; 29: 1599–606.

11 Nayeem MA, Hess ML, Qian YZ, Loesser KE, Kukreja RC. Delayed preconditioning of cultured adult rat cardiac myocytes: role of 70- and 90-kDa heat stress proteins. *Am J Physiol* 1997; 273: H861–8.

12 Zhou X, Zhai X, Ashraf M. Direct evidence that initial oxidative stress triggered by preconditioning contributes to second window of protection by endogenous antioxidant enzyme in myocytes. *Circulation* 1996; 93: 1177–84.

13 Imagawa J, Baxter G, Yellon D. Genistein, a tyrosine kinase inhibitor, blocks the 'second window of protection' 48 h after ischemic preconditioning in the rabbit. *J Mol Cell Cardiol* 1997; 29: 1885–93.

14 Baxter GF, Marber MS, Patel VC, Yellon DM. Adenosine receptor involvement in a delayed phase of myocardial protection 24 hours after ischemic preconditioning. *Circulation* 1994; 90: 2993–3000.

15 Maldonado C, Qiu Y, Tang XL, Cohen MV, Auchampach J, Bolli R. Role of adenosine receptors in late preconditioning against myocardial stunning in conscious rabbits. *Am J Physiol* 1997; 273: H1324–32.

16 Mei D, Elliot G, Gross G. KATP channels mediate late preconditioning against infarction produced by monophosphoryl lipid A. *Am J Physiol* 1996; 271: H2723–9.

17 Vegh A, Szekeres L, Parratt JR. Local intracoronary infusions of bradykinin profoundly reduce the severity of ischaemia-induced arrhythmias in anaesthetized dogs. *Br J Pharmacol* 1991; 104: 294–5.

18 Sekili S, Jeroudi MO, Tang XL, Zughaib M, Sun JZ, Bolli R. Effect of adenosine on myocardial 'stunning' in the dog. *Circ Res* 1995; 76: 82–94.

19 Piot CA, Padmanaban D, Ursell PC, Sievers RE, Wolfe CL. Ischemic preconditioning decreases apoptosis in rat hearts in vivo. *Circulation* 1997; 96: 1598–604.

20 Richard V, Kaeffer N, Tron C, Thuillez C. Ischemic preconditioning protects against coronary endothelial dysfunction induced by ischemia and reperfusion. *Circulation* 1994; 89: 1254–61.

21 Thornton J, Striplin S, Liu GS *et al.* Inhibition of protein synthesis does not block myocardial protection afforded by preconditioning. *Am J Physiol* 1990; 259: H1822–5.

22 Meldrum DR, Cleveland JCJ, Rowland RT, Banerjee A, Harken AH, Meng X. Early and delayed preconditioning: differential mechanisms and additive protection. *Am J Physiol* 1997; 273: 725–33.

23 Liu GS, Jacobson KA, Downey JM. An irreversible A1-selective adenosine agonist preconditions rabbit heart. *Can J Cardiol* 1996; 12: 517–21.

24 Liu GS, Richards SC, Olsson RA, Mullane K, Walsh RS, Downey JM. Evidence that the adenosine A3 receptor may mediate the protection afforded by preconditioning in the isolated rabbit heart. *Cardiovasc Res* 1994; 28: 1057–61.

25 Qian YZ, Levasseur JE, Yoshida K, Kukreja RC. KATP channels in rat heart: blockade of ischemic and acetylcholine-mediated preconditioning by glibenclamide. *Am J Physiol* 1996; 271: H23–8.

26 Cohen MV, Walsh RS, Goto M, Downey JM. Hypoxia preconditions rabbit myocardium via adenosine and catecholamine release. *J Mol Cell Cardiol* 1995; 27: 1527–34.

27 Liu Y, Tsuchida A, Cohen MV, Downey JM. Pretreatment with angiotensin II activates protein kinase C and limits myocardial infarction in isolated rabbit hearts. *J Mol Cell Cardiol* 1995; 27: 883–92.

28 Starkopf J, Bugge E, Ytrehus K. Preischemic bradykinin and ischaemic preconditioning in functional recovery of the globally ischaemic rat heart. *Cardiovasc Res* 1997; 33: 63–70.

29 Schultz JJ, Hsu AK, Gross GJ. Ischemic preconditioning and morphine-induced cardioprotection involve the delta (delta)-opioid receptor in the intact rat heart. *J Mol Cell Cardiol* 1997; 29: 2187–95.

30 Headrick JP. Ischemic preconditioning: bioenergetic and metabolic changes and the role of endogenous adenosine. *J Mol Cell Cardiol* 1996; 28: 1227–40.

31 Ganote CE, Armstrong S, Downey JM. Adenosine and A1 selective agonists offer minimal protection against ischaemic in-

jury to isolated rat cardiomyocytes. *Cardiovasc Res* 1993; 27: 1670–6.

32 Cave AC, Collis CS, Downey JM, Hearse DJ. Improved functional recovery by ischaemic preconditioning is not mediated by adenosine in the globally ischaemic isolated rat heart. *Cardiovasc Res* 1993; 27: 663–8.

33 Miura T, Ishimoto R, Sakamoto J *et al.* Suppression of reperfusion arrhythmia by ischemic preconditioning in the rat: is it mediated by the adenosine receptor, prostaglandin, or bradykinin receptor? *Basic Res Cardiol* 1995; 90: 240–6.

34 Bugge E, Ytrehus K. Ischaemic preconditioning is protein kinase C dependent but not through stimulation of alpha adrenergic or adenosine receptors in the isolated rat heart. *Cardiovasc Res* 1995; 29: 401–6.

35 Asimakis GK, Inners McBride K, Conti VR. Attenuation of postischaemic dysfunction by ischaemic preconditioning is not mediated by adenosine in the isolated rat heart. *Cardiovasc Res* 1993; 27: 1522–30.

36 Li Y, Kloner RA. The cardioprotective effects of ischemic 'preconditioning' are not mediated by adenosine receptors in rat hearts. *Circulation* 1993; 87: 1642–8.

37 Liu Y, Downey JM. Ischemic preconditioning protects against infarction in rat heart. *Am J Physiol* 1992; 32: H1107–12.

38 Goto M, Liu Y, Yang XM, Ardell JL, Cohen MV, Downey JM. Role of bradykinin in protection of ischemic preconditioning in rabbit hearts. *Circ Res* 1995; 77: 611–21.

39 Baxter GF, Kerac M, Zaman MJ, Yellon DM. Protection against global ischemia in the rabbit isolated heart 24 hours after transient adenosine A1 receptor activation. *Cardiovasc Drugs Ther* 1997; 11: 83–5.

40 Bolli R, Bhatti ZA, Tang XL, Qiu Y, Zhang Q, Guo Y, Jadoon AK. Evidence that late preconditioning against myocardial stunning in conscious rabbits is triggered by the generation of nitric oxide. *Circ Res* 1997; 81: 42–52.

41 Schultz J, Hsu A, Nagase H, Gross G. TAN-67, a delta 1-opioid receptor agonist, reduces infarct size via activation of Gi/o proteins and KATP channels. *Am J Physiol* 1998; 274: H909–14.

42 Fryer R, Hsu A, Eells J, Nagase H, Gross G. Opioid-induced second window of cardioprotection: potential role of mitochondrial KATP channels. *Circ Res* 1999; 84: 846–51.

43 Nayeem MA, Elliott GT, Shah MR, Hastillo-Hess SL, Kukreja RC. Monophosphoryl lipid A protects adult rat cardiac myocytes with induction of the 72-kD heat shock protein: a cellular. *J Mol Cell Cardiol* 1997; 29: 2305–10.

44 Zhao L, Weber PA, Smith JR, Comerford ML, Elliott GT. Role of inducible nitric oxide synthase in pharmacological 'preconditioning' with monophosphoryl lipid A. *J Mol Cell Cardiol* 1997; 29: 1567–76.

45 Yoshida K, Maaieh MM, Shipley JB *et al.* Monophosphoryl lipid A induces pharmacologic 'preconditioning' in rabbit hearts without concomitant expression of 70-kDa heat shock protein. *Mol Cell Biochem* 1996; 156: 1–8.

46 Thornton JD, Liu GS, Downey JM. Pretreatment with pertussis toxin blocks the protective effects of preconditioning: evidence for a G-protein mechanism. *J Mol Cell Cardiol* 1993; 25: 311–20.

47 Kehrl J. Heterotrimeric G protein signaling: roles in immune function and fine-tuning by RGS proteins. *Immunity* 1998; 8: 1–10.

48 Downey JM, Cohen MV. Signal transduction in ischemic preconditioning. *Z Kardiol* 1995; 4: 77–86.

49 Ytrehus K, Liu Y, Downey JM. Preconditioning protects ischemic rabbit heart by protein kinase C activation. *Am J Physiol* 1994 266: H1145–52.

50 Speechly Dick ME, Mocanu MM, Yellon DM. Protein kinase C. Its role in ischemic preconditioning in the rat. *Circ Res* 1994; 75: 586–90.

51 Kitakaze M, Node K, Minamino T. Role of activation of protein kinase C in the infarct size-limiting effect of ischemic preconditioning through activation of ecto-5′-nucleotidase. *Circulation* 1996; 93: 781–91.

52 Liu Y, Cohen MV, Downey JM. Chelerythrine, a highly selective protein kinase C inhibitor, blocks the anti-infarct effect of ischemic preconditioning in rabbit hearts [letter]. *Cardiovasc Drugs Ther* 1994; 8: 881–2.

53 Ping P, Zhang J, Qiu Y, Tang XL,

Manchikalapudi S, Bolli R. Repetitive episodes of myocardial ischemia and reperfusion induce translocation of protein kinase C epsilon isoform in conscious rabbits which is associated with late preconditioning against myocardial stunning. *Circulation* 1996; 94 (Suppl.): I-660 (Abstract).

54 Ping P, Zhang J, Qiu Y *et al*. Ischemic preconditioning induces selective translocation of protein kinase C isoforms epsilon and eta in the heart of conscious rabbits without subcellular redistribution of total protein kinase C activity. *Circ Res* 1997; 81: 404–14.

55 Goldberg M, Zhang HL, Steinberg SF. Hypoxia alters the subcellular distribution of protein kinase C isoforms in neonatal rat ventricular myocytes. *J Clin Invest* 1997; 99: 55–61.

56 Armstrong S, Ganote CE. Preconditioning of isolated rabbit cardiomyocytes: effects of glycolytic blockade, phorbol esters, and ischaemia. *Cardiovasc Res* 1994; 28: 1700–6.

57 Gray MO, Karliner JS, Mochly-Rosen D. A selective epsilon-protein kinase C antagonist inhibits protection of cardiac myocytes from hypoxia-induced cell death. *J Biol Chem* 1997; 272: 30945–51.

58 Baines C, Wang L, Cohen M, Downey J. Protein tyrosine kinase is downstream of protein kinase C for ischemic preconditioning's anti-infarct effect in the rabbit heart. *J Mol Cell Cardiol* 1998; 30: 383–92.

59 Dana A, Skarli M, Papakrivopoulou J, Yellon DM. Adenosine A(1) receptor induced delayed preconditioning in rabbits: induction of p38 mitogen-activated protein kinase activation and Hsp27 phosphorylation via a tyrosine kinase- and protein kinase C-dependent mechanism. *Circ Res* 2000; 86: 989–97.

60 Maulik N, Watanabe M, Zu YL *et al*. Ischemic preconditioning triggers the activation of MAP kinases and MAPKAP kinase 2 in rat hearts. *FEBS Lett* 1996; 396: 233–7.

61 Weinbrenner C, Liu G, Cohen MV, Downey JM. Phosphorylation of tyrosine 182 of p38 mitogen-activated protein kinase correlates with the protection of preconditioning in the rabbit heart. *J Mol Cell Cardiol* 1997; 29: 2383–91.

62 Sugden P, Clerk A. 'Stress-responsive'

mitogen-activated protein kinases (c-Jun N-terminal kinases and p38 mitogen-activated protein kinases) in the myocardium. *Circ Res* 1998; 83: 345–52.

63 Sugden P, Clerk A. Regulation of the ERK subgroup of MAP kinase cascades through G protein-coupled receptors. *Cell Signal* 1997; 9: 337–51.

64 Abe MK, Kartha S, Karpova AY *et al*. Hydrogen peroxide activates extracellular signal-regulated kinase via protein kinase C, Raf-1, and MEK1. *Am J Respir Cell Mol Biol* 1998; 18: 562–9.

65 Knight RJ, Buxton DB. Stimulation of c-Jun kinase and mitogen-activated protein kinase by ischemia and reperfusion in the perfused rat heart. *Biochem Biophys Res Commun* 1996; 218: 83–8.

66 Bogoyevitch MA, Gillespie-Brown J, Ketterman AJ *et al*. Stimulation of the stress-activated mitogen-activated protein kinase subfamilies in perfused heart P38/RK. *Circ Res* 1996; 79: 162–73.

67 Ahlers A, Engel K, Sott C, Gaestel M, Herrmann F, Brach M. Interleukin-3 and granulocyte-macrophage colony-stimulating factor induce activation of the MAPKAP kinase 2 resulting. *Blood* 1994; 83: 1791–8.

68 Wolfe CL, Sievers RE, Visseren FL, Donnelly TJ. Loss of myocardial protection after preconditioning correlates with the time course of glycogen recovery within the preconditioned segment. *Circulation* 1993; 87: 881–92.

69 Kida M, Fujiwara H, Ishida M *et al*. Ischemic preconditioning preserves creatine phosphate and intracellular pH. *Circulation* 1991; 84: 2495–503.

70 Steenbergen C, Perlman M, London R, Murphy E. Mechanism of preconditioning. Ionic alterations. *Circ Res* 1993; 72: 112–25.

71 Sanz E, Garcia Dorado D, Oliveras J *et al*. Dissociation between anti-infarct effect and anti-edema effect of ischemic preconditioning. *Am J Physiol* 1995; 268: H233–41.

72 Bugge E, Ytrehus K. Inhibition of sodium-hydrogen exchange reduces infarct size in the isolated rat heart — a protective additive to ischaemic preconditioning. *Cardiovasc Res* 1995; 29: 269–74.

73 Light P, Sabir A, Allen B, Walsh M, French R. Protein kinase C-induced

changes in the stoichiometry of ATP binding activate cardiac ATP-sensitive K$^+$ channels. *Circ Res* 1996; 79: 399–406.

74 Speechly Dick ME, Grover GJ, Yellon DM. Does ischemic preconditioning in the human involve protein kinase C and the ATP-dependent K$^+$ channel? Studies of contractile function after simulated ischemia in an atrial *in vitro* model. *Circ Res* 1995; 77: 1030–5.

75 Mizumura T, Nithipatikom K, Gross GJ. Bimakalim, an ATP-sensitive potassium channel opener, mimics the effects of ischemic preconditioning to reduce infarct size, adenosine release, and neutrophil function in dogs. *Circulation* 1995; 92: 1236–45.

76 Schultz JE, Hsu AK, Gross GJ. Morphine mimics the cardioprotective effect of ischemic preconditioning via a glibenclamide-sensitive mechanism in the rat heart. *Circ Res* 1996; 78: 1100–4.

77 Ferdinandy P, Szilvassy Z, Koltai M, Dux L. Ventricular overdrive pacing-induced preconditioning and no-flow ischemia-induced preconditioning in isolated working rat hearts. *J Cardiovasc Pharmacol* 1995; 25: 97–104.

78 Armstrong SC, Liu GS, Downey JM, Ganote CE. Potassium channels and preconditioning of isolated rabbit cardiomyocytes: effects of glyburide and pinacidil. *J Mol Cell Cardiol* 1995; 27: 1765–74.

79 Walsh RS, Tsuchida A, Daly JJ, Thornton JD, Cohen MV, Downey JM. Ketamine-xylazine anaesthesia permits a KATP channel antagonist to attenuate preconditioning in rabbit myocardium. *Cardiovasc Res* 1994; 28: 1337–41.

80 Auchampach JA, Grover GJ, Gross GJ. Blockade of ischaemic preconditioning in dogs by the novel ATP dependent potassium channel antagonist sodium 5-hydroxydecanoate. *Cardiovasc Res* 1992; 26: 1054–62.

81 Koning MM, Gho BC, van Klaarwater E, Opstal RL, Duncker DJ, Verdouw PD. Rapid ventricular pacing produces myocardial protection by nonischemic activation of KATP channels. *Circulation* 1996; 93: 178–86.

82 Schulz R, Rose J, Heusch G. Involvement of activation of ATP-dependent potassium channels in ischemic preconditioning in swine. *Am J Physiol* 1994; 267: H1341–52.

83 Yao Z, Gross G. Effects of KATP channel opener bimakalim on coronary blood flow, monophasic action potential duration, and infarct size in dogs. *Circulation* 1994; 89: 1769–75.

84 Grover GJ. Pharmacology of ATP-sensitive potassium channel (KATP) openers in models of myocardial ischemia and reperfusion. *Can J Physiol Pharmacol* 1997; 75: 309–15.

85 Liu Y, Sato T, O'Rourke B, Marban E. Mitochondrial ATP-dependent potassium channels: novel effectors of cardioprotection? *Circulation* 1998; 97: 2463–9.

86 Pell TJ, Yellon DM, Goodwin RW, Baxter GF. Myocardial ischemic tolerance following heat stress is abolished by ATP-sensitive potassium channel blockade. *Cardiovasc Drugs Ther* 1997; 11: 679–86.

87 Shinbo A, Iijima T. Potentiation by nitric oxide of the ATP-sensitive K$^+$ current induced by K$^+$ channel openers in guinea-pig ventricular cells. *Br J Pharmacol* 1997; 120: 1568–74.

88 Yamashita N, Nishida M, Hoshida S *et al*. Induction of manganese superoxide dismutase in rat cardiac myocytes increases tolerance to hypoxia 24 hours after preconditioning. *J Clin Invest* 1994; 94: 2193–9.

89 Hoshida S, Kuzuya T, Fuji H *et al*. Sublethal ischemia alters myocardial antioxidant activity in canine heart. *Am J Physiol* 1993; 264: H33–9.

90 Heads RJ, Latchman DS, Yellon DM. Stable high level expression of a transfected human HSP70 gene protects a heart-derived muscle cell line against thermal stress. *J Mol Cell Cardiol* 1994; 26: 695–9.

91 Marber MS, Mestril R, Chi SH, Sayen MR, Yellon DM, Dillmann WH. Overexpression of the rat inducible 70-kD heat stress protein in a transgenic mouse increases the resistance of the heart to ischemic injury. *J Clin Invest* 1995; 95: 1446–56.

92 Guay J, Lambert H, Gingras-Breton G, Lavoie JN, Huot J. Regulation of actin filament dynamics by p38 map kinase-mediated phosphorylation of heat shock protein 27. *J Cell Sci* 1997; 110: 357–68.

93 Benndorf R, Haye K, Ryazantsev S, Wieske M, Behlke J, Lutsch G. Phospho-

rylation and supramolecular organization of murine small heat shock protein HSP25 abolish its actin polymerization-inhibiting activity. *J Biol Chem* 1994; 269: 20780–4.

94 Kukreja RC, Kontos MC, Loesser KE *et al*. Oxidant stress increases heat shock protein 70 mRNA in isolated perfused rat heart. *Am J Physiol* 1994; 267: H2213–9.

95 Simmons WW, Ungureanu-Longrois D, Smith GK, Smith TW, Kelly RA. Glucocorticoids regulate inducible nitric oxide synthase by inhibiting tetrahydro-biopterin synthesis and L-arginine transport. *J Biol Chem* 1996; 271: 23928–37.

96 Vegh A, Papp JG, Parratt JR. Prevention by dexamethasone of the marked anti-arrhythmic effects of preconditioning induced 20 h after rapid cardiac pacing. *Br J Pharmacol* 1994; 113: 1081–2.

97 Imagawa J, Yellon D. Pharmacological evidence that inducible nitric oxide synthase is a mediator of delayed preconditioning. *Br J Pharmacol* 1999; 126: 701–8.

98 Takano H, Manchikalapudi S, Tang XL *et al*. Nitric oxide synthase is the mediator of late preconditioning against myocardial infarction in conscious rabbits. *Circulation* 1998; 98: 441–9.

99 Qiu Y, Rizvi A, Tang XL *et al*. Nitric oxide triggers late preconditioning against myocardial infarction in conscious rabbits. *Am J Physiol* 1997; 273: H2931–6.

100 Murphy ME, Brayden JE. Nitric oxide hyperpolarizes rabbit mesenteric arteries via ATP-sensitive potassium channels. *J Physiol Lond* 1995; 486: 47–58.

101 Xi L, Jarrett N, Hess M, Kukreja R. Essential role of inducible nitric oxide synthase in monophosphoryl lipid A-induced late cardioprotection: evidence from pharmacological inhibition and gene knockout mice. *Circulation* 1999; 99: 2157–63.

102 Fliss H. Accelerated apoptosis in reperfused myocardium: friend of foe? *Basic Res Cardiol* 1998; 93: 90–3.

103 Freude B, Masters TN, Kostin S, Robicsek F, Schaper J. Cardiomyocyte apoptosis in acute and chronic conditions. *Basic Res Cardiol* 1998; 93: 85–89.

104 Gottlieb RA, Gruol DL, Zhu JY, Engler RL. Preconditioning in rabbit cardio-

myocytes: role of pH, vacuolar proton ATPase, and apoptosis. *J Clin Invest* 1996; 97: 2391–8.

105 Maulik N, Yoshida T, Engelman R *et al*. Ischemic preconditioning attenuates apoptotic cell death associated with ischemia/reperfusion. *Mol Cell Biochem* 1998; 186: 139–45.

106 Baghelai KGL, Wechsler AS, Jakoi ER. Delayed myocardial preconditioning by alpha1-adrenoceptors involves inhibition of apoptosis. *J Thorac Cardiovasc Surg* 1999; 117: 980–6.

107 Yellon DM, Alkhulaifi AM, Pugsley WB. Preconditioning the human myocardium. *Lancet* 1993; 342: 276–7.

108 Lee HT, LaFaro RJ, Reed GE. Pretreatment of human myocardium with adenosine during open heart surgery. *J Card Surg* 1995; 10: 665–76.

109 Leesar MA, Stoddard M, Ahmed M, Broadbent J, Bolli R. Preconditioning of human myocardium with adenosine during coronary angioplasty. *Circulation* 1997; 95: 2500–7.

110 Alkhulaifi AM. Preconditioning the human heart. *Ann R Coll Surg Engl* 1997; 79: 49–54.

111 Jenkins DP, Pugsley WB, Alkhulaifi AM, Kemp M, Hooper J, Yellon DM. Ischaemic preconditioning reduces Troponin-T release in patients undergoing cardiac surgery. *Heart* 1997; 77: 314–18.

112 Carroll R, Yellon D. Mechanisms of delayed cardioprotection in a human cardiocyte cell line. *J Mol Cell Cardiol* 1999; 31: A102.

113 Arstall MA, Zhao YZ, Hornberger L *et al*. Human ventricular myocytes *in vitro* exhibit both early and delayed preconditioning responses to simulated ischemia. *J Mol Cell Cardiol* 1998; 30: 1019–25.

114 Hartz AJ, Kuhn EM, Pryor DB *et al*. Mortality after coronary angioplasty and coronary artery bypass surgery (the national Medicare experience). *Am J Cardiol* 1992; 70: 179–85.

115 Vogt AM, Ando H, Arras M, ElsasSeries A. Lack of adenosine causes myocardial refractoriness. *J Am Coll Cardiol* 1998; 31: 1134–41.

116 Tsuchida A, Thompson R, Olsson RA, Downey JM. The anti-infarct effect of an adenosine A1-selective agonist is diminished after prolonged infusion as is the cardioprotective effect of ischaemic pre-

conditioning in rabbit heart. *J Mol Cell Cardiol* 1994; 26: 303–11.

117 Dana A, Baxter GF, Walker JM, Yellon DM. Prolonging the delayed phase of myocardial protection, repetitive adenosine A₁ receptor activation maintains rabbit myocardium in a preconditioned state. *J Am Coll Cardiol* 1998; 31: 1142–9.

118 Ohno Y, Minatoguchi S, Uno Y *et al.* Nicorandil reduces myocardial infarct size by opening the K (ATP) channel in rabbits. *Int J Cardiol* 1997; 62: 181–90.

119 Imagawa J, Baxter GF, Yellon DM. Myocardial protection afforded by nicorandil and ischaemic preconditioning in a rabbit infarct model *in vivo*. *J Cardiovasc Pharmacol* 1998; 31: 74–9.

120 Mizumura T, Nithipatikom K, Gross GJ. Infarct size-reducing effect of nicorandil is mediated by the KATP channel but not by its nitrate-like properties in dogs. *Cardiovasc Res* 1996; 32: 274–85.

121 Sakata Y, Kodama K, Komamura K *et al.* Salutary effect of adjunctive nicorandil administration on restoration of myocardial blood flow and functional improvement in patients with acute myocardial infarction. *Am Heart J* 1997; 133: 616–21.

122 Sen S, Neus H, Berg G, Nitsche K, Goddemeier T, Doring G. Beneficial effects of nicorandil in acute myocadial infarction: a placebo-controlled, double-blind pilot safety study. *Br J Cardiol* 1998; 5: 208–20.

123 PURSUIT Trial Investigators. Inhibition of platelet glycoprotein IIb/IIIa with eptifibatide in patients with acute coronary syndromes. Platelet Glycoprotein I, Ib/IIIa. in Unstable Angina: Receptor Suppression Using Integrilin Therapy. *N Engl J Med* 1998; 339: 436–43.

124 Kloner RA, Shook T, Przyklenk K *et al.* Previous angina alters in-hospital outcome in TIMI 4. A clinical correlate to preconditioning? *Circulation* 1995; 91: 37–45.

125 Kloner RA, Shook T, Antman EM *et al.* Prospective temporal analysis of the onset of preinfarction angina versus outcome: an ancillary study in TIMI-9B. *Circulation* 1998; 97: 1042–5.

126 Napoli C, Liguori A, Chiariello M, Di Ieso N, Condorelli M, Ambrosio G. New-onset angina preceding acute myocardial infarction is associated with improved contractile recovery after thrombolysis. *Eur Heart J* 1998; 19: 411–19.

16: Is myocardial protection effective?

Ravichandran Ramasamy and Steven R. Bergmann

Introduction

Acute myocardial ischaemia can result in diverse outcomes, ranging from asymptomatic (silent) episodes to frank myocardial infarction (MI). Reperfusion therapy has become the mainstay for the treatment of patients with evolving MI and has provided a practical approach for the salvage of ischaemic myocardium. The dramatic reduction in morbidity and mortality from acute ischaemia observed in clinical trials of reperfusion therapy has led to the routine recommendation that recanalization therapy, either by direct angioplasty or with thrombolytic therapy, should be universally employed. Nonetheless, the benefits of reperfusion therapy can be reduced by factors such as the duration and severity of ischaemia prior to reperfusion, the adequacy of reflow, the presence of residual stenosis, and coronary reocclusion. Furthermore, reperfusion can trigger specific biochemical, functional, and ultrastructural changes which may also limit maximal myocardial salvage.

A number of pharmacological adjuncts have been proposed to minimize ischaemic injury and thereby maximize the myocardial salvage achievable upon reperfusion. In this chapter, we will explore strategies designed to protect ischaemic myocardium, based on modifying substrate metabolism as an adjunct to the treatment of acute myocardial ischaemia and evolving infarction. It should be stated at the outset, however, that, while some of the interventions to be discussed have been shown to be beneficial on their own in patients with myocardial infarction, maximal benefit can only be realized when these metabolic adjuncts are combined with reperfusion therapy.

Review of myocardial metabolism

Substrate metabolism under normoxic conditions

In order to discuss specific metabolic therapies, a brief overview of myocardial metabolism is warranted. The heart is an intrinsically aerobic organ, constantly requiring and producing energy to meet the needs of contraction and maintenance of ionic homeostasis. The regulation and utilization of various metabolic substrates to produce adenosine triphosphate (ATP), the high-energy compound needed for contractile function, is complex, redundant, and dependent on the arterial levels of substrate, oxygen, and hormones, as well as on coronary flow and inotropic state [1–3]. Among the various substrates that are available, long-chain fatty acids and glucose provide the majority of energy that is used by the heart. Nonetheless, the heart is remarkably adaptive and can use numerous other substances, such as lactate or ketone bodies, to meet its energy needs. Under normal fasting conditions, long-chain fatty acids serve as the preferred fuel for the heart as they are abundant in arterial blood and provide significant amounts of ATP for each mole of fatty acid oxidized (Fig. 16.1).

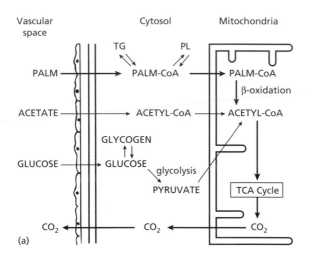

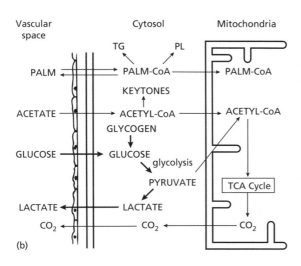

Fig. 16.1 Schematic diagram of myocardial metabolism under normoxic conditions (a), and during ischaemia (b). Under normal physiological conditions, fatty acids, of which palmitate is the major constituent in arterial blood, serve as the major source of substrate for energy production. Alternative fuels can also be used. With ischaemia, beta oxidation of fatty acids is impaired and glucose metabolism is both de-inhibited and up-regulated. Anaerobic metabolism of glucose also becomes an important method of ATP production. Abbreviations: PALM, palmitate; TG, triglyceride; PL, phospholipid; CoA, coenzyme A; TCA, tricarboxylic acid. (Reproduced from Bergmann *et al.* [7]. (Garson MC (ed.) *Cardiac Nuclear Medicine*, 3rd edn, 1997), with permission of the McGraw-Hill companies.)

Oxidative metabolism through the Krebs or tricarboxylic acid (TCA) cycle generates most of the ATP that is required to maintain contractile function, by providing the reducing equivalents for mitochondrial oxidative phosphorylation and generating ATP. All routes of aerobic metabolism shuttle ultimately, by way of the TCA cycle, through acetyl CoA, which is formed from the breakdown of pyruvate (formed from glycolysis as well as from lactate utilization), as well as from beta-oxidation of fatty acids. The rates of these metabolic pathways are tightly coupled to the rate of contractile work and vice versa. Contractile work is coupled to the availability of oxygen and the rate of oxidative phosphorylation.

After a meal, glucose becomes a major source of substrate used for energy. This is because after a carbohydrate load, insulin is released, which results in decreased lipolysis, thereby decreasing arterial fatty acid levels. This decrease in fatty acid stimulates myocardial glucose metabolism indirectly by decreasing the usual inhibitory effect of fatty acids and their intermediates on cardiac glucose utilization.

Myocardial glucose metabolism is dependent on the uptake of extracellular glucose, which is regulated by the transmembrane glucose gradient and the activity of glucose transporters, GLUT-1 and GLUT-4 [4–6]. In the heart, GLUT-1 is insulin-insensitive, and is considered to be responsible for basal glucose uptake in the setting of low fasting insulin concentrations under normal conditions, whereas GLUT-4, which is insulin-sensitive, is confined to the intracellular vesicles under normoxic conditions [4–6]. Upon stimulation by insulin or ischaemia, GLUT-4 is translocated to the sarcolemma, where it mediates increased glucose uptake into the myocyte. In fact, the up-regulation of glucose by the ischaemic heart has become the metabolic signature of viable, but jeopardized (hibernating), myocardium as assessed with Positron Emission Tomography (PET) [7]. Upon entering the myocyte, glucose is rapidly phosphorylated by hexokinase to form glucose-6-phosphate (G-6-P), which can either proceed down the glycolytic pathway or to glycogen synthesis. The rates of glucose uptake, glycogen synthesis and breakdown, and glycolysis are controlled by multiple steps in each of these pathways. Since, under most conditions, the levels of G-6-P remain constant, the activity of phosphofructokinase, and levels of NAD^+ and NADH are primary factors that influence glycolysis [8–10]. Pyruvate, derived from glycolysis and from lactate, can undergo decarboxylation catalysed by pyruvate dehydrogenase (PDH) [2,8] to form acetyl CoA. The activity of cardiac PDH is decreased when fatty acid oxidation is increased. Conversely, PDH activity is increased when fatty acid uptake or oxidation is suppressed. In general, high rates of fatty acid oxidation feed back to inhibit glucose uptake and oxidation [2,8].

Substrate metabolism during ischaemia and the rationale for metabolic protection

During ischaemia, lack of oxygen induces a shift to anaerobic metabolism with rapid stimulation of glucose uptake, glycogenolysis, and glycolytic flux [2,8]. The extent to which glucose contributes to energy production is dependent on the severity of ischaemia. Moderate reductions in blood flow and oxygen supply result in increased glucose extraction and glycolysis, with no changes in glucose uptake. As the severity of ischaemia increases, myocardial glucose uptake, glucose extraction, and glycolysis increase more significantly.

The induction of ischaemia is followed by recruitment of the glucose-transporters GLUT-4 and GLUT-1 from the intracellular stores to the plasma membrane [4–6]. Depending on the severity and duration of ischaemia, the transcription of the glucose transporters also get modified. The stimulation of glucose transport during ischaemia is reflected by the increased glycolytic flux. Activation of phosphofructokinase-1 (PFK-1) by AMP or by decreases in ATP are likely factors increasing glycolytic flux [2,8]. However, prolonged ischaemia results in the inhibition of glycolysis, as a result of increased levels of intermediates such as lactate and protons, and the decreased availability of NAD^+ [9–11].

Sustaining glycolysis during ischaemia is an important source for providing ATP to sustain the activities of sarcolemmal Na^+,K^+-ATPase and the sarcoendoplasmic Ca^{2+}-ATPase [12–14]. There is evidence to suggest that glycolysis preferentially supplies ATP for these critical ionic pumps [13,14], and thus, even if glycolytic metabolism does not provide sufficient energy to provide enough ATP to maintain cardiac contraction, it may provide adequate energy to maintain the ionic homeostasis, and thus preserve viability during the ischaemic insult.

Fatty acids have been shown to be detrimental to ischaemic myocardium. The accumulation of long-chain fatty acids may modify intermediary metabolism unfavourably by: increasing $NADH/NAD^+$ (increasing the lactate : pyruvate ratio, thereby decreasing glucose uptake and oxidation); increasing acetyl-CoA/CoASH, with consequent increases in citrate levels and inhibition of PFK; inhibiting pyruvate dehydrogenase and pyruvate carboxylase; and increasing the amounts of long-chain acyl carnitine (LCA). Experimental studies have suggested that accumulation of LCA may also be toxic to myocardium [15], leading to dysrhythmias by insertion of these lipophilic moieties into sarcolemmal membranes, inhibiting contractile function, perhaps by altering the activity of ATP translocase [16], and, *a priori*, by decreasing glycolytic flux [17,18]. In addition, children with inherited disorders of beta oxidation can develop overt cardiomyopathy when there are high levels of fatty acid in arterial blood [19].

Oliver and colleagues in the 1960s were among the first to demonstrate a relationship between serum fatty acids and morbidity and mortality in patients presenting with acute coronary syndromes [20,21]. They observed that patients with high serum levels of fatty acids had increased incidence of dysrhythmias and death compared with those with lower fatty acid levels. They hypothesized that these may be due to high levels of circulating catecholamines, and suggested the use of β-blocking drugs, blocking fatty acid release from fat by nicotinic acid, and supplying the heart with increased glucose [20–22]. This concept—that ischaemic myocardium could be protected by reducing fatty acid levels and increasing the availability of alternative fuels subsequently—was later championed by Oliver, Opie, and others [20–23].

Numerous experimental studies have convincingly demonstrated that sustenance of glycolytic metabolism by the ischaemic myocardium can preserve viability [24–26], delay ischaemic contracture—a hallmark of glycolytic failure, and prevent irreversible cell damage [27]. Glycolysis appears to support membrane function specifically [12], and, in particular, maintain sodium and calcium homeostasis [13,14]. It has been shown repeatedly that the protection of myocardium during ischaemia, by favourably modifying metabolism, prevents ischaemic injury and improves functional recovery upon reperfusion [2,8,23–26,28–31].

Enhancement of glycolysis and the reduction of circulating fatty acids can be accomplished by numerous and diverse approaches (Fig. 16.2). In addition

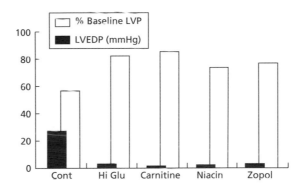

Fig.16.2 Histogram of end-ischaemic levels of left-ventricular end-diastolic pressure (LVEDP, mmHg 7) and of recovery of left ventricular-developed pressure (LVP, expressed as a percentage of baseline, preischaemic, levels) in isolated rat hearts subjected to ischaemia followed by reperfusion. In control, untreated hearts, EDP increases during ischaemia, an index of diastolic and glycolytic failure, and the percent recovery of LVP with reperfusion is only 60%. In contrast, when hearts are treated with agents that enhance myocardial substrate metabolism by diverse pathways during ischaemia, rises in EDP are attenuated, and, with reperfusion, LVP is increased towards baseline. Thus, metabolic manipulation of the myocardium prevents ischaemic damage and thereby enhances the beneficial effects of reperfusion. Abbreviations: Cont, control hearts; Hi Glu, high exogenous glucose in the perfusate; Zopol, zopolrestat—an aldose reductase inhibitor.

to the most widely-tested and direct approach to enhance glucose metabolism, i.e. directly with high levels of exogenous glucose (with or without added exogenous insulin), myocardial glucose metabolism can be stimulated by strategies that reduce serum fatty acids (glucose–insulin–potassium (GIK) infusions; and drugs such as oxfenicine, etomoxir, carnitine and congeners of niacin and nicotinic acid) [18,21–23]; stimulation of adenosine A_1 receptors [25,32]; or agents such as dichloroacetate or ranolazine which stimulate (or deinhibit) specific glycolytic enzymes [26,28,30]. In addition, preconditioning may elicit beneficial effects in ischaemic myocardium in part by enhancing glycolysis [29].

Changes during reperfusion

With reperfusion, mitochondrial oxidative phosphorylation returns to normal levels promptly. In clinical studies using PET, it was shown that recovery of oxidative metabolism occurs over a week after prompt thrombolytic therapy [33], and that the recovery of function, by necessity, requires the recovery of oxidative metabolism [34,35]. It should be mentioned that, even after brief periods of ischaemia, such as occur with balloon inflation during angioplasty, contractile function can take some time to recover, even when blood flow is completely restored—a phenomenon referred to as myocardial stunning. Based on PET scanning, many myocardial segments with contractile dysfunction may in fact be manifesting myocardial stunning from repetitive episodes of ischaemia followed by spontaneous reflow [36]. Thus, adjunctive metabolic therapy may not only benefit patients with acute coronary syndromes, but also those with chronic coronary artery disease—and perhaps even those with non-ischaemic cardiomyopathy.

While, in some studies, fatty acid metabolism is reduced after reperfusion, other studies have suggested normal metabolism early after ischaemia [2,8]. Likewise, there is controversy regarding whether glucose metabolism is normal, enhanced, or deceased early after coronary reperfusion [2,8], with experimental evidence varied, probably as a result of the myriad of protocols and models employed. Thus, no single metabolic pathway clearly appears to supervene in reperfusion. Oxidative metabolism, whether from glycolytic or fatty acid oxidation, is required for ultimate recovery of contractile function [34,35].

Reperfusion injury

Timely reperfusion has been demonstrated to be the most effective means of limiting necrosis and salvaging ischaemic myocardium [37–39]. However, full salvage may also be compromised as a result of reperfusion injury, which reduces the full benefits of recanalization therapy. Principal mediators of reperfusion injury include neutrophils and reactive oxygen species (ROS) (oxygen-centred free radicals). Reactive oxygen species are generated in small amounts under normal metabolic conditions and are inactivated by the presence of scavenger enzyme systems. Reperfusion of ischaemic myocardium is accompanied by increased generation of ROS, which overwhelm cellular scavenger enzymes and induce tissue damage [40–42]. The generation of ROS is influenced by mitochondrial respiration, activation of neutrophils, and xanthine oxidase activity. During ischaemia, xanthine accumulation increases and the mitochondrial redox state is altered, setting up a favourable system for generating ROS on reperfusion. Numerous animal studies have documented the occurrence of myocardial injury caused by ROS generation [40–42]. However, the evidence that ROS contributes to myocardial injury in humans is still lacking, and clinical trials of ROS scavengers have yielded disappointing results [43].

Neutrophil reintroduction in the postischaemic myocardium is accompanied by their activation and adhesion to endothelial surface and migration in tissues [44]. These activated neutrophils can release ROS and proteolytic enzymes that cause tissue necrosis, block capillaries, and reduce blood flow [44]. In addition, activated neutrophils can also release platelet-activating factor, thromboxane, and leukotrienes, which increase inflammation and further increase leucocyte and platelet activities in reperfused tissue. Interventions that reduce neutrophil activation in reperfused tissue have been shown to reduce myocardial reperfusion injury [42,44], but will not be considered further here as the numbers of observations are quite limited.

Protection of ischaemic myocardium with glucose–insulin–potassium

The fact that glucose can effectively be used to limit ischaemic injury has been known for many years. Experimental studies by Opie *et al.* proposed the therapeutic role of glucose for protecting ischaemic myocardium [22,31]. A number of subsequent studies demonstrated that infusions of glucose–insulin–potassium (GIK) decreased infarct size, lessened ultrastructural damage, and improved the contractile function of the heart. In addition, GIK was shown to reduce the frequency and duration of ventricular dysrhythmias and improve both cardiac function and survival of patients after myocardial infarction [45,46], especially when administered in combination with a thrombolytic [47–49].

Although it is obvious that the maximum salvage of ischaemic myocardium occurs only when reperfusion is employed, a recent meta-analysis of placebo-controlled clinical trials of GIK treatment in acute MI demonstrated that the treatment was effective in reducing overall mortality even in the absence of reperfusion therapy [50] (Fig. 16.3). Despite this finding, it is to be expected that the patients who will derive most benefit will be those in whom glucose is combined with reperfusion strategies. Two recent studies have been supportive of this concept. In the Diabetes mellitus Insulin-Glucose infusion in Acute Myocardial Infarction (DIGAMI) study [48], diabetic patients with acute myocardial infarction receiving insulin and glucose (approximately 50% receiving thrombolytic therapy) had a 29% reduction in death at 1 year compared with patients not receiving glucose and insulin (Fig. 16.4). In another recent study, patients with suspected acute myocardial infarction receiving GIK exhibited decreased mortality, heart failure, and dysrhythmias compared with patients not receiving GIK. Results were most favourable in patients receiving thrombolytic therapy (Fig. 16.5). The presumed mechanism of benefit in these studies is the decrease in putatively deleterious fatty acids by the peripheral action of insulin in limiting lipolysis, and the stimulation of myocardial glucose use by deinhibition of metabolism by the lowered fatty acid levels.

Short-term infusion of GIK has also been effectively used in patients with refractory left ventricular failure after revascularization surgery [51]. In these patients, GIK resulted in lower plasma levels of fatty acids, decreased systemic

Study	Mortality rate (%) GIK	Control	O–E	Variance	Odds ratio and CIs* GIK better	Placebo better
Heng	8.3	0	0.6	0.2		
Stanley	7.3	16.4	−2.5	2.8		
Rogers	6.5	12.3	−1.9	2.4		
Satler	0	0	0	0		
Mittra	11.8	28.2	−7.0	6.8		p=0.007
Pilcher	13.9	29.3	−2.6	3.4		
Pentecost	15	16	−0.5	6.5		
MRC	21.4	23.6	−5.1	41.5		
Hjermann	10.6	20	−4.8	6.8		p=0.07
All patients	16.1	21	−24	70.4		p=0.004

0   0.5   1   1.5   2

Fig. 16.3 Comparison of mortality data in patients receiving glucose–insulin–potassium (GIK), compared with those receiving placebo, as summarized in a meta-analysis. Overall, patients receiving GIK exhibited improved survival, even though in most of these studies reperfusion therapy was not used. Abbreviations: O–E, observed minus expected; CIs, confidence intervals. (Reproduced with permission from Fath-Ordoubadi *et al.* [50].)

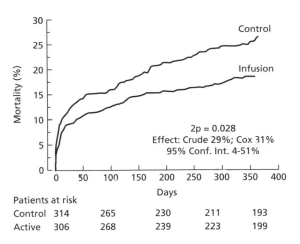

Fig. 16.4 Mortality curve over one year from patients in the Diabetes mellitus Insulin–Glucose infusion in Acute Myocardial Infarction (DIGAMI) study. Those diabetic patients with myocardial infarction receiving glucose and insulin (about half of whom received thrombolytic therapy as well) had superior survival rates compared with those who were not treated with glucose and insulin. (Reproduced with permission from the American College of Cardiology, from Malmberg *et al.* [48].)

Patients at risk					
Control	314	265	230	211	193
Active	306	268	239	223	199

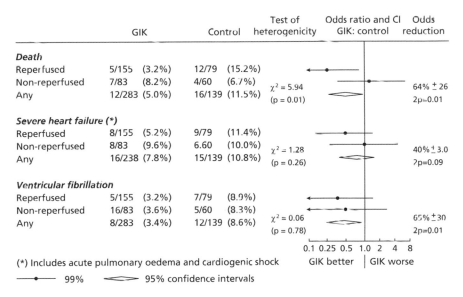

	GIK		Control		Test of heterogenicity	Odds ratio and CI GIK: control	Odds reduction
Death							
Reperfused	5/155	(3.2%)	12/79	(15.2%)			
Non-reperfused	7/83	(8.2%)	4/60	(6.7%)	$\chi^2 = 5.94$		64% ± 26
Any	12/283	(5.0%)	16/139	(11.5%)	(p = 0.01)		2p=0.01
Severe heart failure (*)							
Reperfused	8/155	(5.2%)	9/79	(11.4%)			
Non-reperfused	8/83	(9.6%)	6.60	(10.0%)	$\chi^2 = 1.28$		40% ± 3.0
Any	16/238	(7.8%)	15/139	(10.8%)	(p = 0.26)		2p=0.09
Ventricular fibrillation							
Reperfused	5/155	(3.2%)	7/79	(8.9%)			
Non-reperfused	16/83	(3.6%)	5/60	(8.3%)	$\chi^2 = 0.06$		65% ± 30
Any	8/283	(3.4%)	12/139	(8.6%)	(p = 0.78)		2p=0.01

0.1 0.25 0.5 1.0 2 4 8

GIK better | GIK worse

(*) Includes acute pulmonary oedema and cardiogenic shock

⟶•⟶ 99% ⟨───⟩ 95% confidence intervals

Fig. 16.5 Summary of in-hospital cardiac events in patients enrolled in a study of GIK infusion in patients with suspected myocardial infarction, broken down by those who did and did not receive thrombolytic therapy. The incidence of death, heart failure, and ventricular fibrillation were all decreased in patients receiving GIK, with the greatest benefit seen in those who received thrombolytic therapy concomitantly. (Reproduced, with permission from Lippincott, Williams, & Wilkins, from Diaz *et al.* [49] *Circulation* 1997: 96.)

vascular resistance, and improved cardiac index. Furthermore, in these patients, the requirement for inotropic support, as well as the time on intra-aortic balloon pump and stay in the intensive care unit, were all significantly reduced.

Thus, there is excellent experimental and clinical data to support the concept that increased glycolytic flux, induced by increased exogenous glucose and reduced serum fatty acids, aids in protecting the ischaemic myocardium and improving survival and function after acute ischaemic episodes.

Alternative agents that modulate myocardial metabolism

A number of other agents have the potential of enhancing the salvage of myocardium, based on the modulation of intermediary metabolism. However, as they have not been used clinically as extensively as GIK, they will be presented here only as potential adjuncts, with clinical utility requiring further evaluation in larger numbers of patients.

Aldose reductase inhibitors

One pathway for altered glucose metabolism that has generated interest in the area of myocardial ischaemia is the flux of glucose and other products via the polyol or the aldose reductase pathway. An increase in glucose metabolism via the polyol pathway has been documented in diabetic heart as well as with ischaemia [11]. In this pathway, glucose is reduced to sorbitol by aldose reductase. Inhibition of aldose reductase conserves NADPH, NAD+, and glucose.

Since aldose reductase and the polyol pathway exhibit increased activity under conditions of elevated blood glucose, considerable attention has been focused on studying the benefits of aldose reductase inhibition [10,11]. Experimental studies have demonstrated that aldose reductase inhibition reduced ischaemic injury [9,11], perhaps by lowering the elevated cytosolic redox state, and conserving NAD+ improves glycolysis in both normoxic and ischaemic myocardium [9–11]. Furthermore, it was also observed that aldose reductase inhibition increased myocardial glucose oxidation [10]. Preliminary studies in a small number of human subjects with myocardial infarction, who were treated with the aldose reductase inhibitor zopolrestat, showed modest improvements in ejection fraction. A larger clinical trial is currently under way to test the efficacy of aldose-reductase inhibitors in protecting patients with myocardial infarction.

Pyruvate dehydrogenase (PDH) activation

Stimulation of glucose oxidation during reperfusion has been shown to be beneficial in animal studies. Direct activation of PDH is an effective approach to increasing pyruvate (derived from glycolysis or lactate) oxidation. Dichloroacetate (DCA) and ranolazine have been tested clinically as they activate PDH in ischaemic tissue. In clinical studies, DCA was shown to increase left ventricular stroke volume in patients with coronary artery disease [52]. While animal studies with DCA showed marked increases in glucose oxidation and cardiac work during reperfusion, its success in clinical studies has been limited due to low potency and short half-life [53].

Ranolazine has demonstrated efficacy as an effective protective agent in myocardium in a number of animal studies [54]. In clinical trials, ranolazine has shown efficacy in extending treadmill exercise times in patients with chronic stable angina [55,56]. Of note, the metabolically mediated anti-ischaemic and antianginal effects of ranolazine were as effective as β-blockers without any haemodynamic effect [54–56].

Other agents that enhance myocardial glucose use

A number of other agents have been shown to increase myocardial glucose use, although their mechanisms of action are not fully understood. These include multiple agents that have been developed as antiglycaemic agents, such as oxfenicine and etomoxir, which have been shown in experimental studies to protect ischaemic myocardium [18,22,23]. Whether the newer generation of antiglycaemic agents that bear a structural analogy to these agents have a similar effect is not known. In addition, agents such as niacin and nicotinic acid have been shown to decrease plasma fatty acid levels and enhance myocardial glucose metabolism [2,23]. Their efficacy in protecting ischaemic myocardium is unknown.

Carnitine

An important step in the oxidation of fatty acids is the transport of fatty acids to the mitochondria by the carnitine-mediated shuttle [19]. In addition to transporting fatty acids, carnitine has been shown to increase glucose oxidation [15] by influencing PDH activity. The carnitine analogue propionyl-carnitine has been shown to have similar effects on glucose oxidation. In addition, it may also influence the TCA cycle via anaplerosis [57]. A number of experimental studies have demonstrated protection of ischaemic myocardium by both carnitine and propionyl-carnitine [2,15]. Clinically, carnitine and its congener have been shown to reduce ST segment depression and left ventricular end-diastolic pressure in patients with coronary artery disease [2], as well as to improve exercise capacity and increased ejection fraction in patients with heart failure [2]. In several clinical trials, carnitine treatment early after acute MI was found to attenuate infarct size, decrease left ventricular dilatation, and favourably influence left-ventricular remodelling [2].

β-Adrenergic blockade (β-blockers), angiotensin-converting enzyme inhibitors (ACEI)

Beta-blockers, because of their anti-ischaemic, antiarrhythmic, and antihypertensive effects, have been extremely useful adjunctive agents in the treatment of patients with MI [58]. Clinical trials have demonstrated that β-blockers lower mortality and non-fatal reinfarction [58,59]. While the beneficial properties of β-blockers are at least in part related to decreases in myocardial work, catecholamine environment, and membrane stabilization, some studies have demonstrated that β-blockers reduce plasma fatty acid levels by counteracting β-adrenoreceptor-mediated lipolysis and myocardial fatty acid uptake [24,60–62].

ACE inhibitors have been in use for almost two decades to treat systemic hypertension. They have also been clinically used to reduce morbidity and mortality in patients with congestive heart failure (CHF) and to prevent the progression of CHF in patients with left ventricular dysfunction [58]. The mechanism for the observed beneficial effects of ACE inhibitors is unclear. ACE inhibitors have been shown to exert vasodilation, inhibit the renin–angiotensin–aldosterone system, augment the kinin system, exert an anti-endothelin effect, and inhibit growth of myocardial and vascular tissue [58]. Experimental studies have demonstrated that ACE inhibitors also can stimulate glucose use in ischaemic and reperfused myocardium, thus maintaining energy requirements and enabling the recovery of function in reperfused myocardium [63]. Thus, their beneficial effect may be mediated, in part, by their metabolic effects.

Conclusions

It is clear that favourable modulation of metabolic events during and after ischaemia result in increased myocardial salvage in reperfused myocardium. The use of metabolic adjuncts such as GIK show great potential in enhancing myocardial salvage in patients with MI. The use of GIK is warranted, despite the lack of patent protection and financial incentives. GIK therapy is clearly cost-effective for treatment of patients with acute MI, especially when combined with recanalization. Other metabolic agents show great promise in experimental studies and merit further evaluation in human trials. Metabolic modulation of ischaemic myocardium continues to be a unique and untapped approach to favourably affect ischaemic myocardium.

It is important to restate that only with early, prompt, and full reperfusion is maximum myocardial recovery from acute ischaemic events likely. Metabolic adjuncts can be employed to lessen ischaemic injury and thereby enhance the salutary effects of reperfusion. The coming years are likely to see increasing trials of these agents for maximizing the efficacy of reperfusion therapy in the treatment of coronary artery disease. In addition, the use of metabolic manipulations which enhance glycolytic pathways and inhibit potentially noxious fatty acid intermediates may also offer a novel approach for the protection of transiently ischaemic myocardium in patients with chronic coronary artery disease.

Acknowledgements

Work in authors' laboratories was supported by grants from National Institutes of Health, Heart, Lung, and Blood Institute HL 61783 and HL58408; the Department of Energy, DE-FG02–97ER62433; and from the Jacob and Hilda Blaustein Foundation, JB980049. Dr Ramasamy is an Established Investigator of the American Heart Association.

References

1 Camici P, Ferrannini E., Opie, LH. Myocardial metabolism in ischemic heart disease: basic principles and application to imaging by positron emission tomography. *Prog Cardiovasc Dis* 1989; 32: 217–38.

2 Stanley WC, Lopaschuk GD, Hall JL, McCormack, JG. Regulation of myocardial carbohydrate metabolism under normal and ischemic conditions. Potential for pharmacological interventions. *Cardiovasc Res,* 1997; 33: 243–57.

3 Taegtmeyer H, King LM, Jones BE. Energy substrate metabolism, myocardial ischemia, and targets for pharmacotherapy. [Review]. *Am J Cardiol* 1998; 82: 54K–60K.

4 Sun D, Nguyen N, DeGrado TR, Schwaiger M, Brosius, FC. Ischemia induces translocation of the insulin-responsive glucose transporter GLUT-4 to the plasma membrane of cardiac myocytes. *Circulation* 1994; 89: 793–8.

5 Young LH, Renfu Y, Russell R, Hu X, Caplan M, Ren J, Shulman GI, Sinusas, AJ. Low-flow ischemia leads to translocation of canine heart GLUT-4 and GLUT-1 transporters to the sarcolemma *in vivo*. *Circulation* 1997; 95: 415–22.

6 Charron MJ, Katz, EB. Metabolic and therapeutic lessons from genetic manipulation of GLUT4. *Mol Cell Biochem* 1998; 182: 143–52.

7 Bergmann SR. Positron emission tomography of the heart. In: Gerson MC ed. *Cardiac Nuclear Medicine,* 3rd edn, New York: McGraw-Hill 1997; 267–99.

8 Depre C, Vanoverschelde JL, Taegtmeyer, H. Glucose for the heart. [Review]. *Circulation* 1999; 99: 578–88.

9 Ramasamy R, Trueblood NA, Schaefer S. Metabolic effects of aldose reductase inhibition during low-flow ischemia and reperfusion. *Am J Physiol* 1998; 275: H1195–H1203.

10 Trueblood NA, Ramasamy, R. Aldose reductase inhibition improves the altered glucose metabolism of isolated diabetic rat hearts. *Am J Physiol* 1998; 275: H75–H83.

11 Ramasamy R, Oates PJ, Schaefer S. Aldose reductase inhibition protects diabetic and non-diabetic rat hearts from ischemic injury. *Diabetes* 1997; 46: 292–300.

12 Weiss J, Hiltbrand B. Functional compartmentation of glycolytic versus oxidative metabolism in isolated rabbit heart. *J Clin Invest* 1985; 75: 436–47.

13 Jermey RW, Koretsune Y, Marban E, Becker LC. Relationship between glycolysis and calcium homeostasis in postischemic myocardium. *Circ Res* 1992; 70: 1180–90.

14 Nakamura K, Kusuoka H, Ambrosio G, Becker LC. Glycolysis is necessary to pre-

serve myocardial Ca^{2+} homeostasis during E-adrenergic stimulation. *Am J Physiology—Heart Circulatory Physiology* 1993; 264: H670–H678.

15 Broderick TL, Quinney HA, Barker CC, Lopaschuk GD. Beneficial effect of carnitine on mechanical recovery of rat hearts reperfused after a transient period of global ischemia is accompanied by a stimulation of glucose oxidation. *Circulation* 1993; 87: 972–81.

16 Lerner E, Shug AL, Elson C, Shrago E. Reversible inhibition of adenine nucleotide translocation by long chain fatty acyl coenzyme A esters in liver mitochondria of diabetic and hibernating animals. *J Biol Chemistry* 1972; 247: 1513–19.

17 Molaparast-Saless F, Liedtke AJ, Nellis SH. Effects of the fatty acid blocking agents, oxfenicine and 4-bromocrotonic acid, on performance in aerobic and ischemic myocardium. *J Molec Cell Cardiol* 1987; 19: 509–20.

18 Lopaschuk GD, Wall SR, Olley PM, Davies NJ. Entomoxir, a carnitine palmitoyltransferase I inhibitor, protects hearts from fatty acid induced ischemic injury independent of changes in long chain acylcarnitine. *Circ Res* 1988; 63: 1036–43.

19 Hale DE, Bennett MJ. Fatty acid oxidation disorders: a new class of metabolic diseases. *J Pediatrics* 1992; 121: 1–11.

20 Oliver MF, Kurien VA, Greenwood TW. Relation between serum-free-fatty acids and arrhythmias and death after acute myocardial infarction. *Lancet* 1968; 1: 710–4.

21 Rowe MJ, Neilson JM, Oliver MF. Control of ventricular arrhythmias during myocardial infarction by antilipolytic treatment using a nicotinic-acid analogue. *Lancet* 1975; 1: 295–300.

22 Opie LH, Tansey M, Kennelly BM. Proposed metabolic vicious circle in patients with large myocardial infarcts and high plasma-free-fatty-acid concentrations. *Lancet* 1977; 2: 890–2.

23 Vik-Mo H, Mjos OD, Neely JR, Maroko PR, Ribeiro LG. Limitation of myocardial infarct size by metabolic interventions that reduce accumulation of fatty acid metabolites in ischemic myocardium. *Am Heart J* 1986; 111: 1048–54.

24 Opie LH, Thomas M. Propranolol and experimental myocardial infarction: sub-

strate effects. *Postgrad Med J* 1976; 52 (Suppl. 4): 124–133.

25 Janier MF, Vanoverschelde J-L, Bergmann SR. Adenosine protects ischemic and reperfused myocardium by receptor-mediated mechanisms. *Am J Physiol—Heart Circulatory Physiology* 1993; 264: H163–H170.

26 Vanoverschelde J-LJ, Janier MF, Bakke JE, Marshall DR, Bergmann SR. Rate of glycolysis during ischemia determine extent of ischemic injury and functional recovery after reperfusion. *Am J Physiol* 1994; 267: H1785–H1794.

27 Kingsley PB, Sako EY, Yang MQ, Zimmer SD, Ugurbil K, Foker JE, From AHL. Ischemic contracture begins when anaerobic glycolysis stops: a ^{31}P-NMR study of isolated rat hearts. *Am J Physiol* 1991; 261 (30): H469–H478.

28 McVeigh JJ, Lopaschuk GD. Dichloroacetate stimulation of glucose oxidation improves recovery of ischemic rat hearts. *Am J Physiol* 1990; 259: H1079–H1085.

29 Janier MF, Vanoverschelde J-LJ, Bergmann SR. Ischemic preconditioning stimulates anaerobic glycolysis in the isolated rabbit heart. *Am J Physiol* 1994; 267: H1353–H1360.

30 McCormack JG, Barr RL, Wolff AA, Lopaschuk GD. Ranolazine stimulates glucose oxidation in normoxic, ischemic, and reperfused ischemic rat hearts. *Circulation* 1996; 93: 135–42.

31 King X, Opie X. Glucose and glycogen utilization in myocardial ischaemia—changes in metabolism and consequences for the myocyte. *Mol Cell Biochem* 1998; 180: 3–26.

32 Finegan BA, Clanachan AS, Coulson CS, Lopaschuk GD. Adenosine modification of energy substrate use in isolated hearts perfused with fatty acids. *Am J Physiol* 1992; 262: H1501–H1507.

33 Henes CG, Bergmann SR, Perez JE, Sobel BE, Geltman EM. The time course of restoration of nutritive perfusion, myocardial oxygen consumption, and regional function after coronary thrombolysis. *Coronary Artery Dis* 1990; 1: 687–96.

34 Gropler RJ, Geltman EM, Sampathkumaran K, Perez JE, Moerlein SM, Sobel BE, Bergmann SR, Siegel BA. Functional recovery after coronary revascularization for chronic coronary artery disease is dependent on maintenance of oxidative

metabolism. *J Am Coll Cardiol* 1992; 20: 569–77.

35 Weinheimer CJ, Brown MA, Nohara R, Perez JE, Bergmann SR. Functional recovery after reperfusion is predicated on recovery of myocardial oxidative metabolism. *Am Heart J* 1993; 125: 939–49.

36 Conversano A, Walsh JF, Geltman EM, Perez JE, Bergmann SR, Gropler RJ. Delineation of myocardial stunning and hibernation by positron emission tomography in advanced coronary artery disease. *Am Heart J* 1996; 131: 440–50.

37 Bergmann SR, Lerch RA, Fox KA, Ludbrook PA, Welch MJ, Ter-Pogossian MM, Sobel BE. Temporal dependence of beneficial effects of coronary thrombolysis characterized by positron tomography. *Am J Med* 1982; 73: 573–81.

38 Bergmann SR, Fox KA, Ter-Pogossian MM, Sobel BE, Collen D. Clot-selective coronary thrombolysis with tissue-type plasminogen activator. *Science* 1983; 220: 1181–3.

39 Bergmann SS, Fox KAA, Ludbrook PA. Determinants of salvage of jeopardised myocardium after coronary thrombolysis. *Cardiol Clinics* 1987; 5: 67–77.

40 Zweier JL, Flaherty JT, Weisfeldt ML. Direct measurement of free radical generation following reperfusion of ischemic myocardium. *Proc Natl Acad Sci USA* 1987; 84: 1404–7.

41 Bolli R, Jeroudi MO, Patel BS, DuBose CM, Lai EK, Roberts R, McCay PB. Direct evidence that oxygen-derived free radicals contribute to postischemic myocardial dysfunction in the intact dog. *Proc Natl Acad Sci USA* 1989; 86: 4695–9.

42 Ambrosio G, Tritto I. Reperfusion injury: experimental evidence and clinical implications. [Review]. *Am Heart J* 1999; 138: 69–75.

43 Flaherty JT, Pitt B, Gruber JW, Heuser RR, Rothbaum DA, Burwell LR, George BS, Kereiakes DJ, Deitchman D. Gustafson N. Recombinant human superoxide dismutase (h-SOD) fails to improve recovery of ventricular function in patients undergoing coronary angioplasty for acute myocardial infarction. *Circulation* 1994; 89: 1982–91.

44 Simpson PJ, Fantone JC, Mickelson JK,

Gallagher KP, Lucchesi BR. Identification of a time window for therapy to reduce experimental canine myocardial injury: suppression of neutrophil activation during 72 hours of reperfusion. *Circulation Res* 1988; 63: 1070–9.

45 Whitlow PL, Rogers WJ, Smith LR, McDaniel HG, Papapietro SE, Mantle JA, Logic JR, Russell ROJ, Rackley CE. Enhancement of left ventricular function by glucose-insulin-potassium infusion in acute myocardial infarction. *Am J Cardiol* 982; 49: 811–20.

46 Rogers WJ, Stanley AWJ, Breinig JB, Prather JW, McDaniel HG, Moraski RE, Mantle JA, Russell ROJ, Rackley CE. Reduction of hospital mortality rate of acute myocardial infarction with glucose-insulin-potassium infusion. *Am Heart J* 1976; 92: 441–54.

47 Satler LF, Green CE, Kent KM, Pallas RS, Pearle DL, Rackley CE. Metabolic support during coronary reperfusion. *Am Heart J* 1987; 114: 54–8.

48 Malmberg K, Ryden L, Efendic S, Herlitz J, Nicol P, Waldenstrom A, Wedel H, Welin L. Randomized trial of insulin-glucose infusion followed by subcutaneous insulin treatment in diabetic patients with acute myocardial infarction (DIGAMI study): effects on mortality at 1 year [see comments]. *J Am College Cardiol* 1995; 26: 57–65.

49 Diaz R, Paolasso EA, Piegas LS, Tajer CD, Moreno MG, Corvalan R, Isea JE, Romero G. Metabolic modulation of acute myocardial infarction. The ECLA (Estudios Cardiologicos Latino America) collaborative group. *Circulation* 1998; 98: 2227–34.

50 Fath-Ordoubadi F, Beatt KJ. Glucose-insulin-potassium therapy for treatment of acute myocardial infarction: an overview of randomized placebo-controlled trials. *Circulation* 1997; 96: 1152–6.

51 Gradinac S, Coleman GM, Taegtmeyer H, Sweeney MS, Frazier OH. Improved cardiac function with glucose–insulin–potassium after aortocoronary bypass grafting [see comments]. *Ann Thoracic Surgery* 1989; 48: 484–9.

52 Wargovich TJ, Macdonald RG, Hill JA, Feldman RL, Stacpoole PW, Pepine CJ. Myocardial metabolic and hemodynamic effects of dichloroacetate in coronary

artery disease. *Am J Cardiol* 1988; 61: 65–70.

53 Stacpoole PW. The pharmacology of dichloroacetate. [Review]. *Metabolism: Clin Exp* 1989; 38: 1124–44.

54 Allely MC, Alps BJ. Prevention of myocardial enzyme release by ranolazine in a primate model of ischaemia with reperfusion. *Br J Pharmacol* 1990; 99: 5–6.

55 Cocco G, Rousseau MF, Bouvy T, Cheron P, Williams G, Detry JM, Pouleur H. Effects of a new metabolic modulator, ranolazine, on exercise tolerance in angina pectoris patients treated with beta-blocker or diltiazem. *J Cardiovasc Pharmacol* 1992; 20: 131–8.

56 Thadani U, Ezekowitz M, Fenney L, Chiang YK. Double-blind efficacy and safety study of a novel anti-ischemic agent, ranolazine, versus placebo in patients with chronic stable angina pectoris. Ranolazine Study Group. *Circulation* 1994; 90: 726–34.

57 Schonekess BO, Allard MF, Lopaschuk GD. Propionyl L-carnitine improvement of hypertrophied heart function is accompanied by an increase in carbohydrate oxidation. *Circulation Res* 1995; 77: 726–34.

58 Frishman WH, Cheng A. Secondary pre-

vention of myocardial infarction: role of beta-adrenergic blockers and angiotensin-converting enzyme inhibitors. [Review]. *Am Heart J* 1999; 137: S25–S34.

59 Boissel JP, Leizorovicz A, Picolet H, Ducruet T. Efficacy of acebutolol after acute myocardial infarction (the APSI trial). The APSI Investigators. *Am J Cardiol* 1990; 66: 24C–31C.

60 Marchetti G, Merlo L, Noseda V. Myocardial uptake of free fatty acids and carbohydrates after beta-adrenergic blockade. *Am J Cardiol* 1968; 22: 370–4.

61 Glaviano VV, Masters TN. The effect of intracoronary norepinephrine on cardiac metabolism before and after beta adrenergic blockade. *Feder Proc* 1967; 26: 771–9.

62 Westera G, van der Wall EE, van Eenige MJ, Scholtalbers S, Visser FC, Roos JP. Metabolic consequences of beta-adrenergic receptor blockade for the acutely ischemic dog myocardium. *Nuklearmedizin* 1984; 23: 35–40.

63 Rett K, Wicklmayr M, Dietze GJ, Haring HU. Insulin-induced glucose transporter (GLUT1 and GLUT4) translocation in cardiac muscle tissue is mimicked by bradykinin. *Diabetes* 1996; 45 (Suppl. 1): S66–S69.

17: Catheter-based interventions for treatment of acute coronary syndromes

Philippe L. L'Allier, Stephen G. Ellis and Eric J. Topol

Introduction

The approach to the treatment of acute myocardial infarction changed markedly after it was demonstrated, in mega-trials of reperfusion with fibrinolytic agents, that there is a powerful relationship between time to restoration of complete infarct vessel patency [1–4] and a reduction in mortality [5,6–9]. Fibrinolytic therapy has limited efficacy (35–55%) with regard to restoration of patency (TIMI Grade 3 flow) at 90 min. A high reinfarction rate, as well as intracranial haemorrhage in nearly 1 in 100 patients treated, also limit this approach. Randomized trials have compared primary angioplasty (percutaneous transluminal coronary angioplasty, PTCA) with fibrinolytic therapy in the hope of improving patency rates in the infarct-related vessel, stabilizing the culprit lesion, and lowering the risk of intracranial haemorrhage. More than 2500 patients have been randomized in these trials and there are ample data to support the use of primary angioplasty as a viable alternative to fibrinolysis, and its potential superiority in certain patient subgroups. This chapter will review the available data and discuss the areas of uncertainty and controversy surrounding this topic. Although less extensively evaluated, data on PTCA and stents in acute coronary syndromes without ST segment elevation (unstable angina (UA) and non-Q-wave myocardial infarction (NQMI)) will also be reviewed.

Randomized trials of primary PTCA vs. fibrinolytic drug therapy

Ten major prospective randomized trials compared primary PTCA to an accepted thrombolytic regimen [10–19] (Table 17.1). Patient populations mostly differed with respect to duration of symptoms (6 vs. 12 h) and prespecified infarct location (anterior, inferior, or not specified). The fibrinolytic regimens used in these trials were also significantly different and included intravenous streptokinase 1.2 or 1.5 million U over 1 h, tissue plasminogen activator (t-PA) over 3 h, and front-loaded t-PA over 1.5 h. It is unclear whether differences in the efficacy of the different fibrinolytic agents and regimens have a significant

Table 17.1 Mortality at the end of the study period in trials comparing primary angioplasty (PTCA) with fibrinolytic regimen.

Study	No. (%)		Odds ratio (95% CI)	P
	PTCA	Lytic therapy		
Streptokinase				
Zijlstra et al. [10]	3/152 (2.0)	11/149 (7.4)		
Ribeiro et al. [11]	3/50 (6.0)	1/50 (2.0)		
Grinfeld et al. [12]	5/54 (9.3)	6/58 (10.3)		
Zijlstra et al. [13]	1/45 (2.2)	0/50		
Subtotal	12/301 (4.0)	18/307 (5.9)		0.38
t-PA				
DeWood [14]	3/46 (6.5)	2/44 (4.5)		
Grines et al. [15]	5/195 (2.6)	13/200 (6.5)		
Gibbons et al. [16]	2/47 (4.3)	2/56 (3.6)		
Subtotal	10/288 (3.5)	17/300 (5.7)		0.28
Accelerated t-PA				
Ribichini et al. [17]	0/41	1/42 (2.4)		
Garcia et al. [18]	3/95 (3.2)	10/94 (10.6)		
GUSTO IIb [19]	32/565 (5.7)	40/573 (7.0)		
Subtotal	35/701 (5.0)	51/709 (7.2)		0.10
Total	57/1290 (4.4)	86/1316 (6.5)		0.02

Forest plot axis: 0.0 0.5 1.0 1.5 2.0; PTCA better — Lytic Better

Test for homogeneity: streptokinase trials, $P = 0.08$; t-PA, $P = 0.33$; accelerated t-PA trials, $P = 0.21$; fibrinolytic regimen, $P = 0.96$, and overall, $P = 0.24$. Percentages are pooled results and odds ratios calculated by exact method using all trials. (From Weaver et al. *JAMA* 1997; 278: 2093–8 [20]; copyrighted 1997 American Medical Association.)

impact on overall results. There is, however, a known gradient effect with regard to death and re-MI, with an absolute risk reduction of 7.4% for streptokinase, 4.8% for conventional t-PA, and 3.3% for accelerated t-PA (Table 17.2) [20]. There were also differences in heparin dosage (0–10 000 U initial bolus, and 2–5 days' infusion), and follow-up periods (hospital discharge vs. 30 days). Although approximately 10% of patients randomized to invasive strategies were unsuitable for PTCA, procedural success was high, achieving TIMI Perfusion Grade 3 in 73–93% [15,19,21]. Furthermore, primary angioplasty may have a wider patient applicability (65% vs. 10% of patients screened were excluded from studies evaluating thrombolytic therapy and primary angioplasty, respectively).

Global Utilization of Streptokinase and Tissue Plasminogen Activator for Occluded Coronary Arteries (GUSTO)-IIb [19], the largest of these trials ($n = 1138$), deserves particular attention because the results are thought to be more representative of most clinical settings (best thrombolytic strategy, 57 centres

Table 17.2 Primary PTCA versus thrombolysis: potential size of benefit based on estimated treatment effects.

Study group	Rate (%)		Odds ratio (95% CI)	Absolute risk reduction, % (95% CI)	Number needed to treat
	PTCA	Lytic therapy			
Mortality					
Streptokinase	4.0	5.9	0.66 (0.29–1.50)	1.9 (–2.7–4.1)	52 (24–)
3- to 4-h t-PA	3.5	5.7	0.60 (0.24–1.41)	2.2 (–2.2–4.3)	45 (23–)
Accelerated t-PA	5.0	7.2	0.68 (0.42–1.08)	2.2 (–0.5–4.0)	46 (25–)
Total	4.4	6.5	0.66 (0.46–0.94)	2.1 (0.4 3.4)	47 (29–250)
Death plus non-fatal reinfarction					
Streptokinase	5.6	13.0	0.40 (0.21–0.75)	7.4 (2.9–10.0)	14 (10–34)
3- to 4-h t-PA	5.6	10.3	0.51 (0.26–0.99)	4.8 (0.1–7.4)	21 (14–1000)
Accelerated t-PA	8.7	12.0	0.70 (0.48–1.08)	3.3 (0.0–5.9)	30 (17–)
Total	7.2	11.9	0.58 (0.44–0.76)	4.6 (2.6–6.3)	22 (16–38)
Non-fatal reinfarction					
Total	2.9	5.3	0.53 (0.34–0.80)	2.4 (1.0–3.4)	41 (29–100)

(From Weaver *et al. JAMA* 1997; 278: 2093–8 [20]; copyrighted 1997 American Medical Association.)

in 9 countries, and endpoints rigorously adjudicated by a central committee). The principal end-point of the study was the composite outcome of death, non-fatal reinfarction, or non-fatal disabling stroke at 30 days (Fig. 17.1a). Patients were randomized in a 2 × 2 factorial design (primary PTCA vs. t-PA and heparin vs. hirudin for 1012 patients). Of the 565 patients randomized to the interventional strategy, 94% had angiography and 82% had PTCA (5% received stents); 17% required coronary artery bypass graft (CABG) on the same day. TIMI Grade 3 flow was obtained in 73% of patients. The average time from randomization to treatment for the PTCA group was 114 min. The aggregate outcome occurred significantly less frequently in the PTCA group (9.6 vs. 13.7, $P = 0.033$). The mortality rates in the PTCA and t-PA groups were 5.7 and 7.0%, respectively ($P = 0.37$) (Fig. 17.1b). Overall, there was a modest relative benefit at 30 days with PTCA with respect to all elements of the primary study end point. However, at 6 months, the gap favouring PTCA significantly narrowed, with the incidence of the composite adverse outcome being 13.3% in the PTCA group and 15.7% in the t-PA group ($P = NS$).

Despite marked intertrial heterogeneity, a *meta-analysis* ($n = 2606$) of 10 trials, published by Weaver *et al.* [20], showed that mortality at 30 days or less was 4.4% in the PTCA group and 6.5% in the thrombolysis group (34% reduction, OR 0.66, 95% CI 0.46–0.94; $P = 0.02$). The rates of death or non-fatal reinfarction were 7.2% for PTCA and 11.9% for thrombolysis (OR

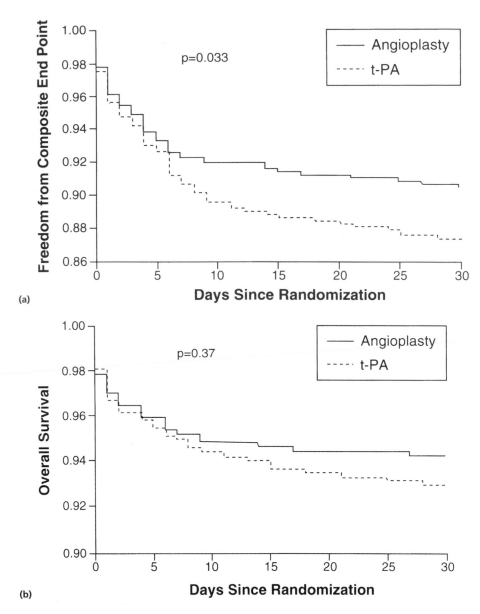

Fig. 17.1 (a) Kaplan–Meier curves for freedom from the composite end-point of death, reinfarction, or disabling stroke; (b) Kaplan–Meier curves for survival. (From the GUSTO IIb Angioplasty Substudy Investigators [19], *N Engl J Med* 1997; 336: 1621–8; copyright © 1997 Massachusetts Medical Society, all rights reserved.)

0.58, 95% CI 0.44–0.76; $P < 0.001$). PTCA was associated with a significantly lower incidence of stroke (0.7% vs. 2.0%, $P = 0.007$). It was concluded, based on outcomes at 30 days or hospital discharge, that primary angioplasty appears to be superior to thrombolytic therapy for treatment of patients with acute myocardial infarction and that data evaluating longer-term outcomes, operator experience, and time delay before treatment are needed before primary PTCA can be universally recommended (where available) as the preferred treatment. It should be noted that the average time to treatment for the PTCA group was 90 min, which is an unachievable goal in many facilities as seen in two large non-randomized studies that showed no benefit of primary angioplasty over fibrinolytic drug therapy [22,23].

The potential mechanisms of benefit are related to greater myocardial salvage initially and/or to better long-term patency of the infarct-related artery. Early reocclusion after fibrinolysis occurs in 5–10% of patients [24], and late reocclusion in 30–40% [25]. The reported results for direct PTCA compare favourably, with up to 90–95% short-term and 87–91% long-term patency [10,21]. The restenosis rate is similar or slightly greater than the rate associated with elective PTCA (30–50% restenosis by angiography, leading to 20% target vessel revascularization (TVR)). The benefit seems to be greater in the sicker subgroup of patients (Killip Class 3, patients ineligible for thrombolysis, patients with previous CABG, and patients with previous contra-lateral infarct, among others). The biggest shortcoming of this treatment is the requirement for a fully equipped and staffed catheterization laboratory that can be activated rapidly and consistently. Moreover, long-term follow-up (6 months) in GUSTO IIb does not suggest a mortality reduction for PTCA as compared with fibrinolytic drug therapy [19].

Recent reports from a French registry of patients ($n = 721$) treated with primary angioplasty or fibrinolysis, indicated no survival benefit for mechanical reperfusion at 1 year (85.5% vs. 89.5%, respectively, $P = 0.18$) (Fig. 17.2). In fact, for patients alive after 5 days, the use of primary PTCA, was found (by multivariate analysis) to be one of the adverse prognostic indicators [26]. However, Grines et al. presented in March 1999 (ESC, Barcelona, Spain) the results of a pooled analysis from 10 randomized trials and showed lower death or re-MI at 6 months (odds ratio 0.55, 95% CI 0.43–0.70).

In summary, although some findings favour primary PTCA over fibrinolytic drug therapy, recent registries suggest the advantage of balloon-mediated reperfusion is at best modest with regard to mortality. This highlights the need for more definitive catheter-based reperfusion.

Stenting vs. balloon angioplasty in acute myocardial infarction

Despite improvements in operator technique and peri-procedural care, primary angioplasty results in recurrent ischaemia before hospital discharge in approximately 4–5% of patient treated with primary PTCA, and this includes approximately 2.8% reinfarction [20,23,26]. Furthermore, the TVR rate during 6-month follow-up remains approximately 20%. Improvements in post-

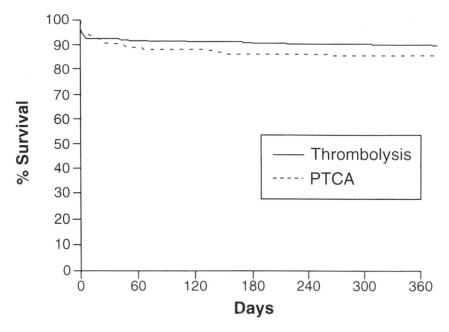

Fig. 17.2 One-year survival in patients treated with intravenous thrombolysis or primary coronary angioplasty. (From Danchin *et al. Circulation* 1999; 99: 2639–44.)

procedural protection against subacute thrombosis paved the way for the use of stents in the setting of acute MI [27]. Results of nine randomized trials comparing coronary stenting with balloon angioplasty in this setting have been presented [28–37].

We performed a meta-analysis of these randomized trials (available data) and found that stenting has a favourable impact on the overall outcome, mainly through a reduction in reinfarction (0.9% vs. 2.5%, $P = 0.002$) (Fig. 17.3) and repeat revascularization (late TVR: 8.6% vs. 17.8%, $P < 0.001$) (Fig. 17.4). None of the individual trials showed a significant difference in mortality at hospital discharge/30 days (meta-analysis, $n = 2484$, also did not reveal a significant difference either: 2.1% vs. 1.7%, $P =$ ns). Furthermore, the effects on mortality at 6–12 months follow-up were quite inconsistent, with some trials demonstrating a small excess with stenting (Figs 17.5 and 17.6). Of note, TIMI-3 flow rates were not improved with stenting, despite better minimal luminal area, suggesting more embolization and distal microvascular obstruction. It is somewhat ironic that stenting in acute myocardial infarction, once thought to be absolutely contraindicated because of the thrombotic nature of the disease, is one of the major advances in catheter-based reperfusion in recent years. Thus, stenting has emerged as the technique of choice for catheter-

RCT: Hosp/30 day RE-MI

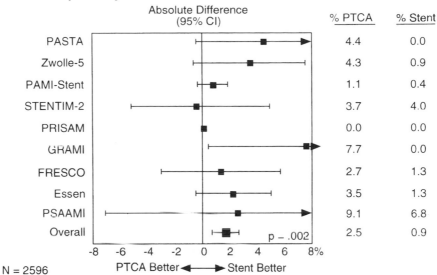

Fig. 17.3 Stenting in acute myocardial infarction: Hospital/30-day reinfarction (absolute difference, including 95% confidence interval). PASTA [28], Zwolle 5 [29], PAMI Stent [30], STENTIM-2 [31], PRISAM [32,33], GRAMI [34], FRESCO [35], Essen [36], PSAAMI [37].

based reperfusion in suitable target lesions, although it remains unclear whether small vessels, long lesions, and other subgroups derive the same benefits. Improvements in adjunctive pharmacotherapy should further amplify the benefits associated with stenting [38,39].

Adjunctive pharmacotherapy for primary coronary interventions

Platelet glycoprotein IIb/IIIa inhibitors

Platelet glycoprotein IIb/IIIa inhibitors have enhanced results of percutaneous coronary interventions, mainly by lowering the peri-procedural ischaemic complications and, to a lesser extent, the need for repeat revascularization. These results have been reproduced in all patients subsets from major trials. The use of these agents in acute myocardial infarction was prompted by a subgroup analysis of the EPIC [39a] trials in which 66 patients with acute MI (primary or rescue PTCA) had an impressive reduction in the combined end-point of death, MI or TVR. The RAPPORT trial (n = 483) [40], a randomized control trial of abciximab vs. placebo with primary PTCA, was conducted to

RCT: Late TVR

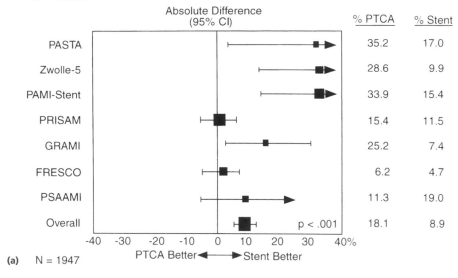

	% PTCA	% Stent
PASTA	35.2	17.0
Zwolle-5	28.6	9.9
PAMI-Stent	33.9	15.4
PRISAM	15.4	11.5
GRAMI	25.2	7.4
FRESCO	6.2	4.7
PSAAMI	11.3	19.0
Overall	18.1	8.9

(a)   N = 1947

Restenosis

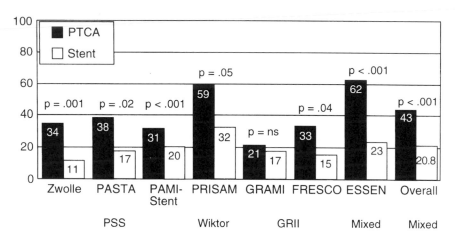

(b) N = 1703

Fig. 17.4 Stenting in acute myocardial infarction: (a) late target vessel revascularization and (b) restenosis (absolute difference, including 95% confidence interval). PSS, Palmaz-Schatz Stent; GR II, Gianturco Rubin stent. (For details of studies see also Fig. 17.3.)

RCT: Hosp/30 day Mortality

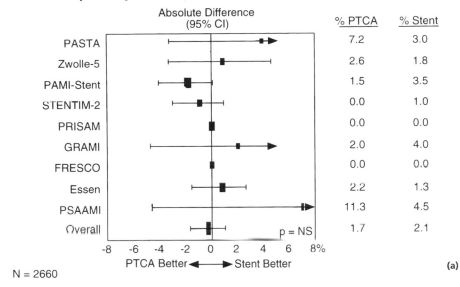

N = 2660

(a)

RCT: 6-12 Month Mortality

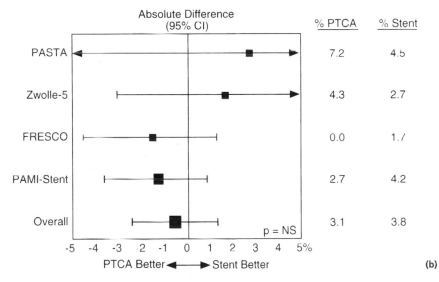

(b)

Fig. 17.5 Stenting in acute myocardial infarction: (a) hospital/30-day mortality and (b) 6–12 months mortality (absolute difference, including 95% confidence interval).

RCT: Hosp/30 day Death, MI, TVR

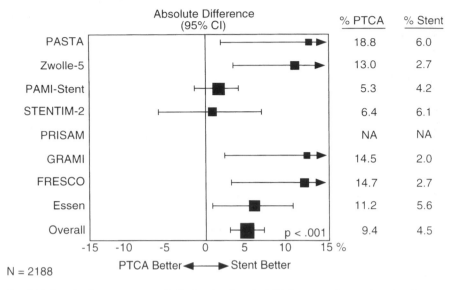

Fig. 17.6 Stenting in acute myocardial infarction: hospital/30-day mortality combined end-point of death, myocardial infarction, or target vessel revascularization (absolute difference, including 95% confidence interval).

evaluate the composite outcome of death/MI/TVR at 6 months. This end-point was not statistically different, mainly because of the expected absence of benefit on restenosis at 6 months (late TVR). However, there was a marked reduction in recurrent ischaemic events at 30 days for balloon angioplasty (death, re-MI, or urgent TVR: 5.8% vs. 11.2%, $P = 0.038$) (Fig. 17.7).

Neumann *et al.* [39] further defined the benefits of abciximab adjunctive therapy in combination with stenting for acute MI. Patients ($n = 200$) were randomized to receive either standard-dose heparin ($n = 98$) or abciximab plus low-dose heparin ($n = 102$). The primary endpoints in the study were the differences in papavirine-induced coronary flow velocity and in wall-motion index between the initial and 14-day follow-up studies. The results showed that the improvements in peak flow velocity and wall-motion index were significantly better in patients assigned to abciximab compared with those assigned to standard heparin (18.1 cm/s vs. 10.4 cm/s, $P = 0.024$; and 0.44 SD/chord vs. 0.15 SD/chord, $P = 0.007$) (Fig. 17.8). Furthermore, there was a significant correlation between the recovery of peak flow velocity and the improvement of wall-motion index. The larger increase in peak velocity with abciximab was attributed to relief of microvascular obstruction, presumably through active disaggregation of platelet-thrombus ('platelet-lysis').

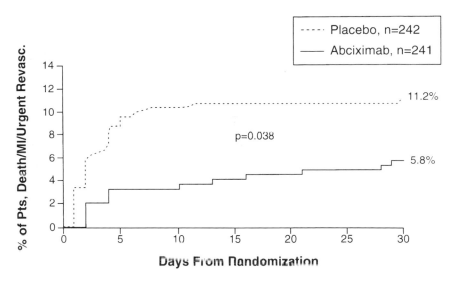

Fig.17.7 Kaplan–Meier curves for death, repeat myocardial infarction, or urgent target vessel revascularization within 30 days in abciximab and placebo group by intention-to-treat analysis. (From Brener *et al. Circulation* 1998; 98: 734–41.)

The strategy of platelet GP IIb/IIIa inhibition in combination with primary angioplasty plus stent implantation was further tested in the ADMIRAL trial [38]. Patients were randomized to either abciximab ($n = 150$) or placebo ($n = 150$) which were administered before the procedure. The primary clinical end-point of the study was the composite of death/re-MI/or urgent TVR at 30 days. The TIMI-3 flow rates were higher before PTCA and stenting (21% vs. 10%, $P < 0.01$) and at 24 h (86% vs. 78%, $P < 0.05$) in the patients assigned to abciximab. Left ventricular ejection fraction was significantly better in patients assigned to abciximab at 24 h (55% vs. 51%) and at 30 days (63% vs. 55%). With regard to the primary end-point of the study (death, MI, or urgent TVR at 30 days), abciximab was associated with a significant risk reduction of 46.5% (10.7% vs. 20.0%, $P < 0.03$). This reduction was consistent in all individual endpoints [1]: death (3.3% vs. 4.7%, $P = 0.35$) [2], re-MI (2.0% vs. 4.7%, $P = 0.09$), and urgent TVR (6.0% vs. 14.0%, $P = 0.03$) (Fig. 17.9). Furthermore, there was no significant difference in major bleeding at 30 days (abciximab 4.0% vs. placebo 2.6%, $P = 0.50$).

With these results, it can be concluded that there is now strong evidence in favour of using the combination of platelet GP IIb/IIIa inhibition with abciximab and stenting whenever possible in patients undergoing primary percutaneous interventions for acute myocardial infarction. As previously discussed, relief of microvascular obstruction in this setting is a newly recognized mechanism of action of abciximab. Mortality reduction may be anticipated in the

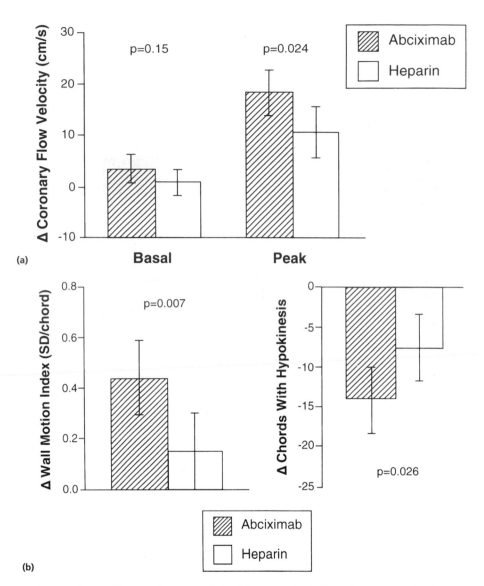

Fig. 17.8 Plot of differences between 14-day follow-up and initial postinterventional studies in (a) basal flow velocity and in papavirine-induced peak flow velocity at treated lesion and in (b) wall-motion index and number of chords within infarct region. Error bars indicate 95% confidence interval. Error bars not including zero indicate that change between initial study and follow-up is statistically significant at 0.05 level. *P*-values above columns refer to differences between two treatment groups. (From Neumann *et al. Circulation* 1998; 98: 2695–701 [39], with permission.)

light of the 1-year findings of the EPISTENT trial. Although this trial was conducted with elective patients undergoing percutaneous revascularization, the combination of abciximab and stents led to a 57% reduction compared with the stent–placebo or balloon–abciximab strategies.

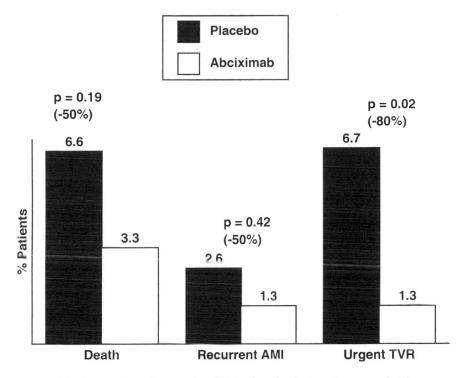

Fig. 17.9 The ADMIRAL trial: comparing abciximab to placebo in patients treated with primary angioplasty and stenting for acute MI, there was a reduction with abciximab in death, recurrent acute myocardial infarction, and urgent target vessel revascularization. (From Montalescot *et al.* [38], with permission.)

Direct thrombin inhibitors

The direct thrombin inhibitor hirudin, was compared with heparin in the GUSTO IIb trial [41], as mentioned above. No difference in clinical outcomes was found (composite of death, non-fatal MI, or re-MI at 30 days was 8.9% vs. 9.8%, *P* = ns). However, direct thrombin inhibitors (hirulog and hirudin) have been shown to improve early outcomes when compared with high-dose heparin in patients treated with PTCA for unstable angina. The concept of combining direct thrombin inhibitors and platelet GP IIb/IIIa inhibitors has theoretical merit and needs to be investigated.

Heparin

The dosage of heparin for primary angioplasty has not been studied adequately and is still somewhat controversial. High doses of heparin (300 U/kg, mean dose 27 000 U) were tested in a randomized trial [42] and failed to show a benefit over standard heparin dosage. None of the lower dose heparin regimens tested in elective procedures has been tested in the setting of primary PTCA for acute myocardial infarction. However, when abciximab is used, a weight adjusted heparin dose (50–70 U/kg) is recommended to achieve an activated clotting time (ACT) of 225–275 s since there is a significant increase in bleeding complications when the ACT is greater than 325 s. Indeed, when this dosage was not used, as was the case in the RAPPORT trial, excess bleeding complications were noted.

Challenging subpopulations of patients

Cardiogenic shock

Historically, cardiogenic shock has been associated with high mortality rate (70–90%). Recent hope that aggressive revascularization in this setting improves outcomes has risen based on results from non-randomized series in which the reported mortality was 26–72% (mean 44%). One of the first randomized trials to address the question of whether early revascularization could reduce mortality was the SHOCK trial (Should We Revascularize Emergently Occluded Coronary Arteries for Cardiogenic Shock, $n = 302$) [43]. Patients who developed cardiogenic shock within 36 h of acute MI, were randomized (within 12 h) to emergency revascularization vs. initial medical stabilization. Patients in both groups underwent intra-aortic counterpulsation (IABP) and were supported pharmacologically. Major exclusion criteria included acute mechanical shock, shock due to cardiac aetiologies other than acute MI, and the presence of other severe systemic illnesses. The primary endpoint of the study was 30-day all-cause mortality. Baseline, clinical, and haemodynamic characteristics were similar in both groups. Of the 152 patients randomized in the early revascularization strategy, 87% had a revascularization procedure (48% PTCA and 38% CABG). At 30 days, the primary end-point was reached in 46% of the early revascularization group and 56% of the initial medical stabilization group, for a 9.3% absolute risk reduction and a 17% relative risk reduction ($P = 0.11$). This difference became statistically significant at 60 days (54% vs. 68%, $P = 0.04$), largely related to benefit in the younger patient subgroup (age < 75 years).

The other randomized trial (S)MASH [44] was conducted in Europe and also failed to show any statistically significant benefit of percutaneous revascularization in this context (mortality at 30 days: 69% invasive group vs. 78% medical group, P = ns). However, this trial was not adequately powered ($n = 55$) because of the small number of patients and premature termination.

Although the results of these two randomized trials were less definitive than expected, the data support the practice of adopting an aggressive approach in this population, including IABP and revascularization procedures, especially if there is potentially salvageable viable myocardium at risk in younger patients.

'Rescue angioplasty' for failed fibrinolytic therapy

One of the difficulties encountered when considering a mechanical intervention (rescue angioplasty) following fibrinolysis, is adequate assessment of failure of the initial therapy. In this regard, complete resolution of chest pain is associated with 80% TIMI 2–3 flow at 90 min in the infarct-related artery (IRA) [45] and >50% resolution of maximal ST segment elevation at 60 min predicts patency of the IRA with 96% sensitivity and 94% specificity [46]. There is, however, significant interpatient variability and practical clinical reperfusion criteria remain elusive [47].

The strategy of performing 'rescue PTCA' of the IRA is certainly feasible, and procedural success rates of >90% have been reported [45,48–51]. Four small, important trials represent the bulk of the randomized data on rescue angioplasty [52–55]. A study performed by Belenkie et al. [52] ($n = 28$) revealed a trend towards reduced mortality (6% vs. 30%, P = ns). The second trial, performed by Ellis et al. (RESCUE trial, $n = 150$) [53], randomly assigned patients with an occluded left anterior descending artery to rescue angioplasty or conservative management. The mortality was reduced from 9.9% to 5.2% (P = ns) and the composite of death or heart failure was diminished from 16.4% to 6.5% ($P = 0.05$). In a study from Maastricht [54], 224 patients presenting at a community hospital with acute MI were randomized to either on-site fibrinolysis with alteplase ($n = 75$), immediate transport to a primary PTCA facility ($n = 75$), or both (fibrinolysis with rescue angioplasty as needed, $n = 74$). Mortality was similar in the three groups (7% vs. 9% vs. 9%, respectively). The main difference between the groups was re-MI (12% vs. 5% vs. 4%, respectively). In the PRAGUE trial [55], the occurrence of the combined endpoint of death, re-MI, urgent revascularization, or heart failure (Killip class III or IV) was less frequent in the primary and rescue angioplasty groups (16% and 20%, respectively) compared with fibrinolytic therapy with streptokinase (45%, $P < 0.05$ vs. primary angioplasty). Mainly lower re-MI, urgent revascularization, and heart failure rates drove this difference.

Recently, results of abciximab administration during early rescue angioplasty in patients enrolled in GUSTO III were presented by Miller et al. [56]. They evaluated patients who had PTCA of the IRA (24 h after receiving fibrinolytic therapy (median 3.5 h). Patients who received abciximab ($n = 81$) were compared with those who did not ($n = 306$). The adjusted 30-day mortality was reduced by administration of abciximab (3.7% vs. 9.8%, $P = 0.04$). There was an associated modest increase in severe bleeding with abciximab (3.7% vs. 1.0%, $P = 0.08$). This involved full-dose fibrinolytic therapy which, combined with heparin and GP IIb/IIIb inhibition, may be fraught with too high a risk of bleeding complications. Furthermore, as discussed subsequently, the combination of low-dose lytic drug therapy plus a GP IIb/IIIa inhibitor offers promising theoretical advantages when compared with full-dose lytic drugs, leading to new hopes for improving outcomes. The benefits associated with stenting in the primary angioplasty setting are expected in rescue angioplasty, and liberal use of stents (when feasible and indicated) is therefore recommended. Accordingly, rescue angioplasty should be considered to be a viable option following treatment with fibrinolytic drug, particularly in high-risk patients (those with heart failure, extensive infarction, previous MI, or a low baseline left ventricular ejection fraction, among others).

Elderly patients

Mortality after acute MI is higher in older patients [57]. Such patients are also at increased risk of intracranial bleeding following the use of fibrinolytic drugs. Therefore, they may derive a greater benefit from primary PTCA. However, results of a subgroup analysis from the largest randomized trial of primary PTCA vs. fibrinolysis (GUSTO IIb) did not reveal any particular incremental benefits of primary PTCA over fibrinolysis [58]. By contrast, the large NRMI-II experience [23,59] and a recent pooled analysis of three randomized trials comparing primary PTCA and fibrinolytic therapy [60] suggested a greater benefit of primary angioplasty over fibrinolytic therapy in patients with advanced age. These results were confirmed in a small single-centre randomized trial comparing primary PTCA and fibrinolytic therapy in elderly patients with acute MI [61]. Patients were randomized to either streptokinase (1.5 million U, $n = 37$) or to primary PTCA ($n = 41$). The primary endpoints of the trial were death and the combined clinical end-point of death, re-MI, or stroke. Baseline characteristics in the two groups were not significantly different. Although the difference in mortality was not statistically different (19% vs. 5%, $P = 0.07$), there was a trend towards a better survival with primary PTCA. The incidence of the predefined combined end-point of death, re-MI, or stroke was significantly lower in the primary PTCA group (27% vs. 5%, $P = 0.01$). Therefore, results of retrospective analyses are somewhat conflicting, but those from the only, albeit small, randomized trial favour primary PTCA in elderly patients with acute MI. Although the optimal requires further elucidation, catheter-based reperfusion is at least as good and, in some cases, superior to fibrinolytic therapy for elderly patients.

Limitations of current catheter-based reperfusion strategies

The first major limitation of primary PTCA for acute MI is the need for

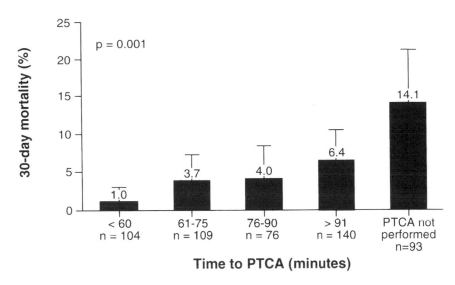

Fig. 17.10 Relationship between 30-day mortality and time from study enrolment to first balloon inflation. Patients assigned to angioplasty in whom angioplasty was not performed are also shown. (From Berger *et al. Circulation* 1999; 100: 14–20 [62], with permission.)

resources: namely skilled operators and personnel, 24-hour availability of a fully equipped catheterization facility, and safe transportation services. These resources have to be available in a timely fashion since there is, as previously discussed, such a strong relationship between time to first balloon inflation and mortality [7,62] (Fig. 17.10). Furthermore, results of randomized trials of primary PTCA may not be applicable in the community setting. Several large registries evaluating outcomes with primary PTCA or fibrinolytic drug therapy in the community setting have not identified differences in mortality between the different strategies [22,26]. Also, resource consumption was higher in the PTCA-treated patients, which raises some questions regarding cost effectiveness of this strategy [63–65].

In most randomized studies, time from 'door to balloon' averaged greater than 90 min (usually >120 min). Therefore, there is a need for a more 'user friendly' strategy, which should include a rapidly administered drug that can open the infarct vessel early and provide a favourable milieu for adjunctive or rescue percutaneous coronary intervention (PCI).

Perspective and future directions

Current data support an *increase in stent utilization* in the setting of primary angioplasty for acute myocardial infarction. There is strong evidence that stents permit the induction of more stable arterial patency in epicardial vessels, and a lower incidence of restenosis (and TVR) rates during follow-up. *Platelet GP IIb/IIIa blockade* clearly yields better outcomes, lowering re-infarction and urgent TVR rates. It also improves patency at the microvascular level, which may correlate better with left ventricular functional improvement. The *combination of the two* has clearly become the preferred strategy for catheter-based reperfusion for treatment of acute myocardial infarction.

Nevertheless, the importance of time to reperfusion cannot be overemphasized. These notions were integrated in the randomized, placebo-controlled PACT trial [66], in which preprocedural low-dose fibrinolytic therapy was evaluated. Patients presenting within 6 h of symptoms were randomized to receive aspirin, heparin, and either t-PA (50 mg, $n = 302$) or placebo ($n = 304$) and brought immediately to coronary angiography. If TIMI Grade 3 flow was present at the initial angiogram, a second bolus of the study medication was administered. If TIMI Grade 0, 1, or 2 was found, the patient was treated with PTCA. In this study, the primary end-point (predischarge left ventricular ejection fraction) was not significantly different. However, the t-PA group had a higher rate of TIMI Grade 3 flow (32.8% vs. 14.8%) on initial angiography. Furthermore, there was no difference in the post-PTCA incidence of TIMI Grade 3 flow.

From these results stemmed the concept of '*combined reperfusion*' or '*facilitated angioplasty*', which is the strategy of initiating reperfusion with the combination of low-dose lytic therapy plus platelet GP IIb/IIIa blockade (intravenously) and then performing a percutaneous intervention to complete the reperfusion process. This strategy has the potential to expedite initiation of reperfusion therapy (both at the epicardial and microvascular levels) while creating a favourable milieu in which to perform a percutaneous intervention to 'complete' the reperfusion process and stabilize the culprit lesion. This strategy could also provide flexibility in the timing of the intervention. In the event of clear reperfusion after medical therapy, the catheter-based intervention could be delayed and done as a more elective procedure while continuing antiplatelet therapy. On the other hand, if medical therapy fails, 'rescue' or early adjunctive mechanical reperfusion could be performed with less risk of prothrombotic complications.

Preliminary results from pilot studies (TIMI 14, SPEED, and INTRO-AMI) evaluating the combination of various platelet inhibitors with low-dose lytic therapy are encouraging with regard to 60 and 90 min patency rates (up to 65% and 79% TIMI 3 flow, respectively), procedural success and clinical outcomes. Rescue angioplasty (TIMI 0–1 flow or TIMI 2–3 flow and ongoing pain) was performed in 122 patients (21% of the study population) randomized to a low-dose lytic plus abciximab regimen in the TIMI 14 trial [67,68]. Outcomes at 30 days were: death 5.7% ($n=7$), re-MI 4.9% ($n=6$), and urgent revascularization 0.8% ($n = 1$). Immediate or rescue percutaneous interventions ($n = 136$, 50.7% of total population) in the INTRO-AMI trial (dose ranging safety and efficacy trial of low-dose t-PA plus eptifibatide) also showed favourable outcomes. Mortality was 3.7% ($n = 5$); re-MI occurred in 3.7% ($n = 5$); and stroke occurred in 0.7% ($n = 1$). Thus, the data from pilot studies are encouraging and phase 3 trials are underway.

Percutaneous coronary interventions for patients with acute coronary syndromes without ST elevation

Unstable angina and non-Q-wave MI patients are evident in a large proportion of patients requiring cardiac hospitalization. Such patients are believed to be at increased risk of recurrent ischaemic events during follow-up if they are treated only medically. However, revascularization procedures in this context are associated with excess adverse events, compared with the incidence in clinically stable patients. The landmark Thrombolysis in Myocardial Infarction (TIMI) IIIB trial ($n = 1473$) evaluated an early invasive strategy and compared it with an early conservative strategy in this setting [69]. The early invasive strategy consisted of coronary angiography in the first 18–48 h after randomization, followed by revascularization when indicated anatomically. The early conservative strategy consisted of angiography and revascularization only if there was evidence of ischaemia (recurrent ischaemic pain with ECG changes, more than 20 min of ischaemic ST deviation on 24-h holter ECG in the hospital, provocable ischaemia before completion of Bruce Stage II or pre-discharge stress test, or post-discharge severe angina at rest or Canadian Class III or IV). Approximately 60% of patients assigned to the early conservative strategy underwent revascularization in the first year [70]. There was no difference in the frequency of death, non-fatal MI, or positive stress test at 6 weeks (primary end-point, early invasive 16.2% vs. early conservative 18.1%, $P = $ ns). However, the incidence of complications was greater in the early invasive group. Nevertheless, a practical conclusion is that an early invasive strategy is suitable in patients without contraindications, and that an early conservative strategy is also suitable but carries a high likelihood of the need for later intervention.

Two other more recent trials evaluated similar strategies. The VAN-QWISH trial (Veterans Affairs Non-Q-Wave Infarction Strategies In-Hospital, $n = 920$) [71] randomly assigned patients to 'invasive' management or conservative management, defined as medical therapy and non-invasive testing, with subsequent invasive management if indicated by the development of spontaneous or stress-induced ischaemia, within 72 h after non-Q-wave infarction. Death or non-fatal infarction made up the combined primary end-point. The average follow up was 23 months. There was no significant difference in the primary end-point. However, this trial has been severely criticized because of a very high event rate in patients who underwent revascularization (especially bypass surgery, with a mortality of 11.6% at 30 days) as part of the early invasive management and because there were similar rates of revascularization in both groups (invasive 44% vs. conservative 33%). Furthermore, this trial did not incorporate the use of platelet GP IIb/IIIa inhibitors, which have been shown to decrease the incidence of ischaemic events in this setting, particularly if a percutaneous intervention is performed.

The FRISC II trial (Fragmin and Revascularization During Instability in Coronary Artery Disease, $n = 2433$) assessed the efficacy of early invasive vs. non-invasive management [72]. Patients were randomized to a non-invasive or invasive strategy. The invasive strategy consisted of coronary angiography any time from day 2 to day 7 of the hospitalization. The non-invasive strategy involved exercise testing and referral to angiography if ischaemia was clinically evident. The primary end-point was 6-month death or MI. Revascularization at 6 months was 78% in the invasive group and 38% in the non-invasive group. The primary combined end-point (death/MI) occurred in 9.5% in the invasive group vs. 12.0% in the non-invasive group ($P = 0.045$). Death alone tended to be less frequent in the invasive group (1.9% vs. 3.0%, $P=0.10$) (Fig. 17.11). Angina was reduced by 50% in the invasive group, as was

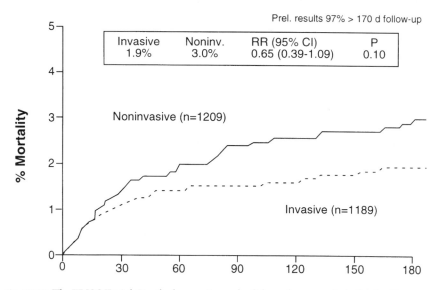

FRISC II: Death

Fig. 17.11 The FRISC II trial: Death alone at 6 months did not show a statistically significant difference but trended toward a benefit in the invasive group [72].

Table 17.3 Composite of death/non-fatal MI at 30 days in unstable angina subanalysis.

Study	n	PCI + ABX (%)	PCI + placebo (%)	P
1. EPIC [74]	489	0.6	11.0	—
2. EPILOG [76]	1328	1.7	9.2	—
3. CAPTURE [75]	1265	4.8	9.0	0.003

PCI: percutaneous coronary intervention.
ABX: abciximab.

readmission. Therefore, it was concluded that an early invasive strategy produced an important benefit with regard to reduction of death or non-fatal MI.

One of the most important recent developments pertinent to interventional cardiology is inhibition of platelet aggregation with GP IIb/IIIa receptor blockers. The first large-scale study with platelet IIb/IIIa inhibitors (EPIC) [73] was with abciximab in the setting of 'high risk' percutaneous coronary interventions (PCI). Subsequently, several studies have been performed to evaluate the efficacy of these agents in a variety of settings (including refractory ischaemia with planned PCI, acute coronary syndromes without ST segment elevation and unplanned PCI) [74–79]. Overall, they reduce periprocedural ischaemic complications and provide long-term clinical benefits (decreased death, re-MI, TVR). Their use in patients with unstable angina undergoing percutaneous revascularization has lowered the risk associated with early revascularization to levels previously seen with stable angina patients [73–75,80] (Table 17.3). In a recently published study by Hamm and colleagues [81], patients with refractory ischaemia (unstable angina) and elevated serum troponin T (a high-risk population) who were treated with abciximab had nearly the same event rate as those without elevated levels (9.5 vs. 9.4%, P = ns). Conversely, in patients who received placebo the risk of death or non-fatal MI was related to troponin levels. As compared with placebo, the relative risk of death or non-fatal MI associated with treatment with abciximab was 0.32 (95% confidence interval, 0.14–0.62; P = 0.002). The major benefit was attributable to a reduction in MI (odds ratio 0.23, 95% confidence interval, 0.12–0.49; P < 0.001) (Fig. 17.12).

Trials evaluating IIb/IIIa receptor blockers as primary medical treatment for unstable angina have provided a unique opportunity to evaluate the safety of early revascularization. In these trials, the subgroup of patients who had the overall best outcomes comprises those who underwent revascularization while 'protected' by a GP IIb/IIIa inhibitor (Table 17.4). The hypothesis developed is being tested in the ongoing TACTICS-TIMI 18 trial, that is re-evaluating the benefits of very early revascularization vs. medical stabilization followed by an ischaemia driven revascularization strategy.

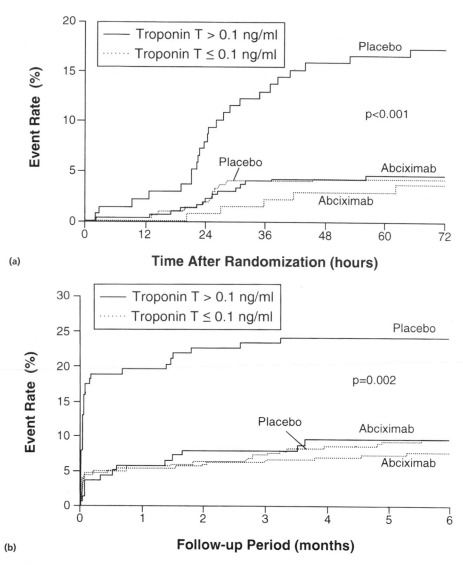

Fig. 17.12 Benefit of abciximab in refractory unstable angina in relation to serum troponin T levels: (a) rates of cardiac events during the first 72 h and (b) during 6-month follow-up. (From Hamm *et al.* [81], with permission.)

Table 17.4 Composite end-point of death/non-fatal MI at 30 days.

Study	Agent	PCI + drug (%)	No PCI + drug (%)
1. PURSUIT [80]	Eptifibatide	11.8	14.6
2. PRISM [78]	Tirofiban	7.2	3.6
3. PRISM-PLUS [79]	Tirofiban	5.9	7.8
4. Overall		9.3	12.1

PCI: percutaneous coronary intervention.

The available evidence favours an early aggressive revascularization strategy for high-risk patients. How early revascularization should be considered remains to be confirmed, but it seems that the stabilization/pretreatment period has been shortened considerably by the availability of novel, powerful antiplatelet agents. Alternatively, the use of low-molecular-weight heparin in a pre-revascularization period of 4–5 days (FRISC-II) was associated with very favourable outcomes using an invasive strategy.

Conclusion

When catheter-based reperfusion therapy for *acute MI* (with ST segment elevation) is performed according to standards developed in randomized trial, there is little controversy that the strategy yields very favourable results. Recent data indicate that increased use of stents and blockade of platelet IIb/IIIa glycoprotein receptors improve results even further. The concept of 'facilitated angioplasty' or 'combined-reperfusion' offers theoretical advantages by initiating pharmacological reperfusion therapy while creating a favourable milieu in which to complete reperfusion with adjunctive or rescue PCI. It remains to be seen whether the theoretical advantages will translate into clinical benefits.

Catheter-based treatments of *acute coronary syndromes without ST segment elevation* (unstable angina and non-Q-wave MI) remain a subject of heated debate. Controversy about whether and when to perform PCI in this setting will undoubtedly continue. However, the enriched pharmacological armamentarium, and strategies of combining new drugs from the different classes (IIb/IIIa inhibitors, ADP receptor antagonists, low-molecular-weight heparins) should lead to progress in the approach to patients with acute coronary syndromes but no ST segment elevation.

Recent promising results increase the likelihood of global improvement of prognosis in patients presenting with acute coronary syndromes in the third millennium. The combination of a tailored anticoagulation/antiplatelet therapy and the increasing use of early revascularization procedures is likely to be impressive.

References

1 Vogt A, von Essen R, Tebbe U, Feuerer W, Appel KF, Neuhaus KL. Impact of early perfusion status of the infarct-related artery on short-term mortality after thrombolysis for acute myocardial infarction: retrospective analysis of four German multicenter Studies. *J Am Coll Cardiol* 1993; 21: 1391–5.

2 Zahger D, Karagounis LA, Cercek B, Anderson JL, Sorensen S, Moreno F *et al.* (TEAM Investigators. Thrombolytic Trial of Eminase in Acute Myocardial Infarction). Incomplete recanalization as an important determinant of Thrombolysis in Myocardial Infarction (TIMI) grade 2 flow after thrombolytic therapy for acute

myocardial infarction. *Am J Cardiol* 1995; 76: 749–52.

3 Karagounis L, Sorensen SG, Menlove RL, Moreno F, Anderson JL. Does thrombolysis in myocardial infarction (TIMI) perfusion grade 2 represent a mostly patent artery or a mostly occluded artery? Enzymatic and electrocardiographic evidence from the TEAM-2 study. Second Multicenter Thrombolysis Trial of Eminase in Acute Myocardial Infarction. *J Am Coll Cardiol* 1992; 19: 1–10.

4 Anderson JL, Karagounis LA, Becker LC, Sorensen SG, Menlove RL. TIMI perfusion grade 3 but not grade 2 results in improved outcome after thrombolysis for myocardial infarction. Ventriculographic, enzymatic, and electrocardiographic evidence from the TEAM-3 Study. *Circulation* 1993; 87: 1829–39.

5 Berger P, Ellis S, Holmes D *et al.* Relationship between delay in performing direct coronary angioplasty and early clinical outcome in patients with acute myocardial infarction: Results from GUSTO-IIb. *Circulation* 1999; 100: 14–20.

6 Berger PB, Stensrud PE, Daly RC *et al.* Time to reperfusion and other procedural characteristics of emergency coronary artery bypass surgery after unsuccessful coronary angioplasty. *Am J Cardiol* 1995; 76 (8): 565–9.

7 Brodie BR, Stuckey TD, Wall TC *et al.* Importance of time to reperfusion for 30-day and late survival and recovery of left ventricular function after primary angioplasty for acute myocardial infarction. *J Am Coll Cardiol* 1998; 32 (5): 1312–9.

8 The European Myocardial Infection Project Group. Prehospital thrombolytic therapy in patients with suspected acute myocardial infarction. *N Engl J Med* 1993; 329 (6): 383–9.

9 Fibrinolytic Therapy Trialists' Group. Indications for fibrinolytic therapy in suspected acute myocardial infarction: collaborative overview of early mortality and major morbidity results from all randomised trials of more than 1000 patients. *Lancet* 1994; 343 (8893): 311–22.

10 Zijlstra F, de Boer JM, Hoorntje JC *et al.* A comparison of immediate coronary angioplasty with intravenous streptokinase in acute myocardial infarction. *N Engl J Med* 1993; 328 (10): 680–4.

11 Ribeiro EE, Silva LA, Carneiro R *et al.* Randomized trial of direct coronary angioplasty versus intravenous streptokinase in acute myocardial infarction. *J Am Coll Cardiol* 1993; 22: 376–80.

12 Grinfeld L, Berrocal D, Belardi J *et al.* Fibrinolytics vs primary angioplasty in acute myocardial infarction (FAP). *J Am Coll Cardiol* 1996; 27 (Abstract): A–222.

13 Zijlstra F, Beukema W, Van't Hof A *et al.* Randomized comparison of primary coronary angioplasty with thrombolytic therapy in low risk patients with acute myocardial infarction. *J Am Coll Cardiol* 1997; 29: 908–12.

14 DeWood MA. Direct PTCA vs intravenous t-PA in acute myocardial infarction: Results from a prospective randomized trial. *Proceedings of the Thrombolysis and Interventional Therapy in Acute Myocardial Infarction Symposium VI*: 28–9, 1990.

15 Grines CL, Browne KF, Marco J *et al.* A comparison of immediate angioplasty with thrombolytic therapy in acute myocardial infarction. (PAMI-I) *N Engl J Med* 1993; 328 (10): 673–9.

16 Gibbons RJ, Holmes DR, Reeder GS *et al.* Immediate angioplasty compared with the administration of a thrombolytic agent followed by conservative treatment for myocardial infarction. *N Engl J Med* 1993; 328 (10): 685–91.

17 Ribichini F, Steffenino G, Dellavalle A *et al.* comparison of thrombolytic therapy and primary coronary angioplasty with liberal stenting for inferior myocardial infarction with precordial st-segment depression. *J Am Coll Cardiol* 1998; 32 (6): 1687–94.

18 Garcia E, Elizaga J, Perez-Castellano N, Serrano JA *et al.* Primary angioplasty versus systemic thrombolysis in anterior myocardial infarction. *J Am Coll Cardiol* 1999; 33 (3): 605–11.

19 GUSTO-I, Ib Angioplasty Substudy Investigators. A clinical trial comparing primary coronary angioplasty with tissue plasminogen activator for acute myocardial infarction. (GUSTO-IIb) *N Engl J Med* 1997; 336 (23): 1621–8.

20 Weaver DW, Simes JR, Betriu A, Grines CL *et al.* Comparison of primary coronary angioplasty and intravenous thrombolytic therapy for acute myocardial infarction:

a quantitative review *JAMA* 1997; 278 (23): 2093–8.

21 Brodie BR, Grines CL, Ivanhoe R *et al.* Six-month clinical and angiographic follow-up after direct angioplasty for acute myocardial infarction. Final results from Primary Angioplasty Registry *Circulation* 1994; 25: 156–62.

22 Every NR, Parsons LS, Hlatky M, Martin JS, Weaver WD. Myocardial infarction triage and intervention investigators. A comparison of thrombolytic therapy with primary coronary angioplasty for acute myocardial infarction. *N Engl J Med* 1996; 335 (17): 1253–60.

23 Tiefenbrunn AJ, Chandra NC, French WJ, Gore JM, Rogers WJ. Clinical experience with primary percutaneous transluminal coronary angioplasty compared with alteplase (recombinant tissue-type plasminogen activator) in patients with acute myocardial infarction: a report from the Second National Registry of Myocardial Infarction (NRMI- 2). *J Am Coll Cardiol* 1998; 31 (6): 1240–5.

24 GUSTO-I, Angiographic Investigators. The effect of tissue plasminogen activator, streptokinase, or both on coronary-artery patency, ventricular function, and survival after acute myocardial infarction. *N Engl J Med* 1993; 329 (22): 1615–22.

25 Meijer A, Verheugt FW, Werter CJ *et al.* Aspirin versus coumadin in the prevention of reocclusion and recurrent ischemia after successful thrombolysis: a prospective placebo-controlled angiographic study: the results of the APRICOT study *Circulation* 1993; 87: 1524–30.

26 Danchin N, Vaur L, Genes N *et al.* Treatment of acute myocardial infarction by primary coronary angioplasty or intravenous thrombolysis in the 'real world': one-year results from a nationwide French survey. *Circulation* 1999; 99 (20): 2639–44.

27 Schomig A, Neumann FJ, Walter H *et al.* Coronary stent placement in patients with acute myocardial infarction: comparison of clinical and angiographic outcome after randomization to antiplatelet or anticoagulant therapy. *J Am Coll Cardiol* 1997; 29 (1): 28–34.

28 PASTA Trial Investigators. Primary stent implantation is superior to balloon angioplasty in acute myocardial infarction: final results of the primary angioplasty versus stent implantation in acute myocardial infarction (PASTA) trial. *Catheter Cardiovasc Interv* 1999; 48 (3): 262–8.

29 Suryapranata H, Van't Hof A, Hoorntje J, de Boer M, Zijlstra F. Randomized comparison of coronary stenting with balloon angioplasty in selected patients with acute myocardial infarction. *Circulation* 1998; 97: 2502–5.

30 Grines CL, Cox DA, Srone GW *et al.* Stent Primary Angioplasty in Myocardial Infarction Study Group. Coronary angioplasty with or without stent implantation for acute myocardial infarction. *N Engl J Med* 1999; 341 (26): 1949–56.

31 Maillard L, Hamon M, Khalife K, Steg PG *et al.* STENTIM-2 Investigators. A comparison of systematic stenting and conventional balloon angioplasty during primary percutaneous transluminal coronary angioplasty for acute myocardial infarction. *J Am Coll Cardiol* 2000; 35 (7): 1729–36.

32 Nishida Y, Nonaka H, Ueda K *et al.* In-Hospital Outcome of Primary Stenting for Acute Myo-cardial Infarction Using Wiktor Coil Stent: Results from a Multicenter Randomized PRISAM Study. *Circulation* 1997; 96: I–397.

33 Ueda K, Nishida Y, Iwase T *et al.* Quantitative angiographic restenosis of primary stenting using wiktor coil stent for acute myocardial infarction: results from a multicenter randomized prisam study. *Circulation* 1997; 96: I–531.

34 Rodriguez A, Bernardi V, Fernandez M *et al.* In-hospital and late results of coronary stents versus conventional balloon angioplasty in acute myocardial infarction (GRAMI trial). Gianturco-Roubin Acute Myocardial Infarction *Am J Cardiol* 1998; 81 (11): 1286–91.

35 Antoniucci D, Santoro GM, Bolognese L, Valenti R, Trapani M, Fazzini PF. A clinical trial comparing primary stenting of the infarct-related artery with optimal primary angioplasty for acute myocardial infarction: results from the Florence Randomized Elective Stenting in Acute Coronary Occlusions (FRESCO) trial. *J Am Coll Cardiol* 1998; 31 (6): 1234–9.

36 Jacksch R, Niehues R, Knobloch W, Schiele T. PTCA versus stenting in acute myocardial infarction: single center pros. (Abstract.) *Eur Heart J* 1998; 19 (Suppl): 239.

37 Scheller B, Hennen B, Severin-Kneib S *et al.* Follow-up of the PSAAMI study population (primary stenting vs. angioplasty in acute myocardial infarction). *J Am Coll Cardiol* 1999; 33 (2): 29A.

38 Montalescot G. ADMIRAL. Abciximab with PTCA and stent in acute myocardial infarction. Presented at the American College of Cardiology (ACC) Annual Scientific Sessions, March 7–10, New Orleans, LA, USA, 1999.

39 Neumann F, Blasini R, Schmitt C *et al.* Effect of glycoprotein iib/iiia receptor blockade on recovery of coronary flow and left ventricular function after the placement of coronary-artery stents in acute myocardial infarction. *Circulation* 1998; 98: 2695–701.

39a EPIC Investigators. Use of a monoclonal antibody directed against the platelet glycoprotein IIb/IIIA receptor in high-risk coronary angioplasty. *N Engl J Med* 1994; 330 (14): 956–61.

40 Brener S, Barr L, Burchenal J *et al.* Randomized, placebo-controlled trial of platelet glycoprotein iib/iiia blockade with primary angioplasty for acute myocardial infarction. *Circulation* 1998; 98: 734–41.

41 The Global Use of Strategies to Open Occluded Coronary Arteries (GUSTO) IIb investigators. A comparison of recombinant hirudin with heparin for the treatment of acute coronary syndromes. *N Engl J Med* 1996; 335 (11): 775–82.

42 Verheugt FW, Liem A, Zijlstra F, Marsh RC, Veen G, Bronzwaer JG. High dose bolus heparin as initial therapy before primary angioplasty for acute myocardial infarction: results of the Heparin in Early Patency (HEAP) pilot study. *J Am Coll Cardiol* 1998; 31 (2): 289–93.

43 Hochman J, Sleeper LA, Webb JG *et al.* Early revascularization in acute myocardial infarction complicated by cardiogenic shock. SHOCK Investigators. Should we emergently revascularize occluded coronaries for cardiogenic shock? *N Engl J Med* 1999; 26: 341 (9): 625–34.

44 Urban P, Stauffer J, Bleed D *et al.* A randomized evaluation of early revascularization to treat shock complicating acute myocardial infarction. The (Swiss) Multicenter Trial of Angioplasty for Shock-(S) MASH. *Eur Heart J* 1999; 20: 1030–8.

45 Califf RM, O'Neil W, Stack RS *et al.* Failure of simple clinical measurements to predict perfusion status after intravenous thrombolysis. *Ann Intern Med* 1988; 108 (5): 658–62.

46 Fernandez AR, Sequeira RF, Chakko S *et al.* ST segment tracking for rapid determination of patency of the infarct-related artery in acute myocardial infarction. *J Am Coll Cardiol* 1995; 26 (3): 675–83.

47 Kircher BJ, Topol EJ, O'Neill WW *et al.* Prediction of infarct coronary artery recanalization after intravenous thrombolytic therapy. *Am J Cardiol* 1987; 59 (6): 513–15.

48 Fung AY, Lai P, Topol EJ *et al.* Value of percutaneous transluminal coronary angioplasty after unsuccessful intravenous streptokinase therapy in acute myocardial infarction. *Am J Cardiol* 1986; 58 (9): 686–91.

49 Gibson CM, Cannon CP, Greene RM *et al.* Rescue angioplasty in the thrombolysis in myocardial infarction (TIMI) 4 trial. *Am J Cardiol* 1997; 80 (1): 21–6.

50 Holmes DR Jr, Gersh BJ, Bailey KR *et al.* Emergency 'rescue' percutaneous transluminal coronary angioplasty after failed thrombolysis with streptokinase. Early and late results. *Circulation* 1990; 81 (3 Suppl.): IV51–6.

51 McKendall GR, Forman S, Sopko G *et al.* Value of rescue percutaneous transluminal coronary angioplasty following unsuccessful thrombolytic therapy in patients with acute myocardial infarction. (TIMI). *Am J Cardiol* 1995; 46: 1108–11.

52 Belenkie I, Traboulsi M, Hall CA *et al.* Rescue angioplasty during myocardial infarction has a beneficial effect on mortality: a tenable hypothesis. *Can J Cardiol* 1992; 8 (4): 357–62.

53 Ellis SG, Ribeiro E, Heyndrickx G *et al.* Randomized comparison of rescue angioplasty with conservative management of patients with early failure of thrombolysis for acute anterior myocardial infarction. (RESCUE Trial) *Circulation* 1994; 90 (5): 2280–4.

54 Vermeer F, Brunninkhuis L, van de Berg E *et al.* Prospective randomized comparison between thrombolysis, rescue PTCA and primary PTCA in patients with extensive myocardial infarction admitted to a hospital without PTCA facilities. *Eur Heart J* 1998; 19 (Abstract, Suppl.): 57.

55 Widimsky P, Groch L, Zelizko M, Aschermann M, Bednar F, Suryapranata H. Multicentre randomized trial comparing transport to primary angioplasty vs immediate thrombolysis vs combined strategy for patients with acute myocardial infarction presenting to a community hospital without a catheterization laboratory. The PRAGUE Study. *Eur Heart J* 2000; 21 (10): 823–31.

56 Miller JM, Smalling R, Ohman EM *et al.* Effectiveness of early coronary angioplasty and abciximab for failed thrombolysis (reteplase or alteplase) during acute myocardial infarction (results from the GUSTO-III trial). Global use of strategies to open occluded coronary arteries. *Am J Cardiol* 1999; 1: 84 (7): 779–84.

57 Stone GW, Grines CL, Browne KF, Marco J, Rothbaum D, O'Keefe J *et al.* Predictors of in-hospital and 6-month outcome after acute myocardial infarction in the reperfusion era: the primary angioplasty in myocardial infarction (pami) trail. *J Am Coll Cardiol* 1995; 25 (2): 370–7.

58 Holmes DR Jr, White IID, Pieper KS, Ellis SG, Califf RM, Topol EJ. Effect of age on outcome with primary angioplasty versus thrombolysis. *J Am Coll Cardiol* 1999; 33 (2): 412–19.

59 Becker RC, Burns M, Gore JM *et al.* The National Registry of Myocardial Infarction (NRMI-2) Participants. Early assessment and in-hospital management of patients with acute myocardial infarction at increased risk for adverse outcomes: a nationwide perspective of current clinical practice. *Am Heart J* 1998; 135 (5 Part; 1): 786–96.

60 O'Neill W, de Boer M, Gibbons R *et al.* Lessons from the Pooled outcome of the PAMI, Zwolle, and Mayo Clinic Randomized Trials of primary angioplasty versus thrombolytic therapy of acute myocardial infarction. *J Invasive Cardiol* 1998; 10: 4–10.

61 de Boer M, Zijlstra F, Liem A, Van't Hof A, Hoorntje J, Suryapranata H. A randomized comparison of primary angioplasty and thrombolytic therapy in elderly patients with acute myocardial infarction. *Circulation* 1998; 98 (17): I-772.

62 Berger P, Ellis S, Holmes D *et al.* Relationship between delay in performing direct coronary angioplasty and early clinical outcome in patients with acute myocardial infarction: results from the global use of strategies to open occluded arteries in acute coronary syndromes (GUSTO-IIb) trial. *Circulation* 1999; 100: 14–20.

63 de Boer MJ, van Hout BA, Liem AL, Suryapranata H, Hoorntje JC, Zijlstra F. A cost-effective analysis of primary coronary angioplasty versus thrombolysis for acute myocardial infarction. *Am J Cardiol* 1995; 76 (11): 830–3.

64 Lieu TA, Lundstrom RJ, Ray GT, Fireman BH, Gurley RJ, Parmley WW. Initial cost of primary angioplasty for acute myocardial infarction. *J Am Coll Cardiol* 1996; 28 (4): 882–9.

65 Stone GW, Grines CL, Rothbaum D, Browne KF, O'Keefe J *et al.* The PAMI Trial investigators. Analysis of the relative costs and effectiveness of primary angioplasty versus tissue-type plasminogen activator: the Primary Angioplasty in Myocardial Infarction (PAMI) trial. *J Am Coll Cardiol* 1997; 29 (5): 901–7.

66 Ross AM, Coyne KS, Reiner JS *et al.* (PACT investigators. Plasminogen-activator Angioplasty Compatibility Trial). A randomized trial comparing primary angioplasty with a strategy of short-acting thrombolysis and immediate planned rescue angioplasty in acute myocardial infarction: the PACT trial. *J Am Coll Cardiol* 1999; 34 (7): 1954–62.

67 Antman EM, Giugliano RP, Gibson CM *et al.* Abciximab facilitates the rate and extent of thrombolysis: results of the thrombolysis In myocardial infarction (TIMI) 14 trial. *Circulation* 1999; 99 (21): 2720–32.

68 Schweiger M, Antman E, Piana R, Giugliano R, Burkott B, Van de Werf F. Effect of Abciximab (ReoPro) on early rescue angioplasty in TIMI 14. *Circulation* 1998; 98 (17): I-17.

69 Effects of tissue plasminogen activator and a comparison of early invasive and conservative strategies in unstable angina and non-Q-wave myocardial infarction. Results of the TIMI IIIB Trial: Thrombolysis In Myocardial Ischemia *Circulation* 1994; 89 (4): 1545–56.

70 Anderson HV, Cannon CP, Stone PH, Williams DO, McCabe CH, Knatterud GL *et al.* One-year results of the Thrombolysis in Myocardial Infarction (TIMI) IIIB clini-

cal trial. A randomized comparison of tissue-type plasminogen activator versus placebo and early invasive versus early conservative strategies in unstable angina and non-Q wave myocardial infarction. *J Am Coll Cardiol* 1995; 26 (7): 1643–50.

71 Boden WE, O'Rourke RA, Crawford MH *et al.* (Veterans Affairs Non-Q-Wave Infarction Strategies in Hospital (VANQWISH) Trial Investigators). Outcomes in patients with acute non-Q-wave myocardial infarction randomly assigned to an invasive as compared with a conservative management strategy. *N Engl J Med* 1998; 338 (25): 1785–92.

72 Invasive compared with non-invasive treatment in unstable coronary-artery disease. FRagmin and Fast Revascularisation during InStability in Coronary artery disease Investigators. FRISC II prospective randomised multicentre study. *Lancet* 1999; 28: 354 (9180): 708–15.

73 EPIC-Investigators. Use of a monoclonal antibody directed against the platelet glycoprotein IIb/IIIa receptor in high-risk coronary angioplasty. The EPIC Investigation. *N Engl J Med* 1994; 330 (14): 956–61.

74 CAPTURE-Investigators. Randomised placebo-controlled trial of abciximab before and during coronary intervention in refractory unstable angina: the CAPTURE Study. *Lancet* 1997; 349 (9063): 1429–35.

75 EPILOG-Investigators. Platelet glycoprotein IIb/IIIa receptor blockade and low-dose heparin during percutaneous coronary revascularization. The EPILOG Investigators. *N Engl J Med* 1997; 336 (24): 1689–96.

76 PARAGON-Investigators. International, randomized, controlled trial of lamifiban (a platelet glycoprotein IIb/IIIa inhibitor), heparin, or both in unstable angina.

Platelet IIb/IIIa Antagonism for the Reduction of Acute coronary syndrome events in a Global Organization Network. *Circulation* 1998; 97 (24): 2386–95.

77 PRISM-Investigators. (Platelet Receptor Inhibition in Ischemic Syndrome Management (PRISM) Study.) A comparison of aspirin plus tirofiban with aspirin plus heparin for unstable angina. *N Engl J Med* 1998; 338 (21): 1498–505.

78 PRISM-PLUS Investigators (Platelet Receptor Inhibition in Ischemic Syndrome Management in Patients Limited by Unstable Signs and Symptoms). Inhibition of the platelet glycoprotein IIb/IIIa receptor with tirofiban in unstable angina and non-Q-wave myocardial infarction. *N Engl J Med* 1998; 338 (21): 1488–97.

79 PURSUIT-Investigators (Platelet Glycoprotein IIb/IIIa in Unstable Angina: Receptor Suppression Using Integrilin Therapy). Inhibition of platelet glycoprotein IIb/IIIa with eptifibatide in patients with acute coronary syndromes. *N Engl J Med* 1998; 339 (7): 436–43.

80 Lincoff AM, Califf RM, Anderson KM *et al.* (EPIC Investigators. Evaluation of 7E3 in Preventing Ischemic Complications.) Evidence for prevention of death and myocardial infarction with platelet membrane glycoprotein IIb/IIIa receptor blockade by abciximab (c7E3 Fab) among patients with unstable angina undergoing percutaneous coronary revascularization. *J Am Coll Cardiol* 1997; 30 (1): 149–56.

81 Hamm CW, Heeschen C, Goldmann B *et al.* (c7E3 Fab Antiplatelet Therapy in Unstable Refractory Angina (CAPTURE) Study Investigators). Benefit of abciximab in patients with refractory unstable angina in relation to serum troponin T levels. *N Engl J Med* 1999; 340 (21): 1623–982.

Index